Raising the Living Dead

Raising the Living Dead

Rehabilitative Corrections in Puerto Rico and the Caribbean

ALBERTO ORTIZ DÍAZ

The University of Chicago Press
Chicago and London

The University of Chicago Press, Chicago 60637
The University of Chicago Press, Ltd., London
© 2023 by The University of Chicago
All rights reserved. No part of this book may be used or reproduced in any
manner whatsoever without written permission, except in the case of brief
quotations in critical articles and reviews. For more information, contact
the University of Chicago Press, 1427 E. 60th St., Chicago, IL 60637.
Published 2023
Printed in the United States of America

32 31 30 29 28 27 26 25 24 23   1 2 3 4 5

ISBN-13: 978-0-226-82449-9 (cloth)
ISBN-13: 978-0-226-82451-2 (paper)
ISBN-13: 978-0-226-82450-5 (e-book)
DOI: https://doi.org/10.7208/chicago/9780226824505.001.0001

Library of Congress Cataloging-in-Publication Data

Names: Ortiz Díaz, Alberto, author.
Title: Raising the living dead : rehabilitative corrections in Puerto Rico and
    the Caribbean / Alberto Ortiz Díaz.
Other titles: Rehabilitative corrections in Puerto Rico and the Caribbean
Description: Chicago ; London : The University of Chicago Press, 2023. |
    Includes bibliographical references and index.
Identifiers: LCCN 2022026309 | ISBN 9780226824499 (cloth) |
    ISBN 9780226824512 (paperback) | ISBN 9780226824505 (e-book)
Subjects: LCSH: Corrections—Puerto Rico—History—20th century. |
    Imprisonment—Puerto Rico—History—20th century. | Criminals—
    Rehabilitation—Puerto Rico—History.
Classification: LCC HV9572.O78 2023 | DDC 365/.97295—dc23/eng/20220716
LC record available at https://lccn.loc.gov/2022026309

♾ This paper meets the requirements of ANSI/NISO Z39.48-1992
(Permanence of Paper).

Contents

Preface

While conducting final research for this book in March 2021, my colleague and friend Javier Almeyda Loucil sent me an email with the subject heading "Los muertos vivos 2021" (The living dead 2021). In light of our ongoing conversations about the history of incarceration in Puerto Rico, Javier mentioned in his message that I just had to watch a recently published interview with the notorious Puerto Rican ex–drug dealer Alex Capó Carrillo, better known as Alex Trujillo. That March week, Telemundo aired a multiepisode series about Capó Carrillo that detailed his criminal and personal histories, his experiences behind prison walls, and his carceral predicament at the time. Early in the series, Capó Carrillo describes his state of mind on the eve of his arrest. He discusses how, far from liberating him, an underground lifestyle had instead dehumanized him. As a result, he felt "dead inside."[1] The day authorities finally took him into custody was the day "God started working on me. I told him, 'God, I feel, like, dead.' Because I felt that feeling. I felt alive, and I would even pinch myself and ask, 'Am I dead?' because I felt devoid of all human sentiment [dead as a person] . . . I had no emotions for anything or anyone."[2] Throughout the Telemundo series, Capó Carrillo narrates his conversion to Christianity, and by its end, he delivers a sermon to a multiracial congregation at the 501 correctional facility in Bayamón in which he elaborates on how becoming a new creature in Jesus Christ has raised him "from death to life."[3]

Capó Carrillo, who has since been paroled, says redemption matters to him and that it is relevant to his individual life process.[4] Therefore, not only should his testimony be taken seriously—it must be taken seriously. The redemptive arc of Capó Carrillo's story is significant in itself but it also predates his own encounter with incarceration by several generations. Indeed, it can be traced to an era of imperfect penal reforms and the rapid maturation of rehabilitative corrections in Puerto Rico in the mid-twentieth century. When this history is put into dialogue with Capó Carrillo's story and his adamant insistence that he has conquered living death by way of spirituality, it becomes clear that living death is an intricate cultural artifact, a condition with multiple meanings. Although Capó Carrillo has been, by his standards, spiritually liberated, before being paroled he remained "living dead" by virtue of his subjection to a physical incarceration beyond his control. In a way, his living death will linger as he completes parole, too, for he will be formally tied to Puerto Rico's carceral system through at least 2024.

Capó Carrillo's story is several generations removed from the rise of medico-religious rehabilitative carcerality in the mid-twentieth century, but both his experience and the history of midcentury Puerto Rican corrections are, to a considerable degree, about the fruits and the pitfalls of prison reform. For many scholars, particularly in the United States, the history of prison reform sits between more consequential facets of the history of incarceration. This history is believed to commence with racial enslavement in the nineteenth century, to progress into the postemancipation era, the humanization of punishment and the failures of reform for much of the twentieth century, and finally lands in post-1970s phenomena—namely, our current preoccupation with racialized mass incarceration and the emergence of present-day movements that seek to reimagine policing, prisons, and related systems. What Capó Carrillo's experience and this book illustrate, however, is that the era of prison reform has staying power that requires explanation and must be better integrated into current debates about carceral history and conversations about the pluralistic forging of pathways forward.

A decade's worth of research on midcentury Puerto Rican corrections, and a lifetime of personal experience as the "collateral damage" of incarceration has taught me that the reform-abolition dyad used to (in)directly frame much of the scholarship on the modern carceral state can perpetuate misimpressions.[5] This is so, in part, because many such narratives fall into a US-centric analytical trap. Observing the prevalence of US-centricity should not be taken to mean that Puerto Rico somehow sidestepped becoming a node in the development of the US carceral state.[6] Rather, it is meant to draw attention to the fact that there are many other meaningful ways of understanding and narrating Puerto Rico's carceral history.

To be clear, and as this book attests, I am not diminishing the salience of global currents or US colonial empire in twentieth-century Puerto Rican history. Puerto Rico has a long colonial relationship with the United States, dating to the War of 1898. Its legal status would not be "resolved" until the US Supreme Court decided Puerto Rico was an "unincorporated territory" (possessed by but separate from the US mainland) and US citizenship was imposed on Puerto Ricans in 1917.[7] While Puerto Rico remains a US colony, it has also acquired considerable domestic autonomy. The Puerto Rican government had pursued a new colonial pact with the United States by midcentury, resulting in commonwealth status in 1952. Free associated statehood has been a double-edged sword, though. Puerto Ricans dictate the terms of politics and culture locally, but government corruption and neoliberal economics are rampant, and increasingly, so are other kinds of tyranny. Through it all, millions of Puerto Ricans have, for a variety of reasons, migrated to the US mainland and nourished diasporic communities while simultaneously holding on to their Puerto Ricanness, generating and intensifying transnational consciousness, and in some cases eventually returning to the Caribbean.[8]

Explicit and subtle racial assumptions have also marked Puerto Ricans' ambivalent colonial relationship with the United States. Most certainly, as many scholars have made clear over the years, race itself is a tool of othering that furthers and naturalizes colonial subordination. However, it is just as crucial to recognize that by the 1940s and 1950s, a half century of US rule and cultural transmission did not magically dissipate the four centuries' worth of flexible caste configurations of race (the "colorism") that previously prevailed in Puerto Rico under Spanish dominion.[9] Some scholars rightly point to how blackness has been denigrated and silenced in Puerto Rican history, yet it is also undeniable that people of color in Puerto Rico could escape racial slavery by marronage, purchase, or testament, exploited migratory, military, socioeconomic, and other opportunities as free people, mingled with and could even enjoy higher status than white peasants, and were immersed in a polyracial culture that cannot be reduced to contemporary assertions that race mixing was and is merely an expression of a color-blind mestizo mythology.[10] The classification of bodies in Spanish colonial Puerto Rico, María del Carmen Baerga has written, involved "genealogy, the legitimacy or illegitimacy of a person's birth, the appropriate marital ties, the sexual behavior of men and women, and the private and public conduct of individuals and families," all of which is suggestive of "remarkably porous" racial identity formation.[11] These and other factors resulted in less rigid race relations than in other parts of the Caribbean and the United States.[12] We must take seriously these nuanced racial legacies when considering Puerto Rican history in the first half of the twentieth century, when the Jim Crow racism that accompanied the US presence had an impact on but did not totally dictate understandings of nation and identity in Puerto Rico.

Complex racial legacies bled into the categorizations used by officials in midcentury Puerto Rican corrections. These were not incompatible with the racial labels then emanating from the US mainland. Between 1917 and the 1950s, Puerto Rico's Justice Department classified the Puerto Rican prison population mostly into the categories of white, mulatto, and black. When these categories are assessed individually, we find that white people in adult prisons (i.e., the penitentiary and district jails) were always incarcerated at higher rates than people of color.[13] Another story emerges when the mulatto and black categories are collapsed, however. Prisoners of color are collectively overrepresented in the prison system relative to their total share of the entire Puerto Rican population, and they even constituted most prisoners in adult institutions certain years (in the penitentiary, 1917–19, 1921–22, 1929; and in district jails, 1917–18). Meanwhile, at the Industrial School for Boys in Mayagüez, most youths incarcerated there between 1918–32 and 1935–45 were of color, but the population was whiter at specific junctures (1917, 1933–34, 1956–57).[14] By the early 1960s, the Puerto Rico Corrections Division reported that 70 percent of the total prison populace was white.[15] The statistical inconsistencies visible in Puerto Rican corrections data over time complicate findings drawn from broader census analyses.[16] Puerto Rico's prison population whitened in the mid-twentieth century not just because the social definition of whiteness expanded (this was already the case in light of long-standing miscegenation and fluidity between racial categories) but also because those incarcerated were literally light skinned, at least in the eyes of the multiracial stakeholders responsible for tabulating the numbers.

The notion that the demographic composition of Puerto Rico's midcentury carceral population was primarily black or of color is therefore incorrect and indicative of the limits of examining this history with a US-centric gaze. For such an assumption to stand, the existence of what I call a broken whiteness (meaning a whiteness fused to class dynamics, experiential deviations, spatial location, and race mixing) must be assumed and also deemed a manifestation of blackness. As several scholars have insinuated, this is not a far-fetched proposition, particularly given how on the US mainland, light-skinned Puerto Ricans have been racialized as black due to their spatial and cultural proximity to African Americans and their embrace of black cosmopolitanism since the early to mid-twentieth century.[17] In Puerto Rico, the administrative adoption of ambiguous racial language in the prison system, such as the category *blanco-trigueño* (white with sun-toasted skin, white-wheat, or racially mixed), is also suggestive of broken whiteness. For Puerto Ricans on the US mainland and in the Caribbean, then, having light skin is not always a marker of whiteness or privilege. The majority presence of incarcerated "white" people in midcentury Puerto Rico amounts to a cautionary tale about the limits of applying an exclusively epidermal notion of race to the history in question, for the Puerto Rican case is one that befuddles tidy understandings of race.

The historically bewildering racial formulations and relations attributed to Latin America and the Caribbean are well documented and defy the seamless transfer of a black-white US model to the rest of the Americas. In Puerto Rico and the wider Caribbean, current political debates about mass incarceration, racial (in)justice, and reform-abolitionism tensions matter but do not entirely reflect binary race relations either. Within the United States, these discussions often overlook Latino and other inmates and where they anchor themselves on the racial spectrum.[18] *Raising the Living Dead* highlights Puerto Rican carceral experiences and in so doing creates an opening to a dialogue about how racially mixed people both fit into and frustrate the US monopoly on conceptualizing carcerality, which is itself an exercise in cultural imperialism.

It is just as crucial to acknowledge that many (though not all) mid-twentieth-century Puerto Ricans embraced a socially constructed and contradictory but ultimately shared mixed-race identity. The remaking of Puerto Ricanness in terms of racialized racelessness amid ongoing US colonialism unfolded in different venues, including the criminal-legal system. There, health professionals, convicts, and others of all racial backgrounds upheld aspects of the underbelly of confinement but also rescripted corrections for their own purposes: rehumanization, healing, and empowerment, to name a few. *Raising the Living Dead* is about incarcerated people and lays bare their racialized marginalization and vulnerability in kaleidoscopic fashion, but it is more interested in showcasing how they were "raised" from their predicaments than in locking them into the static category of "racialized colonial subjects," as if colonialism has not evolved or ordinary people have not been able to negotiate or subvert it.

Much like today's reformists and abolitionists, in addition to imperfectly aspiring to problem solve incarceration, the architects and proponents of midcentury rehabilitative corrections in Puerto Rico facilitated the progress of state and professional research into the causes of crime (e.g., unemployment, housing inadequacies, unstable upbringings, health disequilibrium) and their rectification through proto–"reformless reforms," chiefly the refinement of reentry structures and technologies such as parole and probation, comprehensive health care, technical (vocational) training, social work, and diverse humanities programming and services. These and other analogous interventions attempted to ameliorate existing prison conditions, what today we would call conventional prison reform. Yet they also confirm that people from all walks of life assembled and committed to forging and supporting alternatives to the problem of managing violence in society. Fernando Picó's postcarceral utopia, or "community of learning," started to take form during the era of rehabilitative corrections.[19] *Raising the Living Dead* shows that the desire to reimagine incarceration and mitigate harm by building a layered, responsive system of rehabilitation preceded contemporary abolitionism. Reform has since looped into abolition and the two create a helix around each other in our present. Nothing is new under the sun other than how we go about things, not necessarily what we go about doing.

It would be a mistake for readers to interpret my giving the history of reform a fair analytical shake as unfair, as hostile toward newfangled abolitionism, or as nostalgic pining for a bygone era of rehabilitative corrections. I take this approach precisely because I seek to balance a reckoning of violence, trauma, and harm with celebration, futurities, and desire, at least in terms of how these manifested in the mid-twentieth century. As a photographer active in midcentury Puerto Rico named Jack Delano recalled in the early 1990s, these two realities need not be incompatible. Living conditions in Puerto Rico's impoverished countryside and urban slums—where many incarcerated people had roots—were horrendous back then. But what most impressed Delano and several of his Farm Security Administration colleagues was the dignity, hospitality, gentleness, patience, and indomitable spirit of the people "in the face of the most appalling adversity."[20] I extend Delano's insight to parallel contemporaneous scenarios, including those unfolding in Puerto Rico's prison system. Tracing the slightest ripples of life in what seems to have been an expansive, insuperable sea of death is a key step in decolonizing our understanding of this history. This also, in turn, requires tempering narratives of pain and damage and putting them into substantive dialogue with narratives of repair.

That a generous, sympathetic, or optimistic, if not mellifluous, reading of this history could surface in today's academic and "high" political climate is a glaring reminder that we must not only check and balance our own moral posturing but also take seriously variabilities of human agency. Historically, the human agency channeled into reformist carcerality has affirmed asymmetrical power relations and structural violence; crucially, however, this agency also has been multivalent and capable of defacing or annulling much of what has cascaded downhill "from above." Still, despite the synergy between human agencies and structures, recent literature about the carceral state emphasizes structural culpability. Agency is entertained insofar as it gets us to where we really need to go—a critique of capitalist, white supremacist structures. Within these parameters, institutions like prisons are depicted as machines that operate in black or white ways and have black or white outcomes. But while prisons are violent and produce conditions of violence, they do not exist for their own sake. They mirror the times and are shaped by a cacophony of ideas and actions emanating from characters of flesh and blood. Like celestial bodies, systems may incline, but they do not oblige. In the end, I do not belabor a structural analysis in this book because, first, I assume structural violence is entrenched in "the violence of everyday life," which is something that predates Western colonialism and imperialism, and second, I am interested in clarifying the intricacies of entangled agencies, which in practice blur the relevance of structures.[21]

In tracing the problem-solving dimensions of midcentury corrections in Puerto Rico, I hope that revisiting them, their potential, and their ceiling will spark scholars, activists, and others to meaningfully integrate histories and voices that do not square with their bottom-line preferences and stances. The tendency to preach to the choir in an echo chamber is one of several reasons contemporary abolitionism is perceived of as an event or a utopian dream state. Recent additions to the emerging neoabolitionist canon correctly contend that today's abolition is more than this—that it is a theory of structural (though apparently not total legal) change and about eliminating the reasons people think they need police and prisons.[22] But even this framing is problematic, for who gets to strip someone of their reasons, decide when those become expendable, deem them myopic, or name them myths? Assuring people that they will eventually see the light and convert to the correct position neglects that there are manifold kinds of growth when it comes to carceral issues and causes. Such a premise also denies the possibility that epiphanies and "unlearning" can happen in reverse, which is to say that people with "radical" sensibilities might become reformists, indifferent, or something else entirely. Contrary to mainstream belief, these types of cases exist and are far more numerous than many scholars and activists care to admit.

I pose these questions and write these words because this is not a theoretical exercise for me. It hits too close to home. My father served twenty-five years for several violent offenses that caused real harm to himself, our family, and our communities. When he was released in the mid-2010s, he both admitted and denied the accusations made against him, but he never solely blamed structures for his trajectory. One of the people on his warpath, my mother, was happy about his second chance. She has since underscored to me how important it was for her safety and well-being that there were barriers in place at the time of his arrest that could protect her, even if only partially. Otherwise, she or someone else would probably be dead. Suggesting that my parents are so colonized that they cannot see the oppressive systems that were *really* at fault for their predicaments erases their agency and subjects them to further violence, only this time at the hands of those professing to be in solidarity with them. Doing so also dodges the individual decision-making—the desires for and clashes over power at the microlevel—that co-sparked the confrontations and exchanges that landed my father in prison in the first place. The spectrum of violence on which cases like my parents' rest and their self-diagnoses must be accepted on their own terms—not trivialized, dismissed, or subsumed by "greater" truths and priorities.[23] This begins with recognizing that power is not just about structures. Power is also about what all kinds of individual people (authorities and others) choose to do with it and why. It is about human nature and fragile egos. And while systems of power certainly structure people's choices, the range of choices people make in their lives is not always dependent on the contexts that we, as scholars, signal as the most significant.

History shows that justice, accountability, and safety issues can be tackled in several ways. Solidarity, restoration, and reconciliation work inside and beyond prison walls with affected groups have been some of the better-known expressions since the latter decades of the twentieth century.[24] Whether we like it or not, incarceration remains one of those ways, too. Granted, we must be careful about how incarceration is deployed. But questioning whether incarceration has run its course does not invalidate that many people accept and value it for their own reasons. My mother and other people I care about are very much alive because my father went to prison. Many formerly incarcerated people with whom I still build speak of varieties of rehabilitation, and more broadly, of the changes they made in their lives for the better because they served time. Whether they are part of a pattern or exceptions is not their focus. For many of them, systemic realities were and are secondary to their individual lived experiences. This has less to do with their alleged inability to "imagine another world," and more to do with what is practical for them.

While grassroots communal responses to ego and harm may help undo or transform ego, erect accountable institutions, and forge new worlds, they also can and *will* generate novel divisions, exclusions, and inequities because human beings can try to but never will be universally just or righteous. New asymmetries perpetually emerge and fuse themselves to the rhetorics surrounding policing and prisons. This was the case before and during the era of rehabilitative corrections, remains so, and is all too visible in academic scholarship, op-eds, social media feeds, and elsewhere. If we are going to bask in optimism about our current abolitionist moment (which clearly is only a moment for some) and emphasize the courage it takes to reimagine structures and our world without entirely uprooting the rule of law itself or substantively preparing for what comes next, then we must hold previous epochs to the same standard.[25] Human fallibility is visible across all human history, not only in those histories we find disagreeable. The same is true of human aspirations, not only when we see them in histories with which we already agree.

This brief meditation is not meant to be an exhaustive overview of race in Puerto Rican history or an argument for or against present-day abolitionism. Quite simply, it is meant to shed light on why I approach the history of carcerality in a "counterintuitive" fashion, to make my intentions clear, and to illustrate that there is a lot more collective and, by extension, restorative relationship work to do when it comes to problem solving incarceration and related phenomena. Part of that work involves completing and complicating our understanding of rehabilitative corrections so that it is deeply incorporated into the "long" history of crime and punishment. *Raising the Living Dead* represents a modest contribution in this regard. It discloses that rehabilitative care formed part of a broader penal reform movement and accompanied significant shifts in modern Puerto Rico's criminal-legal system. Rehabilitation was complex, contested, shifting terrain and subject to multiple applications, interpretations, and meanings. Sometimes its advocates and adherents were successful in implementing the rehabilitative ideal, and sometimes they were not. The people who animate this history—their lives, internal histories, and politics—merit tomes, not tweets.

Finally, I am aware of the power of humanizing language in telling this story and choose to use the term "incarcerated people" when discussing individuals ensnared by Puerto Rico's criminal-legal system. However, the historical record also refers to incarcerated people as "criminals," "convicts," "offenders," "prisoners," and "the living dead," among other terms. To stay true to that history as it unfolded, I deploy this nomenclature, too. Exclusively imposing the politically correct terminology of our own times onto the past would be disingenuous. To strike a balance between the yearnings of the present and the realities of the past, however, I interchangeably utilize all eligible vocabulary.

Introduction:
Toward a Holistic History of Incarceration

In a summer 2018 op-ed published in the *Washington Examiner*, Erik Y. Rolón Suárez, then secretary of the Corrections and Rehabilitation Department, claimed that the administration of Governor Ricardo Rosselló Nevares could be credited with introducing rehabilitative corrections to Puerto Rico.[1] He underscored that governments were responsible for providing convicts with meaningful lives while incarcerated, and he lauded the US Congress for boosting education and rehabilitation programming in the federal prison system through the First Step Act.[2] Rolón Suárez also urged Congress to mimic fruit-bearing Puerto Rican penal reforms on the US mainland, including family integration initiatives, vocational training in auto mechanics, and civic participation. "We need to start preparing them [prisoners] to lead healthy, constructive lives once they are back in society," Rolón Suárez insisted.[3]

More than a year later, Rolón Suárez was no longer leading Puerto Rico's Corrections and Rehabilitation Department. Javier Colón Dávila reported in *El Nuevo Día* that the departures of Rolón Suárez and his deputy in September 2019 coincided with a spate of inmate deaths in the US territory's deteriorating and neglected prisons. Their departures also played out against the backdrop of a battle for access to the departmental budget within Corrections and Rehabilitation and by Puerto Rico's Financial Oversight and Management Board.[4] By October, condemnatory accounts of prison health care in Puerto Rico were published in *El Nuevo Día*. In two consecutive stories, anonymous prisoners, their family members, government officials, and activists described the precarious living and health conditions still plaguing the prison system more than forty years after convicts like Carlos Morales Feliciano and their communities mobilized to demand state action to address such grievances.[5] Several patterns emerge in the 2019 newspaper articles: low budgets, professional staff constraints, and a public perception of incarcerated people as not entirely human, all of which impeded inmates' access to health services, life-extending or life-saving medicine, and physical and mental health in general.

Although the realities documented by *El Nuevo Día* are grim, once upon a time in Puerto Rico the state aspired to be responsive to the health-care needs of incarcerated people. In turn, incarcerated people and their social networks took this prospect seriously. Less than a century ago, between the 1930s and 1960s, years that witnessed the rise and fall of a rehabilitative era and a reformed colonialism in Puerto Rico under colonial-populist rule, prison health-care professionals promulgated a contradictory form of nonviolent health politics during a violent historical moment.[6] The (in)direct colonial-populist promulgation of a scientific praxis that was cognizant of prisoners' humanity illustrates that colonized health professionals created their own scientific expertise and deployed it for rehabilitative purposes in the midst of unequal power relations with the United States.[7] Their politics of care hinged on physically, psychosocially, and spiritually resurrecting pathologized, incarcerated Puerto Ricans of all class, race, space, gender, sexual, ideological, and age backgrounds.[8] Together with incarcerated people and others, health professionals co-enacted a carceral culture of uplift anchored in socialized medicine, in the process articulating a comprehensive science of rehabilitative corrections that tempered and neutralized the extent to which social difference factored into whether prisoners were deemed rehabilitable or qualified to reenter society. In the mid-twentieth century, Puerto Rico's colonial-populist state and its (in)formal collaborators working in the prison system had a more holistic, albeit imperfect, understanding of prison health care than they do now. Beyond invoking a rehabilitative ideal, a culture of rehabilitative corrections existed and to a degree flourished in Puerto Rico long before it dawned upon Rolón Suárez and the Rosselló Nevares administration.

Raising the Living Dead examines this taken-for-granted history. It explores the fundamental roles that health professionals, incarcerated people, and their families and wider communities have played in shaping medical, transnational, and local histories in Puerto Rico and the broader Caribbean. By "health professionals," I mean intersecting communities of care across the rehabilitative spectrum—physicians, psychiatrists and psychologists, social workers, and people of faith, for example. I zoom in and out on the experiences of these different groups to offer a different way of viewing the history of prison health care in the Caribbean and Latin America, most notably from the "middle" and "below" (middle-class and subaltern—or vernacular—perspectives) rather than exclusively "from above" (elites).

Histories of incarceration framed with a holistic (physical, mental, social, and spiritual) understanding of health can provide a window into not only the lives of prisoners but also the communities in which they are embedded. Centering the incarcerated people involved in the colonial-populist remaking of Puerto Rican society in the mid-twentieth century (1917–64), instead of highlighting the development and abuses of the US-influenced carceral state, distinguishes *Raising the Living Dead* from similar studies.[9] Tracing the history of rehabilitation in Puerto Rico and the Caribbean shows how multiple communities of care endeavored to uplift incarcerated people despite the structure that brought them together. They imagined and instituted correctional cultures that fused seemingly incommensurable approaches to health to secure convict and, by extension, societal well-being. In this context, rehabilitative corrections meant the ideology and practice of salvaging infirm incarcerated people through medicine, applied knowledge exposure and training, social orientation, and moral and humanistic dialogue and activities. It was a project with implications beyond prison walls. Ideally, for mid-century convicts, rehabilitation signaled a potential return to life and all that entailed personally, interpersonally, socioeconomically, and civically while also speaking to their functionality in relation to others, broader contexts, and their ability to sculpt themselves.[10]

The case of Puerto Rico's largest prison, the Insular Penitentiary at Río Piedras (popularly known as Oso Blanco, or White Bear), allows for a meticulous assessment of convict well-being and health practitioners and practices in a gray zone of medicine. The Insular Penitentiary opened in 1933 and was considered a place for the physical, mental, and social regeneration of delinquent people, as well as a place where they could receive educational, industrial, and agricultural instruction.[11] Oso Blanco replaced the antiquated La Princesa (Princess) penitentiary located in Old San Juan, which was founded in the 1830s and had a less pedagogical orientation than its successor.[12] As historians of Latin America have argued, such "transitions" unfolded across the region in the nineteenth and early twentieth centuries and served social control purposes.[13] *Raising the Living Dead*, however, goes beyond narratives of social control that have largely examined the discourses of actors who fit well within traditional histories of the prison (e.g., those of criminologists, penal administrators, police, other similarly positioned legal authorities).[14] With rare exceptions, historians have treated rehabilitative corrections as an aberration or anomaly in the history of incarceration, instead of engaging its medico-humanistic cast of characters and their commitment to interdisciplinary approaches to healing over time.[15] *Raising the Living Dead* underscores a powerful case study (Oso Blanco) and the complicated worlds of other Puerto Rican prisons, and it situates them in pan-Caribbean and inter-American contexts to produce a layered history of incarceration from the points of view of health professionals, convicts, and their wider communities.

Crime, Punishment, and the New History of Medicine

Despite incarceration's antiquity, scholars have mostly connected the phenomenon to early modern and modern history.[16] In modern histories, capitalism and labor exploitation are foregrounded in analyses of prisons, given their role in creating disciplined and productive work forces and the accrual of profits for stakeholders.[17] Scholarship about settler colonialism, racial capitalism, and the "transition" from enslavement to the prison, particularly in the Americas, has expanded considerably.[18] A key insight of the recent literature is that the class and race identities of coerced laborers and other groups are structurally normalized as inferior and expendable. Furthermore, scholars are tracing the "afterlives" of slavery to drive home the point that, despite abolition at different junctures in the nineteenth-century Americas for instance, the legacies of enslavement persisted well into the twentieth century and remain relevant today.[19] This book assumes the importance of the labor power of incarcerated people and makes clear that economic and scientific endeavors were tethered to one another, but its focus is on knowledge production, rehabilitative therapeutics, and the social exchanges that defined them.

Of the many frameworks used to write the history of incarceration, Michel Foucault's has probably affected academics the most. The birth of the modern prison heralded a first wave of penal reform, Foucault postulated, and represented a seismic shift from primitive, religiously inspired forms of punishment toward modern, scientific approaches that taught carceral subjects how to self-police.[20] Inspired by Enlightenment thinkers like Cesare Beccaria and others who clamored for changes in criminal justice, prison reformers in the eighteenth century started encouraging the abandonment of cruel and ineffective punishments in favor of more humane alternatives.[21] Foucault understood the modern prison as part of a vast web of similar institutions, including schools, factories, and military barracks. Collectively, these institutions helped produce and sustain modern panoptic societies, meaning societies that internalized and mimicked the precepts of the all-seeing panopticon—Jeremy Bentham's eighteenth-century notion of an institutional building and a system of control that allows subjects to be watched without their knowing it.[22] According to Foucault, asylums and clinics served as sites of corporeal control and scientific knowledge production as well, ensuring "the capillary functioning of power" and offering complementary authoritative epistemologies for the naturalization of discipline and the prison as everyday forms of modern life.[23] *Raising the Living Dead* highlights the prison, but in a colonial scenario, not through a Eurocentric lens. And although Oso Blanco was the capstone of an integrated complex of welfare institutions—a sanitary city—where boundaries were porous and exchanges frequent irrespective of who occupied the central tower of the panopticon, my intention is not to display the sanitary city in abstract operation but to account for the open medico-humanistic experiences of incarcerated people and their relations.[24] In the chapters that follow I blend the insights of Foucault's power theories with the socioreligious concepts of Emile Durkheim, like the purification of the criminal and the sanctification of the individual, to better understand the modern Puerto Rican state's self-assigned duty to preserve the dignity of prisoners through redemptive carcerality.[25]

Mary Gibson's recent work on Western liberal reformers has identified a second wave of prison reform in the late 1800s and early 1900s.[26] In her book on Italian prisons, she shows how rehabilitative labor was central to the development of a renewed national identity.[27] In the United States, this second wave commenced earlier in the nineteenth century and was characterized by competing models of reform that combined religious instruction and forced labor in different ways.[28] This is where historians and sociologists of Latin America have principally augmented the scholarly literature. Ricardo D. Salvatore and Carlos Aguirre, for instance, led the charge with *The Birth of the Penitentiary in Latin America*, an edited volume focusing on modernization and prison reform in postcolonial Latin America. In this foundational text, they called for deeper social histories of incarceration attentive to class, race, and gender dynamics, studies that center processes of cultural and ideological contention, and narratives that account for the experiences of incarcerated people within and beyond their prison orders.[29] Aguirre's own magnum opus, *The Criminals of Lima and Their Worlds*, did exactly this for the history of incarceration in modern Peru.[30] Scholars of Mexico and Brazil also contributed, covering everything from prisons across time to social life, sexuality, civic education, and parole hearings behind bars.[31] Regrettably, few scholars have followed up on this initial wave of scholarship, and even fewer have transcended constructivist, intersectional analysis of the traditional sort.[32] *Raising the Living Dead*, however, unpacks carceral intersectionality differently by undoing a palimpsest of medicine, belief, and death and awakening during a third moment of reform in the middle decades of the twentieth century, when progressive prison philosophy ascended and overlapped with the expansion of welfare states.[33]

While the traditional centers of colonial and postcolonial power in Latin America are well represented in this cumulative literature, scholarship on the

Caribbean remains sparse.[34] For the case of Puerto Rico, there are works that focus on crime, juvenile offenders, incarcerated labor migrants, enslaved people, vagrants, women, and political prisoners.[35] Solsiree del Moral is developing several projects that probe race, class, childhood, and punishment in the early to mid-twentieth century.[36] These studies, however, do not reckon with the dynamism of rehabilitative corrections. *Raising the Living Dead* helps fill the geographic gap for scholarship on the modern period, answers Salvatore and Aguirre's call for critical yet nuanced social and cultural histories of incarceration "from the inside out," and rejects an analytic lens that simply hyperbolizes the raw hegemony or sins of the carceral state. Moreover, although *Raising the Living Dead* focuses on Oso Blanco, it also considers other Caribbean prisons.

Caribbean societies were among the last in the Americas to erect modern penitentiaries in the early to mid-twentieth century.[37] Their construction accompanied US empire building in the region, but as fully operational institutions they reflected the goals of (neo)colonial and national governments. In the Greater Antilles under US rule, penitentiaries emerged in the following order: roughly at the same time in Haiti and the Dominican Republic (the Pénitencier National and Nigua, respectively), the Presidio Modelo in Cuba, and Oso Blanco in Puerto Rico.[38] The proliferation of modern penitentiaries in the Caribbean, then, was connected to US-driven state-building projects. These materialized across the first decades of the twentieth century everywhere from Hispaniola to Panama and can be comprehended as part of an extended and geographically expansive process of colonial macrostructuring.[39] The premise for framing *Raising the Living Dead* in the Caribbean context is also practical. Again, this book is chiefly about Puerto Rico's carceral archipelago and, within it, Oso Blanco penitentiary. But I strategically incorporate other corners of the Caribbean and American worlds to spotlight what was shared in a midcentury Caribbean marked by national differences yet still experientially integrated. A Caribbean scope is necessary given the degree to which ideas, people, and goods (e.g., penal principles, prison blueprints, convict bodies, health professionals, medicines, therapeutic models, literature) moved around the region and broader Atlantic world at the time.[40] This reflected the radiating vibrancy of holistic prison health care, all of which could not be sourced or worked through in Puerto Rico alone. Thus, *Raising the Living Dead* is not meant to be a balanced comparative study. Rather, it is organically Caribbean and Atlantic facing. Consequently, such an approach unearths local forms of comparison while unveiling the political desires and overlapping geographic and sociocultural circuits that shaped midcentury carcerality in Puerto Rico and elsewhere.

Scholars have also combined the lenses of science, medicine, and technology to write the history of incarceration in Latin America. Lila Caimari and Julia Rodríguez, for example, illustrate how in early twentieth-century Argentina scientific and state authorities advanced a medicalized political culture that defined social problems such as poverty and violent crime as illnesses to be contained and treated through carceral social hygiene. The scientific knowledge bolstering this political culture diagnosed what exactly ailed the Argentine national body and offered prescriptions to improve the majority-white body politic.[41] Turn-of-the-century Argentine hygiene efforts behind bars blended science and religion and were, for all intents and purposes, a protoversion of rehabilitative corrections.[42] Aguirre, for his part, is skeptical of rehabilitation's impact. Prisons in racially mixed Peru were not sites of regeneration, he argues, but "bastions of authoritarianism and exclusion" that reproduced and maintained an "unjust and exclusionary social order."[43]

In *Raising the Living Dead*, I do not entirely disavow or shy away from the discourses and practices surrounding rehabilitation and how they could be inclusive. Instead, I borrow conceptual tools from new histories of medicine and medical humanities to understand incarceration in Puerto Rico and the Caribbean in ways that trouble the usual emphasis on uneven power relations, flat or one-sided biopower and violence, and romanticized notions of resistance and freedom.[44] Recent histories of medical incarceration, especially, unveil how ordinary people have infused institutions with their own anxieties and hopes, as well as alternative, competing, and unanticipated meanings.[45] These new histories challenge scholars to consider knowledge production and its circulation from the ground up to elucidate patients' experiences of illness, their narratives of suffering and healing, and how these relate to politics and other topics.[46] Diego Armus and Pablo Gómez's notion of the gray zones of medicine is particularly central to the framework of *Raising the Living Dead*, for it loosens the mortar agglutinating the bricks of the "impenetrable" panopticon, specifically the Foucauldian idea that the penitentiary is principally an insulated laboratory of power where different experiments are contemplated and realized.[47] If we view the penitentiary and similar carceral spaces as epistemic and interactive gray zones, however, it becomes evident that the variable health practitioners based in these institutions and incarcerated people themselves defied being easily boxed into rigid and stable systems of knowledge about the human body, mind, and behavior. The prison itself can be dissected to lay bare the (in)formal marketplace of health care behind the walls, reciprocity between service providers and inmates, and the sociocultural tendencies of the multiple communities enmeshed in constituting and negotiating penitentiary science.

In the Atlantic and Caribbean worlds, the different ways of knowing and being that have breathed life into medical gray zones include the senses and pleasure, but for many of the incarcerated people in this book, their bodies or flesh (whether deemed agreeable or wicked by authorities) were but a single aspect of their multidimensionality. Convict notions of the spirit, their social imperatives and intellects, their humanistic preferences and sensibilities, their knowledge of place, and their kin networks were also relevant to how they endured and tried to overcome incarceration. In this context, injustice, racialization, eugenic science, and structural violence—while salient and pervasive— were never preordained nor insurmountable. Nor are they enough to explain this history. Therefore, *Raising the Living Dead* disentangles colonialism and medicine to the extent this is possible and subdivides carceral medicine by considering how medical and social science, social work, the therapeutic humanities, and health activism were slippery and contested terrain constantly in flux. The shifting tectonics of multivalent, diffuse medico-humanistic knowledge production and care, rather than laboratorial knowledge inescapably tied to an unfazed juridical-medical system, are my focus.[48] "Unthinkable" structural nuance defined and swayed by incessant waves of human agency characterized midcentury rehabilitative corrections in Puerto Rico and other corners of the Caribbean. To shed light on this paradox, I track a history of situations and micropower inside and outside of prisons that amplify the factors and fusions that enchained individual prisoners, their wider communities, and the groups of health professionals with whom they interacted.

A Brief Genealogy of Living Death

Multiple communities of care worked within the architecture of midcentury rehabilitative corrections in Puerto Rico to advance a system that sought to restore and protect individuals and larger communities. They aspired to raise the "living dead"—a resurrection trope with roots in antiquity, medieval times, and Atlantic racial slavery that reemerged in the mid-twentieth century to capture what it meant to be incarcerated.[49] The project of raising the living dead was connected to the broader liberal-progressive, colonial-populist goal of securing a reformed colonialism, which in part meant rehabilitating a society that was reeling from a series of political, economic, social, and environmental crises through New Deal, emergency, and reconstruction policies.[50] Prisoners eligible for healing (understood here as corporally, socially, and spiritually infirm beings *with potential*) were to be diagnosed and treated so that they might become capable, responsible, and productive caretakers, providers, and citizens with middle-class sensibilities. Living death in modern

Puerto Rico did not preclude civic rebirth. It merged the resurrection accounts of antiquity (principally Jesus Christ's conquest of death); medieval ideas about evil spirits and restless corpses tormenting the living through chaos, disease, and violence (the problem of crime in times of privation, sickness, and tension); and legacies of Atlantic racial slavery (in particular, the resocialization of traumatized, conscienceless, and kinless bodies for the purposes of coercive labor exploitation and their insertion into conformist politics).[51]

Ancient accounts of living death can be traced to the resurrection stories of Kemet, Israel, and other parts of the "Old World." The ancient Egyptians, for instance, worshipped a pantheon of gods, chief among them Osiris—a god of fertility, agriculture, vegetation, death, resurrection, and life. Osiris was killed and dismembered by his brother Set and salvaged by his sister-wife Isis, who collected his scattered body parts and wrapped him up, enabling his reanimation. Isis temporarily resurrected Osiris so they could conceive a child—Horus, the falcon god of kingship and the sky, the all-seeing or spiritual eye. In terms of human cultural practices, ancient Egyptians lived with the dead by venerating their ancestors and reserving spaces, occasions, and times to interact with them.[52]

The Bible also develops the concept of living death. Israel's constant spiritual and physical fornication with other gods and peoples, especially their embrace of pagan customs, marks their relationship with Jehovah generation after generation. This results in a spiritual death (separation from God as a result of disobedience) that has corporeal consequences but does not rule out the possibility of redemption should Israel stop rebelling, genuinely repent, and return to God with a contrite, humble heart. The dry bones of the people of Israel can be rehydrated and they can escape their predicament, just as followers of Jesus Christ can be raised from living death if they let the word of God cleanse them, repent, believe that Jesus is God manifested in the flesh and convert, and take other required steps to live in righteousness (e.g., ritual baptism, receiving the Holy Spirit and bearing its fruit, serving others). A major difference between Old and New Testament renderings of living death was who mediated for sinners—the Levitical priesthood, on the one hand, and a new pact with Melchizedek (Jesus himself), on the other.

In medieval Europe, people accorded living death a vital role in the community. They called upon saints and the dead to aid them in conflict resolution.[53] The dead crisscrossed at will the imagined impermeable border between the world of the living and the afterlife.[54] Medieval French and English literature used dying, death, and the dead to think about life's problems—political, social, ethical, philosophical, existential. In these literary texts, ghosts, revenants, and isolated living people who long to perish straddle life and death. The dead place demands on the living, and the living envision and put into motion their own deaths.[55] Centuries later, English romantics revived the trope of living death in their own literary tradition through vampires and the Frankenstein monster to explain the dilemmas associated with interpersonal relations.[56]

As European Romantics attempted to revive emotional and intuitive medievalism to escape the population growth, early urban sprawl, industrialism, rationalism, and classicism of the Enlightenment, living death itself shed its old skin for a new one in the Atlantic colonies. The era of transatlantic racial slavery transformed the meaning of living death and in the process created the figure of the modern zombie. A probable ancestor of the zombie migrated from the Kongolese and Angolan regions of Africa to the Caribbean beginning in the seventeenth century, assuming definitive form in French Saint-Domingue during the Haitian Revolution, an eighteenth-century slave rebellion that became a war of independence. In its transatlantic and French-Haitian configuration, living death was inseparable from enslavement and insurgency. The zombie figure represented the ills of the time, including destruction, disease, and death, but it also served as a symbolic conflict zone where a cultural war was waged between cannibalistic imperialism and Afro-diasporic cultural preservation.[57] Death had resuscitative dimensions as well, however. These were apparent in everyday funerary practices and mortuary politics—those activities and social meanings derived from beliefs and practices associated with dying and death that people employed toward specific ends. As Vincent Brown has argued, these were key facets of black life and its remaking in an era of lethal racial slavery. Death announced endings in one sense, and sowed seeds of renewal in another.[58]

The zombie and, by extension, living death entered US public consciousness through the US occupation of Haiti (1915–34) and American literature and visual arts.[59] The middle decades of the twentieth century witnessed a renaissance in this regard, particularly concerning the penal colony of Cayenne (commonly known as Devil's Island), which operated for more than a century in French Guiana.[60] The Canadian journalist Gordon Sinclair, a reporter for the *Toronto Star* who filed stories from exotic locations around the world during these years, wrote a travel literature series about Devil's Island that he published as the book *Loose among Devils*.[61] The French Guiana portions of this book disclose the various struggles of the living dead: mistreatment at the hands of guards, poor food quality, and deficient medical care. Puerto Rican journalists reprinted excerpts of this series in the magazine *Puerto Rico Ilustrado* throughout 1935.[62]

At about the same time, the former convict René Belbenoît published *Dry Guillotine*, a memoir about his imprisonment in French Guiana. Like Sinclair,

Belbenoît also provided readers with ethnographic accounts of the living dead. His descriptions of convict labor and solitary confinement, among other themes, clarify the expendability of incarcerated people. Prison authorities in French Guiana distributed inmates among different labor camps in the tropical jungle. Labor assignments included installing radio stations, downing mahogany trees, cleaning living quarters, growing crops, and road construction. As for solitary confinement, it was "unendurable" and could be worse than the death penalty.[63] According to Belbenoît, solitary confinement meant entombment in a dimly lit or otherwise dark, unsanitary cell while susceptible to disease and mental persecution: "The convicts call it . . . the dry guillotine!"[64] His narrative of solitary confinement points to convicts enduring the punishment of slow rot. Prisoners' minds were obliterated even if their bodies managed to survive the tombs of the living.

Although understandings of modern living death revolve around the French Caribbean for good reason, Puerto Rico has figured into the articulation of living death in the broader trans-American imagination as well. The Puerto Rican case similarly affirms the labor coercion, social rupture, dehumanization, and fugitivity linked to the trope, but also its literary repackaging as an allegory referring to incarcerated people and their shared condition. Shortly after Oso Blanco's inauguration in 1933, the Puerto Rican poet, playwright, and journalist Carlos Carreras published an important story about penitentiary convicts, their collective psyche, and their labor power in *Puerto Rico Ilustrado*.[65] His May 1934 photojournalistic account "Un día tras las rejas" (A Day behind Bars) captured the "living dead, as [Spanish-Cuban writer Eduardo] Zamacois would call them," in action.[66] In one image, prisoners till the soil surrounding Oso Blanco for the cultivation of sugarcane and other crops. Other images present them as they are shepherded by guards to and from classrooms, industrial workshops, and their cells.[67] Carreras's references to pedagogical imperatives hinted that living death could be defeated, but it would be another decade or so before the vision was sufficiently scaled up to help address the structural deficiencies of Puerto Rico's prison system. His description of the solitary cell known as "Dungeon 116" sheds light on the social death and mental disequilibrium provoked by solitary confinement in "hermetically closed" cells with "the appearance of a coffin or a niche."[68] It also exposes the spark of hope incarcerated people preserve through fleeting social interaction with trusted prison staff and visitors. The nameless inhabitant of Dungeon 116 exclaimed penitentiary warden Sixto Saldaña's name "with a touch of affection" when he realized light had entered his cell and who was visiting.[69]

As these different Caribbean scenarios involving solitary confinement confirm, and as Lisa Guenther has argued for the US case, prolonged solitary confinement reduces the lives of those incarcerated to a living death of the worst kind by driving presumably healthy prisoners insane and making the mentally ill more infirm.[70] This reflects the broader necropolitics in which modern states often traffic, for they are more than capable of imposing physical, social, and civic death on their citizenries.[71] Caleb Smith similarly shows how incarceration engenders social death but importantly also spiritual rebirth.[72] The angle of rebirth is central to *Raising the Living Dead*, for in mid-twentieth-century Puerto Rico living death came to insinuate probable social and civic resurrection. Although penal reformers the world over at the time struggled or failed to implement policies that bore fruit, resulting in the reinforcement of understanding prisons as "tombs of the living," the Puerto Rican case exposes the centrality of a multidirectional and multilayered rehabilitative ideal imbued with an urgency to reimagine punishment that was, for a time, put into practice.[73] From Puerto Rico to places as far away as China, as Frank Dikötter has contended, penal reforms were linked to social and civic imperatives achievable by way of pedagogical carcerality, an inclusive project for which everyone—from young offenders and adult criminals to prostitutes and political dissidents—qualified.[74]

Overall, while this book is broadly concerned with the experiences of the "living dead," its emphasis is really on the less-explored phenomenon of how incarcerated people perceived to be physically, socially, and spiritually infirm were "raised," whether by their own doing or in conjunction with others.[75] *Raising the Living Dead* is about incarcerated people's navigation of a culture of rehabilitative corrections dressed in medical language, their varied responses to human caging and warehousing, and how they and those in their respective circumferences endured, contested, and sought to overcome uneven health interventions. They did so not only by resisting but also by adopting, borrowing from, and rescripting the epistemologies undergirding the forms of carcerality to which they were subjected. Focusing on processes of consciousness raising in the history of modern corrections decenters violence without casting it as trivial while allowing us to flesh out quotidian ways of living and making relation.

The Inspired Archive

An underlying tension in Puerto Rican historiography, and by extension most historical scholarship produced since the social and cultural turns of the 1970s and 1980s, is whether analyses of structures or individuals more accurately convey historical truth(s). Nowhere is this tension more evident than in the vast, irreplicable scholarship of Francisco Scarano and Fernando Picó.

Scarano has written perceptively about structures, systems, and historical causality, whereas Picó is known for studies of local context and characters of flesh and blood.[76] Neither Scarano nor Picó have stressed the importance of medico-humanistic knowledge production as a mechanism of mediation between structures and people, however. *Raising the Living Dead* blends their respective approaches, but it admittedly emphasizes the histories of individuals, in this case the incarcerated and their extended communities, to the extent that these lives, voices, and experiences are visible and decipherable. It builds on Picó's study of Puerto Rican prisoners by painting a focused picture of rehabilitative corrections across multiple decades rather than a general history of convicts spanning centuries. Rehabilitative corrections in Puerto Rico was marked not only by an aspirational pedagogy, as Picó has noted and as I corroborate in this book, but also by varieties of medicine and belief that crashed into one another in compelling and contingent ways.[77]

Questions about whether ordinary lives are truly accessible have shaped historical debates since at least the appearance of subaltern studies.[78] Documentary archives grant access to the intricate worlds of disadvantaged, marginalized, and dispossessed people, but even this access is limited and not always transparent. These days many scholars distrust archives in large part because of the violence associated with the making of archival data, the assumption that archive building frequently occurs within a vindication ethos, and the perceived codependence of colonialism and the traditional archive itself.[79] More often than not, archives are viewed as sites of racialized knowledge production where asymmetrical power relations are imagined, normalized, and reproduced. And for better or worse, scholars utilize the speculative tools of the present to reassemble history and come to terms with what is (un)written in the documentary record.

Several decades ago, Natalie Zemon Davis called for treating archives as part of the research process rather than just mining the documents therein.[80] Michel-Rolph Trouillot took this insight further and argued that power shapes every stage of historical production, silencing certain intentions and voices more than others and distorting history as a result.[81] To demystify the power of the colonial state in this regard, Ann Laura Stoler followed in the footsteps of those responsible for archival production. To trace their affective registers and identify the knowledge(s) that guided their perceptions and practices, she read along the archival grain, uncovering racialized biases that confused the construction of epistemic spaces.[82] More recently, Marisa Fuentes has artfully read into the silences and senses of the slavery archive to critique archival knowledge production and its deleterious effects, such as the deliberate erasure of blackness.[83] In Puerto Rican Studies, scholars are

increasingly engaging "alternative" and "ideational" archives to tease out the
hidden histories and power dynamics of policing and workers' movements,
for instance.[84]

The problem with sacrificing the archive on the altar of theory is that the
serious, decades- and centuries-long work that went into forging the archive
is buried to prioritize the somehow more honest and moral knowledge production of the contemporary scholar extracting data from it. This is not to say
that archival practice is devoid of social context or contradiction. Nor that a
"naïve" reading of archival materials suffices.[85] Rather, what I am proposing is
that scholars be as cynical and suspicious of our own semantic gymnastics as
we are of the documentary record. Despite the contemporary assertion that
archives conspire to silence and erase certain voices and people, the reality is
that archives have never been or claimed to be more than partial. Archives
we have inherited may be elusive and even illusory, but the truths of ordinary
people constitute their foundation. This is especially evident in criminal-legal
records, which would not exist as such without vernacular raw material.

On one level, the criminal-legal archive that forms the backbone of *Raising the Living Dead* was crafted from the fabric of ordinary, surveilled lives.
On another level, this archive can divulge as much about the intellects, inge-
nuity, priorities, and social circles of incarcerated people inside and outside
of institutions as it can about the entropy of their circumstances, suffering,
and victimization.[86] As Adria Imada has suggested for the case of Hawai'i,
"colonial-carceral" records divulge an alienating archive of skin (individualized "raced-sexed bodies"), but also an archive of kin ("affective approaches"
to "connection").[87] In the context of midcentury Puerto Rico, convicts and
their kin were not merely devastated by structural violence through the criminal-
legal system. They *lived*, even under the direst of circumstances, and their
lives, no matter how defaced or mutilated, dictated what ended up preserved
in Puerto Rico's criminal-legal archive. Such understanding is possible by
standing firm on the square of the traditional archival record. Bearing witness to how ordinary people have lived does not automatically require turning the archive into an analytical straw man, nor does it mean deifying "secret" knowledge, oral histories, shoebox record keeping, or other so-called
counterarchives.

To trace the history of the living dead in mid-twentieth-century Puerto
Rico and the Caribbean, I rely on deep archival and library research. I am
careful to not bite the hand that feeds me and inflate my own interpretations over what the archival record says for two primary reasons. First and
foremost, notwithstanding having read thousands of pages over the years for
this project, my framing and interpretations are as fallible as those that went

into producing the criminal-legal archive I depend on in this book. Second, privileging the theory of our own times in my reading of this archive would be an anachronistic exercise. In other words, I do not ask the past, or the archive, for what it cannot provide me. Even if human beings have taken moral positions or defined harm across time and place, this does not mean that the options, choices, and contexts informing people's moral positions and experiences of harm have been the same across time and place.[88] *Raising the Living Dead* does not aim to serve "gotcha" history. It instead reveals the stories, challenges, and successes specific to rehabilitative corrections during the period in question—aspirations, warts, and all.

For these reasons, rather than merely critique rehabilitative corrections by identifying and hovering over a spectrum of silences, reading against the archival grain, or purportedly going *through* the archive altogether, I appreciate what I find in the archive. This is the golden rule of my method. It rests on two experiential pillars. First, I previously worked as an archivist and respect the craft and its specialists beyond the "truth seeking" and wresting rituals at the core of writing history. Second, I can personally attest to an example of when an archive gets a story (more or less) right.[89] Still, it is true that criminal-legal records are bred under class, race, and gender duress (e.g., police interrogation, trial cross-examination, forced observation in prison). As Kirsten Weld notes in *Paper Cadavers*, archives are sites of both social struggle and social control.[90] However, no matter how hurtful the narratives buried in archives may be, the resulting materials remain a product of inspired, collective exchange. Regardless of their mood, tone, and intent, pieces of everyone involved in knowledge production processes configure them, not only those pertaining to people in authority who have a monopoly on violence, and not only the fictions and strategies inherent in people's narratives. Most modern records are often reflections of convoluted human interactions despite who frames them and how they do so.

Collections housed at the General Archive of Puerto Rico in Puerta de Tierra, San Juan, are the core sources for *Raising the Living Dead*. I dive deep into relevant materials within Puerto Rico's criminal-legal archive and, to a lesser extent, other Caribbean societies. Inmate files; parole records; biomedical, psychiatric, and psychological evaluations; social workers' field notes and observations; clemency petitions; the private letters of inmates and their kin; the mainstream and religious press; prisoners' writings; historical journals and texts; and photographs—among other sources, these enable me to tell the story I propose. These sources were interdisciplinary in their production as well as in their consequent consumption. The brew of sources that animate *Raising the Living Dead* indicates that health professionals, prisoners, and many others co-forged a comprehensive human science (rehabilitative corrections) that positioned convicts to navigate and negotiate their time behind bars (living death), and to maintain and even amplify their interpersonal and societal relevance beyond bars.

Because the sources in this book comprise a thick archival vein, I had to make choices about which case files or stories to include. What gives me solace in this regard is one of Picó's insights—that history would be impossible without the names that constitute it and everything those names entail: the details of people's lives.[91] *Raising the Living Dead* cannot elaborate on every name that haunts Puerto Rico's criminal-legal archive, an unrealistic task for a single book in today's laconic publication climate. Beginning or continuing the effort, however, can establish or stretch interpretive parameters, unknot conflicting patterns, and showcase how snapshots of individual lives can speak to broader processes if we dare to critically embrace "the facts" as preserved in the historical record without subjecting them to the gravitational pull of our times. Valorizing the everyday embedded in archival sources about individuals that were produced under fraught conditions illuminates a wealth of knowledge, belief, and meaning making. Works drawn from few or otherwise concentrated sources provide models for what it looks like to write rich histories of the complex principles, forces, and scenarios animating the lives of (extra)ordinary people often deemed wretched of the earth by virtue of their unglorified circumstances.[92] Similarly, *Raising the Living Dead* engages the archival record in a granular, face-to-face format. By looking at "biased" sources from the "inside out," as Claire Edington has put it, this book synthesizes the annals of little-known historical actors across races, classes, professions, genders, ideologies, sexualities, ages, and other markers of difference into a cohesive narrative.[93] I center names and situations while acknowledging how systemic realities framed people's options and experiences, and treat individual case files as their own lifeworlds because, first, that is what they are, and second, because I intend to bring more of them to the fore in due course. In *Raising the Living Dead*, though, archival slices cut from multiple criminal-legal record series are enough to detect the substance and flow of Puerto Rican rehabilitative corrections.

Compartmentalizing Rehabilitative Corrections

Raising the Living Dead is a book of six chapters that spans nearly five decades (1917–1964) but is concentrated between the 1930s and 1960s. This period covers the waning years of US colonial rule proper and the emergence of a colonial populism in Puerto Rico dispatched by Luis Muñoz Marín and the

Partido Popular Democrático (PPD). My focus is not on the PPD or US colonialism, however. Other scholars, such as Ángel Quintero Rivera, Michael Lapp, and José Luis Méndez, have already clearly established that socioscientific institutionalization was a key, driving component of populist ideology in mid-twentieth-century Puerto Rico. Quintero Rivera, for example, beautifully illustrates how cross-class, social justice–oriented, and public service–minded populism went hand in hand with "objective," scientific, and technocratic planification. The two, in fact, were indissolubly interrelated and fundamental to lodging social science in Puerto Rican statecraft.[94] *Raising the Living Dead* is mindful of the areas of research advanced by colonial populists (e.g., industrialization, manpower, psychosocial dynamics, social stratification and mobility, cultural change) and rehabilitation's connection to them, but its emphasis is on how prison reform unraveled on their watch, if not within their immediate purview, and even more so on the interactions of incarcerated people, health professionals, and other critical actors.[95]

Put another way, US colonialism and the PPD emerge in this history as a necessary part of the backdrop, but do not necessarily constitute the bulk of the analysis that follows. Nonetheless, a brief description of the evolution of prison administration in Puerto Rico under US and colonial-populist auspices is in order. These signposts will allow readers to situate individual chapters into broader context without letting the usual suspects take over the narrative. Under US military rule (1898–1900), a prison board supervised Puerto Rico's prisons. A civilian director of prisons assumed control of penal institutions in 1901. By 1904, the Office of the Director of Health, Charity, and Corrections replaced the director of prisons. In 1912, the Labor, Charity, and Corrections Department inherited prison administration. A watershed moment finally occurred in 1917, when Puerto Rico's Justice Department took over carceral facilities. It was at this moment that flashes of an institutionalized rehabilitative future surfaced in Puerto Rican corrections.[96]

Although a modern penitentiary materialized in Puerto Rico by the early 1930s, flawed but meaningful prison reform would not germinate until the mid-1940s through early 1950s. Changes in the prison system reflected and responded to the transformation of Puerto Rico's judicial system.[97] During these decades, the Bureau of Prisons was nested in the Justice Department, with growing personnel noted in the 1945–46 fiscal year.[98] In 1946–47, the Bureau of Prisons was reorganized into the Bureau of Corrections and split between an administrative unit and a division of classification and treatment.[99] This same year a Prison Industries Corporation was set up, ensuring that carceral capitalism and rehabilitation existed side by side and in harmony.[100] The industrial emphasis of the corporation coincided with government efforts to modernize and industrialize Puerto Rico via Operation Bootstrap.[101] These changes came on the heels of a federal evaluation of Puerto Rico's penal and correctional program, carried out by the US prison official Frank Loveland and Puerto Rican partners beginning in 1944.[102] Loveland's was the first of several external studies, which would continue into the next decade. Muñoz Marín's first attorney general Vicente Géigel Polanco executed several major penal reforms while he was in office (1949–51) by using administrative authority in the absence of legal mechanisms.[103]

By the early 1950s, the Bureau of Corrections was interchangeably referred to as the Division of Corrections. Perhaps most important, Puerto Rico's 1952 commonwealth constitution negotiated by colonial populists finally encoded what had been transpiring since the mid-1940s—that the government shall, "within the scope of the means available, aim the treatment of offenders toward making their moral and social rehabilitation possible."[104] In light of constitutional enshrinement, the Division of Corrections underwent an administrative overhaul in 1953–54, while the Prison Industries Corporation faced its first major setback and sustained a financial deficit before rebounding in subsequent years.[105] In 1956–57, prison officials proposed the consolidation of run-down municipal jails into the commonwealth penal system and created the Penal Reform Committee.[106] A Department of Corrections proper (or Corrections Administration) would not be founded until 1974.[107]

The individual chapters of *Raising the Living Dead*, however, are less concerned with peeling away the layers of the criminal justice and prison bureaucracy to which I just alluded than with highlighting the entanglement of physical, mental, and social health and religiousness, spirituality, and other humanistic impulses and embodiments in the history of Puerto Rican corrections. *Raising the Living Dead* demonstrates that medical and social scientists and social workers deployed the tools of science and medicine to raise convicts from bodily, social, and civic death. Convicts, their families, and their communities often tapped into religion, the humanities, and health activism to prevent, cope with, or recover from all manner of infirmity. Together, the different chapters showcase the tensions between and cross-pollination of popular mortuary politics and state necropolitics. Notwithstanding the death dealing of the Puerto Rican state, the government also had occasion to productively respond to prisoners, their needs and demands, and those of their wider communities.

Each chapter of this book examines rehabilitative corrections from a different point of view. Combined, they home in on the relationship between incarcerated people and (extra)institutional communities of care. The first chapter, "Under a Microscope," traces Puerto Rico's turn toward rehabilitative corrections in the wake of US citizenship in 1917. Biomedicine that targeted infectious disease set the health-care tone in Puerto Rican prisons in the 1920s and 1930s and continued to play a significant but secondary role in the 1940s and 1950s. It was a first, physical step toward rehabilitation. Incarcerated people benefited from improved health-care infrastructure in terms of access to physicians and other service providers, medical diagnostics, and treatments, but vertical health integration could also come at a price and harm as much heal.

Chapter 2, "To Classify and Treat," probes when Oso Blanco became more of a psychosocial health institution in the 1940s and early 1950s. This second layer of the penitentiary mission coincided with the birth of Oso Blanco's Classification and Treatment Board, an interdisciplinary entity that studied convicts and imagined rehabilitative programs for them. Mental health professionals helped set the pace of the board, using psychometrics, observations, and interviews to pathologize convicts while insisting that they were treatable and salvageable intellectually and vocationally.

In the third chapter, "Interactional Care," I explore the contributions of social workers and parole officers to Oso Blanco's culture of rehabilitation in the 1940s and 1950s. Using comprehensive interviews, social workers assembled socioeconomic histories of prisoners for the Classification and Treatment Board. These helped determine the social health of convicts and their prospects for societal reincorporation. Parole officers investigated prisoner recidivism ethnographically to problem solve rehabilitative failure. Social health professionals served as carceral gatekeepers but aimed to return incarcerated people to their kin and communities as well.

Chapter 4, "More Than Flesh," moves away from credentialed biopsychosocial medicine and documents other ways of knowing and experiencing health and healing. Between the 1930s and early 1960s, convicts tapped into a variety of edifying and empowering religious and spiritual options. Belief was integral but peripheral to corporeal rehabilitative efforts. Still, prisoners immersed themselves in the sacred to achieve self-improvement, healing, and degrees of freedom en route to an illuminated citizenship.

The fifth chapter, "In Pursuit of Awakening," centers incarcerated people's engagement with the therapeutic humanities at the high point of rehabilitative corrections. In the late 1940s and 1950s, literature, the fine and performing arts, and inmate-produced magazines provided Puerto Rican prisoners with opportunities to substantively shape their own consciousness raising. These activities positioned them to critique the system while extolling and working within it to sharpen their civic swords and attain rehabilitation.

Chapter 6, "Health Activism," demonstrates how Puerto Rican and Dominican prisoners, their families, and their communities attempted to mitigate the worst effects of incarceration through executive clemency. Between the 1930s and midcentury, incarcerated people and those linked to them utilized clemency to shed light on their health predicaments and stretch the rigidity of the criminal-legal system. Health relationships and movements were as important to inmates as the scientific and humanities knowledges and practices circulating inside prisons.

The conclusion details the decline and collapse of the rehabilitative ideal in Puerto Rico and how it became a punitive nightmare, starting with the nationalist purge and transnationalization of rehabilitation in the 1950s but particularly after the late 1960s. I draw attention to the emergence of a prisoner rights organization (the Ñetas) and a major legal case that set a precedent for the health rights of incarcerated people (*Morales Feliciano v. Romero Barceló*).[108] The conclusion also touches on the closing of Oso Blanco in the early twenty-first century and discourses surrounding its demolition in 2014.

Raising the Living Dead redirects existing scholarship on incarceration by encouraging scholars to contemplate the entwined histories of medicine and belief in penitentiaries and prisons before the punitive (re)turn in carceral studies. Skewing this history challenges the stories many scholars and others tell themselves about incarceration, enabling us to see the familiar from different and inconvenient angles. Critically examining rehabilitative corrections invites readers to take seriously how imprisoned people have worked within and on the margins of criminal-legal systems to deal with uneven power relations and inequalities. Indeed, *Raising the Living Dead* shows how imperfect communities of care and rehabilitation coalesced and mutually problem solved incarceration in Puerto Rico in the mid-twentieth century.

Under a Microscope:
Convict Bodies and Prison Biomedicine

On October 28, 1933, the United States federal court in San Juan sentenced a forty-five-year-old white entrepreneur named Juan Sampayo López to two years in prison for producing and disseminating counterfeit money.[1] Shortly after he entered the Insular Penitentiary, medical professionals examined him.[2] They found he was infected with sexual diseases and therefore unhealthy. A year later the Catholic physician Leandro López de la Rosa, a graduate of Jefferson Medical College in Philadelphia, reexamined the still-ailing Sampayo López.[3] The convict's condition had improved "except for syphilis, probably cerebral spinal."[4] Subsequently, Sampayo López rejected a lumbar puncture, a procedure that collects and analyzes the fluid surrounding the brain and spine, as well as follow-up treatment for his sexually transmitted infections.

Sampayo López's inmate file fails to disclose exactly why he rejected a spinal tap and additional treatment. If we attempt to walk in his shoes, however, it is clear he was not enamored of physicians or their assistants violating the sanctity of his body with a large needle beyond his immediate line of vision. Although medical experts had used the puncture technique for diagnostic and treatment purposes since the late nineteenth century, between the 1920s and 1970s it was also employed to conduct what are now obsolete X-ray imaging studies of the brain.[5] During the painful procedure, cerebrospinal fluid was drained from around the brain and replaced with air, oxygen, or helium to enhance its appearance on radiographs. Also, Sampayo López likely rejected treatment in general because he was aware that the "cure" could be worse than syphilis itself. By the 1930s, medical professionals in Oso Blanco (and beyond Puerto Rico for that matter) treated syphilis with salvarsan, an arsenic-based drug that could have toxic and other negative effects on patients, such as pain, rashes, liver damage, and risks of life and limb.[6] Sampayo López presumably experienced, witnessed, or heard about these cumulative effects firsthand.[7]

In conjunction with somehow having been personally exposed to the motions of toxic treatment, Sampayo López was a practicing Spiritist. He formed part of the social circle and fraud network of the Cuban "occult" physician Antonio Lezcano Prado, who the journalist Carlos Carreras discovered among Oso Blanco's "living dead" while touring the institution for a magazine story he published in May 1934.[8] Sampayo López's spiritual identity and the company he kept suggests he trusted other forms of knowledge and ritual to secure his health—for example, knowledge of plants, bark, baths, metals, and minerals, which in the deep and recent past were believed to alleviate and even cure syphilis, or the invocation of spirits that could reveal the social basis of causality and treatment possibilities.[9] While penitentiary physicians like López de la Rosa hoped to treat Sampayo López according to their epistemological and ontological standards, the prisoner's rejection of their framing and methods indicates that he had another understanding of how to go about demystifying his condition and getting better. To federal and penitentiary health officials, such audacity was organic to the inmate, guided his misbelief and original crime, and was reflective of the place he occupied in a fraud network as fishy as bouillabaisse.[10]

Using government reports, health bulletins, and other sources, this chapter examines the emergence and consolidation of a medicalized science of prisoners and their bodies in Puerto Rico in which the lines between the medical diagnosis and treatment of the person and anthropological ranking of the human were blurred. To a lesser degree, it considers how convicts like Sampayo López interpreted the logics and practices of bodily regeneration. In the 1920s and 1930s, physicians and their collaborators subjected convicts to microscopic scrutiny, relying on their flesh to understand disease and advance tropical medicine. The inauguration of Oso Blanco in 1933 and the institution's initial biomedical orientation opened rehabilitative levees that channeled incarcerated Puerto Ricans into state-building efforts. For physicians, the process of rehabilitation began with rescuing convicts from physical death and deterioration through vertical health intervention, which entailed mapping the external markers and internal workings of their bodies and diagnosing and curing them of disease. Biomedical intervention allowed for increased surveillance and clinical judgment about incarcerated people while directing them into a political economy transitioning from agriculture to modern industries.

From Criminal Anthropology to Biomedicine

Acquiring knowledge about prisoners in Oso Blanco commenced during central booking, when new convicts entered the penitentiary for the first time. As prisoners stepped into the prison, two stone engravings representing the law and justice and a nineteenth-century slogan pioneered by the Spanish writer-activist Concepción Arenal greeted them: "Hate the crime and pity the criminal," a spin on the notion of "Hate the sin and not the sinner."[11] Once inside, prisoners were questioned, searched, stripped of possessions, and outfitted.[12] Their demographic data was compiled, they were assigned to a cell block, and their photographs were taken. Mug shots identified their features—birthmarks, deformities, scars, skin color, and so on—and offered front and side views of their faces and skulls. According to prevailing socioscientific intellectual currents, these hinted at their criminal inclinations.

By the time Sampayo López and hundreds of other convicts entered Oso Blanco in the 1930s, mug shots had been in use in Puerto Rico for about a half century. Widespread usage of mug shots helped centralize law enforcement and consolidate criminal-legal systems in the late nineteenth century the world over. The French biometrics researcher Alphonse Bertillon is credited with the expansion of identification systems based on mug shots and physical measurements. In the early 1880s, he founded a laboratory in Paris where anthropological measurements and observations were used to identify criminals, whom he classified according to the length, width, and diameter of their skulls and other body parts. Bertillon also stressed the importance of logging additional physical characteristics, such as eye, hair, and skin color and indicators of ethnicity like scars.[13] Spanish colonial authorities in Puerto Rico depended on physical descriptions in response to the abolition of racial slavery and resistance to postemancipation forms of coerced labor in the 1870s, as well as the proliferation of interpersonal violence thereafter. While formulaic written descriptions and visual sketches of rebellious and surveilled populations were initially essential components of the modern security apparatus that bridged enslavement and the prison on Puerto Rico's big or main island, these templates were complemented by mug shots as the nineteenth century ended and the twentieth began.[14]

Spanish colonial officials procured not only images of convicts but also rudimentary assessments of their physiques to produce knowledge about deviance, infirmity, and the body's reaction to adverse land, labor, and social conditions. This happened in a context of infectious and parasitic disease, high infant mortality and malnutrition, privation, and overall despair for Puerto Rico's majority

rural population.[15] Mug shots emerged alongside criminal anthropology, a pseudoscience about "inherent criminality" popularized by the Italian physician Cesare Lombroso in the late nineteenth century. According to Lombroso, "born
criminals" could be identified by their visible "atavistic deficiencies."[16] These became perceptible through anthropometry—the measurement of certain parts of
the human body. Across Latin America, the confluence of positivist medical and
human science helped birth criminal anthropology. Latin American intellectuals and health professionals absorbed and reconfigured Lombroso's musings,
with some parroting him and others complicating his ideas.[17]

Criminal anthropology reached Spanish Caribbean shores in the 1870s and
1880s.[18] During this period in Cuba, Rebecca Scott writes, members of the prop-
ertied and educated classes embraced a racialized variant of anthropology. They
thought it showed "the differences between whites and blacks and that, in times
of great turmoil, blacks historically reverted to barbarism and human sacrifice."[19] Similar developments occurred in Puerto Rico, where creole intellectuals shared the Eurocentric and custodial-punitive grammar of positivist science.
They emphasized the "natural immoralities" of mixed-race and white peasants,
free people of color, the enslaved and formerly enslaved, and convicts.[20] Many
of the scholars who assessed disadvantaged people portrayed them as beings
in need of regeneration and socialization. To repair and orient these individuals, physician-anthropologists informed by Atlantic intellectual currents steered
them toward verifiable knowledge and practices that could fix their glitches.

Scientific laboratory medicine transformed Puerto Rico's medical profession in the early twentieth century. Physicians trained in Spain and France
often clashed with their US-American counterparts after the War of 1898 precisely because Americans were more laboratory-oriented (or detached) than
the former, who were more concerned with socioeconomic contexts. This
apparent shift tempered the interpretive power of criminal anthropology but
did not eliminate the pseudoscience altogether. Rather than abate, positivist
science fused into everyday medico-legal practice. In the first decades of the
twentieth century, Puerto Rican authorities progressively turned to laboratory medicine without entirely abandoning Lombrosian precepts. These were
deployed to understand and probe the bodies of criminals and convicts, and
subsequently, to physically rehabilitate them.

Physicians tried to treat individuals for infirmities that could have legal
and societal ramifications, including alcoholism, prostitution, mental illness,
criminality, superstition, and quackery. All of these, Reinaldo Román asserts,
were believed to cause the degradation of genetic types.[21] Lombrosian ideas
influenced not only physicians but also criminologists and even Spiritists,
convincing many of them that positivist science was crucial for physical and

social "regeneration" at the individual and national levels.[22] Eugenics-tinged interventionist discourses of rescue, family, and sexuality fueled US imperial projects and organized US colonialism in Puerto Rico more broadly.[23]

Rescuing and regenerating Puerto Rico depended on the intersecting efforts of US administrators, creole elites, and competing grassroots groups. The redemptive work of physicians, for example, was carried out on individual bodies. According to Nicole Trujillo-Pagán, medical experts constructed rural light-skinned peasant (*jíbaro*) bodies as both a "symbol and myth of Puerto Rico as a sick nation." Under Spanish rule, *jíbaros* were anemic patients requiring care. Under US rule, the *jíbaro* symbolized Puerto Ricans' "primitive nature" and "lack of capacity for self-government."[24] Exclusively focusing on disease, prophylactic hygiene, and the redemption of certain bodies, however, ignored the obstacles posed by factors such as unemployment, hunger, natural disasters, and hopelessness.[25] Although varied constituencies approached regeneration and salvation in early twentieth-century Puerto Rico in different ways, they shared a common destination of national progress and uplift.[26] By the 1930s, prisons were increasingly viewed as sites where the project of rehabilitation could be fruitfully advanced. This occurred on the heels of the introduction of New Deal–era emergency relief and reconstruction policies.[27]

While criminal anthropology and its technologies crystallized in Puerto Rico in the late 1800s and early 1900s, and tropical medicine gained a foothold in the first decades of the twentieth century, by the 1930s and 1940s physicians in Puerto Rican prisons were primarily concerned with the body and sought to map its complexity biomedically. They made rigorous attempts to bring convicts back from the physical health brink by diagnosing and treating them for all manner of disease. This fascination with and aspiration to raise prisoners from biological death played out in Oso Blanco as soon as the penitentiary opened in 1933.[28] Physicians were among the institution's most active health professionals. Importantly, they also set a moral standard, as many of them identified with Christianity, Freemasonry, or some combination of these or other ritualistic belief systems. Prison medical experts advanced a kind of biological determinism but also helped pave the way for the colonial-populist carceral social science of the 1940s.

Prison Health Care

In the late nineteenth century, prison health care in Puerto Rico revolved around what transpired in Spanish military hospitals.[29] Sick and dying convicts enjoyed access to rudimentary diagnostic infrastructure at the time. Still, medical personnel reported inmate causes of death on a regular basis.

These causes included injuries related to grueling labor, interpersonal violence, strokes, fevers, infections, tuberculosis, and other diseases. Diagnostics
grew more sophisticated and demonstrably successful prophylaxis was added
to prison therapeutic regimens under US rule, culminating in unprecedented
health interventions by the late 1910s and 1920s.

Justice and health authorities carried out a major health operation in and
near a Santurce army camp (Las Casas) during the latter bookend of World
War I, for instance. The undertaking targeted diseased prostitutes, adulter-
ers, and intoxicating liquors.[30] More than 850 women of all colors (at least
422 whites, 304 mulattas, and 65 blacks) were convicted and confined during
the operation. The Arecibo district jail was refitted for the introduction of 300
of these women. The Ponce district jail was converted into a hospital and held
some 450 women.[31] The Mayagüez district jail soon followed and received the
180 remaining, but a devastating earthquake rendered the facility unsafe, and
authorities were obliged to send the women to Arecibo and San Juan.[32]

The venereal disease officer Lieutenant Hermann Goodman reported that
all these women were checked for syphilis with the Wassermann reaction, an
antibody blood test, revealing a 62 percent rate of infection across participating district jails. The field director of the American Red Cross for Puerto
Rico and the Virgin Islands furnished five hundred tubes of arsenobenzol
606 (salvarsan) and arranged transportation for Goodman to administer the
drug. More than 1,400 intravenous injections and 5,000 injections of mercury
were given to incarcerated women. "We gave the most intensive treatments
possible [on a daily basis] and followed up each course of salvarsan with the
necessary mercury to a degree that we are certain that cures are permanent
in most cases," Goodman asserted.[33] Examinations of imprisoned prostitutes
also disclosed that several of them were infected with gonorrhea, yaws, scabies, ringworm, hookworm, lice, influenza, and ulcerating granuloma of the
pudenda. An organic salt of antimony—tartar emetic—purportedly proved
efficacious in treating the latter condition but took too long to produce results.[34] Health authorities vaccinated female prisoners against typhoid and
smallpox as well, with the idea of preempting future public health crises.[35]

Prison health-care infrastructure in Puerto Rico improved in the 1920s
despite ongoing health challenges. When the legislature approved $750,000
for the construction of a new penitentiary in 1923 in the midst of an influenza epidemic, the Insular Sanatorium at Río Piedras assigned cottages to
tubercular prisoners, where they received "attendance and treatment of the
same kind as all other patients."[36] The "degrading and inhuman" wooden
board beds used in La Princesa penitentiary in Old San Juan and district jails
around the big island were substituted by "comfortable, cool, and sanitary"

cots.[37] By 1925, La Princesa prisoners received special medical attention in the form of surgeries and in the treatment of syphilis and hookworm. About half of the five hundred convicts residing there were given salvarsan.[38] Through 1929, medico-legal officials persisted in treating convicts infected with syphilis, hookworm, and to a lesser extent tuberculosis. Many inmates suffered from at least one of these diseases when they entered prisons. Surgeries of various kinds continued to be performed as well.[39]

As Oso Blanco neared completion, prison health care became more potent. In penitentiaries, lengthy sentences kept convicts under medical surveillance for longer periods of time. Thousands of convicts made their way through prison hospitals on a regular basis in the 1930s. Most of them consulted doctors and received treatment. Dozens benefited from surgeries. Prison health professionals submitted thousands of biological and other samples to the Health Department laboratory for examination. They used diagrams to make lung disease legible to justice officials and nonexperts. Visual aids also served as guides for penitentiary and sanatorium medical staff to explain diagnostics, X-ray evidence, and potential surgical interventions. Warden Saldaña and López de la Rosa hoped to transfer Luciano Ayala Ramos, a forty-year-old mulatto day laborer from Fajardo serving three years for breaking and entering, for example, to the nearby Insular Sanatorium in June 1931. He was suffering from tuberculosis, sprue, and ulcers. López de la Rosa submitted diagrams of Ayala Ramos's lungs and paperwork detailing his symptomology (chest pain, the coughing up of blood, diarrhea, weight loss, and physical weakness) to sanatorium colleagues. His sputum tested positive for advanced "Koch bacillus," or mycobacterium tuberculosis, a species of pathogenic bacteria that causes the disease. Given his "decadent health state," however, he could not be transferred and died in the penitentiary tuberculosis ward the next month.[40]

Improved medical capacity equated diagnostic clarity. In 1931, the superintendent of prisons Martín Ergui, who had been active in reimagining Puerto Rican corrections since 1917, identified the conditions for which most prisoners were treated. He named uncinariasis, weakness (linked to being anemic and therefore hookworm), syphilis, pretuberculosis, and pyorrhea (advanced gingivitis). A flu epidemic also affected the prison population this particular year.[41] Through Oso Blanco's inauguration in 1933, inmates were most vulnerable to venereal, parasitic, and bacterial diseases and natural disasters (e.g., Hurricane San Ciprián devastated the penitentiary food supply in 1932).[42]

United States and Puerto Rican officials stressed the penitentiary's multifaceted health potential. According to Ergui, Oso Blanco had a dual objective: to "reform" and physically and mentally "regenerate" prisoners while using labor therapy to advance self-sustaining carceral capitalism.[43] The activist journalist

Ángela Negrón Muñoz, who toured the model penitentiary alongside Ergui in 1934, went a step further and called the prison "a temple" of moral and social regeneration.[44] Mainstream newspapers reported that the new penitentiary substituted the antiquated La Princesa in Old San Juan. During inaugural festivities, the colonial governor James R. Beverley of Texas and other officials received guests, delivered speeches, and led a tour of the institution, emphasizing Oso Blanco's state-of-the-art medical facilities.[45] Authorities hoped the Insular Penitentiary would provide in-house medical services to all convicts who needed or required them, but if for some reason that was not possible, convicts could be transferred to hospitals in San Juan and Bayamón.[46]

The Insular Penitentiary formed part of an interconnected, tri-institutional medical complex that also included a mental asylum and a tuberculosis hospital. Each institution was tasked with pathologizing and healing a specific sector of Puerto Rico's incarcerated population—lunatics, tuberculosis patients, and criminals. During Oso Blanco's inauguration, state officials highlighted how mental, biomedical, and behavioral treatment regimens reinforced one another inside the penitentiary.[47] The deputy warden Pedro Toledo Márquez explained Oso Blanco's health organization to visitors. He led a tour of the prison's psychiatric, surgical, and dental facilities. These were under the supervision of López de la Rosa and dentist Ángel C. Cortés. Toledo Márquez then showed visitors the tuberculosis infirmary, a miniature version of the nearby Insular Sanatorium visible from penitentiary sentry boxes. He also introduced them to Miguel Quiñones, an inmate who helped carry out "sanitation service" for the surgery department.[48]

Since the late 1920s, dozens of convicts were encamped on Oso Blanco grounds to prepare the site and building for habitation. They were responsible for cleaning and sanitizing the nearby mental asylum and tuberculosis hospital, and for producing and sustaining the food and milk supplies of these institutions.[49] Notably, they endured their own health crises, such as an outbreak of acute diarrhea documented by the physician Oscar Costa Mandry, a University of Maryland graduate, in 1928.[50] The labor contributions of convicts to health and medical enterprise shows that the penitentiary was not meant to be isolated and inward looking. There was a great deal of movement and exchange between the three institutions. In fact, in the 1930s and 1940s the Health Department reliably employed prisoners and put them to work gardening, draining lowlands to control malaria, destroying tubercular sputum, as well as cleaning streets, parks, and government offices.[51] Through labor assignments that improved the common good, then, many inmates received a public health education. Certain tasks put them at risk, however, demonstrating that, in the end, they were deemed disposable and replaceable.

Oso Blanco's hospital, located at the back of the imposing structure, quickly became a focal point for health and medicine. It was a beehive of activity in the 1930s and 1940s. The hospital space included a surgical hall stocked with relevant technologies and medicines.[52] There, health-care professionals studied, treated, and in some cases even trained or entrusted responsibilities to inmates.[53] This represented a shift from the 1920s, when the closest most convicts got to administering health care was by serving as foot soldiers during public health crusades and national emergencies.[54] Later in the 1920s, and especially by the 1930s, convicts mainly interfaced with medicine as objects of research. Urine, blood, serological, bacteriological, and agglutination and precipitation exams now formed part of the diagnostic arsenal of prison health professionals, as did a variety of preventive medicines, including inoculations, vaccinations, injections, and antileutic and spinal syphilis treatments. These developments contrasted sharply with the poor health-care infrastructure, services, and conditions prevailing in Puerto Rico's municipal jails during the same period.[55] District jails were located between these two extremes. The physician Ernesto Quintero, another University of Maryland graduate, mentioned the use of bismuth, arsenicals, and mapharsen to treat venereal disease in district jails in the late 1930s and early 1940s, for example.[56]

After Oso Blanco opened, its medical capacity expanded, and with it the rate of sick prisoners. In 1934, the daily average number of infirm convicts was 125; by 1947, it rose to 222.[57] Physicals, body fluid and fecal exams, X-rays, treatments, and surgeries all increased substantially from their levels the previous decade.[58] Despite this progress in medical capacity building and a steady decline in Puerto Rico's general mortality rate—from 22 percent in 1933 to between 10 and 20 percent at midcentury—venereal, parasitic, and bacterial ailments continued to plague inmates through the early 1940s.[59] Across the entire Puerto Rican prison system (the penitentiary, district jails, youth institutions, and penal encampments), dozens of prisoners died each year between 1927 and 1951.[60] The number of deaths in prisons ebbed and flowed through the early 1940s, hitting a high of sixty-five in 1935–36.[61] The high number that specific year reflected, in part, the prevalence of the "white plague" (tuberculosis), which was a leading cause of death in Puerto Rico at the height of the Great Depression (about 17 percent of the total).[62] Throughout the 1940s, prison mortality decreased and stabilized, with authorities reporting a low of eleven total deaths in 1950–51.[63]

The workflow bottleneck that developed at the Health Department laboratory in 1936 because of the spread of tuberculosis and other diseases justified the installation of a modest laboratory inside the penitentiary hospital for routine and urgent cases.[64] By 1937, distinct duos of physicians and surgeons began administering health services in Oso Blanco and Puerto Rico's seven district jails.[65] They conducted tuberculosis surveys to shield uninfected prisoners from their tubercular counterparts, which had the effect of preserving their labor power for state projects.[66] Additionally, in the mid-1930s, medical experts and others even called for the creation an insular eugenic board that would allow prison staff and health professionals to sterilize incarcerated people deemed unfit for procreation due to hereditary disease or physical and mental "defects."[67]

Many of these patterns persisted through the latter years of World War II, when the concerns of justice officials shifted toward the most basic elements of convict well-being, chiefly Oso Blanco's food supply and strained human resources. In 1943, the interim attorney general Manuel Rodríguez Ramos noted that the prison system faced food expense and personnel problems triggered by wartime conditions.[68] Such concerns circulated until the end of the global conflagration. Biomedical exclusivity itself began waning in Oso Blanco around 1945, when a psychiatrist became the penitentiary's informal resident physician, signaling the ascendance of integrated carceral medical practice.[69] Congruent medical practice also percolated at the district jail level and is perhaps best captured by the University of Maryland graduate and Catholic physician Julio R. Rolenson's 1947 examination of an "insane" nineteen-year-old convict-patient from Cabo Rojo named Ángel Montalvo. Rolenson, who was based at the San Juan district jail, found Montalvo to be "physically healthy" but showing symptoms of "acute violent dementia," bad memory, and abnormal behavior.[70] As Puerto Ricans inched toward changes in prison administration and biomedicine, US officials equipped with what they believed were cutting-edge ideas and methods encouraged them to hasten their efforts.

Prison Conditions and Oso Blanco's Hospital

Linked to the magnification of integrated medicine in Oso Blanco was the publication of the first of several federal studies that focused on both the shortcomings and promising future of Puerto Rican rehabilitative corrections. A 1947 report by the Federal Bureau of Prisons official Frank Loveland outlined recommendations that justice and prison authorities in Puerto Rico hoped to immediately implement, although many of them would not be entertained until the 1950s.[71] At the request of governor Rexford G. Tugwell, who as early as 1942 told local legislators that they could no longer "neglect to improve the condition of the men and women confined in the prison and correctional system," Loveland visited Puerto Rico for eight days in January 1944 to evaluate the commitment of juvenile offenders.[72] On the ground, however, he cast a wider net that included the main island's broader carceral archipelago and recommended the construction of facilities for young men and women and camps or farms for men serving short sentences.[73]

While visiting adult prisons, Loveland identified areas of concern in the biomedical health aspect. Overcrowded conditions complicated the allocation of resources.[74] A "modernized kitchen," a "better diet for the inmates," and an "improved medical program" were needed at Oso Blanco, all of which would facilitate the extraction of efficient labor from prisoners, avoid riots and strikes, and rehabilitate and release convicts in "good physical and mental health."[75] Concerning Oso Blanco's medical capacity, Loveland was not impressed. Despite proximity to a mental asylum and a tuberculosis hospital, insane and tubercular convicts remained confined inside Oso Blanco, where adequate facilities and supervision were not available. In 1945, the budget for penitentiary medical staff more than doubled ($16,132) to contract a tuberculosis specialist, a laboratory X-ray assistant (to be drawn from an applicant pool of returning war veterans), and eight male nurses. However, there was no indication that a resident physician or medical director would be included in the budget.[76] Stabilizing these positions and services required bringing interns and students into the mix, which would save the government money and provide apprentices with field experience.

San Juan district jail, where Rolenson often worked, was another story. There, medical services were inadequate from a public health perspective. Noticeable odors indicating poor sanitation marked the olfactory ambiance. Bowls used for food were greasy and unsanitary given the lack of hot water. Syphilitic and tubercular inmates mingled with healthy peers, sharing the same utensils and facilities. The resident physician was constantly missing in action. Dirty and bedraggled prisoners walked around barefoot and scrubbed their clothes on the brick floor. Older inmates routinely sexually assaulted younger prisoners. The experience prisoners received at this "disgraceful" and seemingly "hopeless" jail, Loveland noted, was "demoralizing."[77] Indeed, district jails around the big island, except for Arecibo, were generally unhygienic, overcrowded, and idle in terms of productive manpower—a "menace to health," according to Loveland.[78] As for living conditions in municipal jails, they were so deplorable that even short sentences bred misery, ill health, and further criminality rather than rehabilitation. Loveland therefore echoed the findings of attorney general Rodríguez Ramos, who recommended that municipal jails be "abolished."[79] Remarkable by today's standards, both officials pointed to decarceration, with Loveland suggesting that "delinquents and adult offenders need not [always] be committed to institutions."[80]

Before Loveland's visit and critiques, however, thousands of Puerto Rican inmates received medical attention in prison hospitals. They were among the infirm masses in need of rescue and rehabilitation, as the independence-populist politician and later attorney general Vicente Géigel Polanco asserted at the 1943 meeting of Puerto Rico's Medical Association.[81] Notwithstanding Géigel Polanco's statement and the development of medical infrastructure within the prison system, incarcerated people still died between the 1930s and midcentury. They came from all walks of life and succumbed to all manner of death, including communicable and noncommunicable diseases, acquired and congenital conditions, and human-inflicted injuries.[82] A twenty-eight-year-old black day laborer from San Cristóbal, Dominican Republic, named Octavio Montilla, for example, entered Oso Blanco in a poor state of health in April 1938. López de la Rosa and the physician J. B. Kodesh examined and treated him for neurosyphilis and a chronic gonorrheal urethritis.[83] Treatment was administered via "neosalvarsan, tryparsamide, bismuth, mercury, and iodide injections."[84] Montilla spent more than year in Oso Blanco's hospital before expiring in June 1939.

External observers such as Loveland reported that the penitentiary's infectious disease capacity had all but collapsed by the mid-1940s, especially in terms of the potential spread of tuberculosis. But the penitentiary archive and other sources reveal that in the 1940s and early 1950s, Oso Blanco's hospital continued to teem with medical activity, social interactions, and experimentation even as the institution continued to face health challenges. Implementing preventive medicine consumed the collective energy of a limited number of prison health professionals. As a result, the daily average number of sick convicts swelled. Systematizing and standardizing diagnostic procedures and treatments professionalized and subdivided medicine and improved the health of prisoners while normalizing vertical interventions on their bodies.

Loveland claimed that in 1945–46, Oso Blanco's hospital lacked most of the equipment recognized as necessary in a modern hospital. He called for clinical diagnostic procedures and preventive medicine, the creation of an outpatient center, the hospitalization of chronically ill patients, and the elimination of sanitation hazards.[85] Yet hundreds of penitentiary inmates were fluorographed (X-rayed) in 1944–45 alone, and more than a thousand by the end of the decade.[86] In 1946, Oso Blanco hospital care included the services of eye doctors and ear, nose, and throat specialists. This contrasted with the district jails, where such specialists were proverbial unicorns given their rarity.[87] Microscopic analyses of blood and fecal samples in the penitentiary hospital laboratory contributed to extirpating filarial and other parasitic worms from convicts.[88] Despite these strides, the penitentiary hospital housed at times as many as two hundred patients, far more than it could handle in 1946–47. Supplies like shoes, clothing, bedding, utensils, soap, towels, toothbrushes, and tooth powder or paste were in short supply.[89] Although penitentiary medical care intensified and the tuberculosis ward was expanded in 1948, diseases long on the radars of prison physicians, such as hookworm, syphilis, and tuberculosis, persisted in impairing inmate bodies, while others without the same reputations, like arthritis, bilharzia, hepatitis, and skin infections, increasingly packed a punch.[90] Officials welcomed pesticide-armed health brigades to the penitentiary when plagues of flies and mosquitoes erupted.[91] Changes in the penitentiary drug regimen were enacted as well. By the 1950s, penicillin replaced the toxic drug salvarsan in Oso Blanco.[92] This did not always mean that prisoners could readily access medications, however.[93] Oftentimes, aspirin was the best they could get.[94]

Incarcerated people reflected on prison health care in *El Despertar*, a mimeographed magazine they produced in collaboration with Oso Blanco authorities.[95] Some wrote columns while hospitalized and deemed their reflections "balm" for their peers.[96] Others mapped Oso Blanco's medical geography. An inmate named Joaquín B., Jr., published a report on the penitentiary hospital and its "magnificent reforms" in June 1949, for example.[97] The hospital spanned several floors. The main floor (located on the second level of an annex behind the penitentiary) was equipped with a pharmacy supervised by a trusted convict, an infirmary and curative facilities for patients with minor emergencies, a sanitary station for medical staff, a small room for convicts to receive weekend visits, and a petite dining room for patients and health-care workers alike. There were four large rooms with hygienic facilities and twelve to fifteen beds inside each one. These rooms would have looked like the one depicted in figure 1.1. Clinicians or trusted prisoners supervised these rooms and monitored convict diets.[98] The third level of Oso Blanco's hospital accommodated physicians, dentists, and their diagnosis and treatment efforts. It housed specialists' offices, a laboratory with microscopes, X-ray machines, an operating room, and tools related to pneumothorax (collapsed lung) treatment.[99] Employees aided by convicts managed these spaces and technologies. The fourth level of the hospital housed record-keeping offices and a "modern" tuberculosis ward where prisoners with the bacterial disease were isolated.[100]

Upon arriving at Oso Blanco, all prisoners visited the hospital to receive a physical (fig. 1.2). Physicians used stethoscopes to listen to the heartbeats and lungs of convicts. The physical exam determined whether inmates were contagious, whether they could handle hard labor, or whether they had another problem meriting attention. If necessary, prisoners also received vaccinations and had their blood drawn. The specialists working in Oso Blanco's hospital around midcentury included Ceferino A. Méndez Polo, a Cuban surgeon who had studied at Tulane University.[101] He served as hospital director and

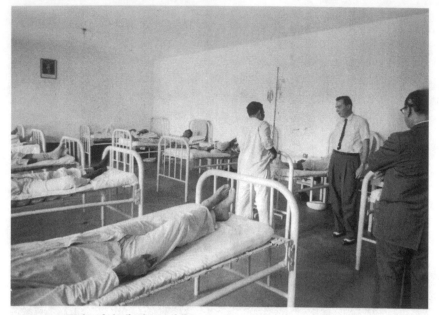

FIGURE 1.1 Unidentified officials visit full penitentiary infirmary room. September 1960. Proyecto El Mundo/Biblioteca Digital Puertorriqueña, Universidad de Puerto Rico–Río Piedras.

was assisted by the Catholic tuberculosis expert Fernando Luis Buxeda Vélez, a graduate of Hahnemann Medical College in Philadelphia; the Emory University graduate and eyes, ears, nose, and throat specialist Miguel A. Mariani; and the bacteriologist José M. Dobal, among others.[102] An anonymous prisoner observed in fall 1949 that specialist care (e.g., physicians, eye doctors) made a real difference for the more than "ninety percent" of impoverished convicts who entered Oso Blanco with anemia, malaria, eyesight problems, or broken molars and suffering from fevers, vomiting, and influenza.[103] Abject poverty reduced many prisoners to bare life before they even entered the penitentiary. For example, Méndez Polo utilized the term "cachexia" to describe the axiomatic condition in which he found a nineteen-year-old mulatto day laborer named Manuel Medina Hernández from Barceloneta, who was serving a short sentence for multiple counts of theft.[104] This inmate weakened and decayed so quickly that when he died he looked wasted, or living dead, as if he had been rotting away for some time.

Joaquín R.B.V. also contemplated Oso Blanco's hospital in *El Despertar*. In his piece, the convict chronicled the activities of Méndez Polo and company. Méndez Polo inspected facilities, periodically examined convicts, and made individual treatment recommendations given his role on the penitentiary's

Classification and Treatment Board. Buxeda Vélez cared for tuberculosis patients, providing them with pneumothorax and pneumoperitoneum treatment. The surgery technician Pedro R. Astor administered Oso Blanco's hospital on a day-to-day basis. He was Méndez Polo's main assistant, lending a hand with major surgical procedures and carrying out minor ones by himself. Dobal supervised the penitentiary laboratory. His daily routine included collecting blood, fecal, urine, and skin samples. He also oversaw the X-ray process. Dobal's work revealed whether convicts suffered from skin conditions or were infected with hookworm, syphilis, and tuberculosis.[105]

To understand the bodies of convicts, Oso Blanco doctors and hospital staff compiled inmate medical histories. Echoing how nineteenth-century physician-anthropologists chronicled their patients, these narratives had

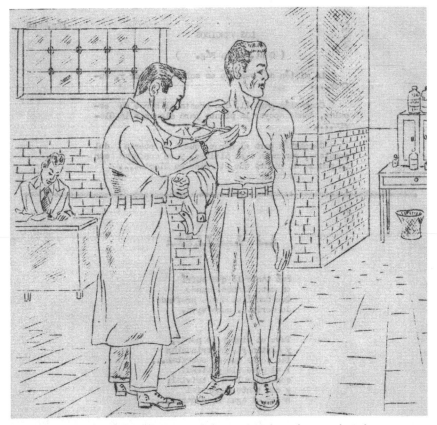

FIGURE 1.2 Convict depiction of physician Ceferino Méndez Polo conducting a physical in penitentiary medical space. *El Despertar* 2, no. 1 (April 1950). Biblioteca y Hemeroteca Puertorriqueña, Universidad de Puerto Rico–Río Piedras.

communal and individual components. According to Méndez Polo, considering domestic arrangements showed whether convict families had histories of "hereditary" or contractible disease (e.g., syphilis, tuberculosis, cancer, diabetes, epilepsy, mental illness), which in turn might explain the predicaments of certain inmates. The portions of medical histories focusing on individual pathologies described the illnesses, surgeries, and vaccinations prisoners experienced and received as children, adolescents, and adults. A physical exam followed the completion of the medical history.[106]

During physicals, physicians logged height, weight, general appearance, skin condition, and body system functionality (e.g., cardiovascular, respiratory, digestive, lymphatic, nervous, genitourinary). They inspected convicts' ears, noses, throats, eyes, muscles, and tendons. Doctors noted lesions or contusions and evidence of vice due to alcohol (ab)use, narcotics (ab)use, or venereal disease. Extremities warranted attention as well, especially if the prisoner had varicose veins, deformities, or was flat-footed.[107] The results of physicals prompted physicians to order chest X-rays, laboratory work, blood tests for cell counts and syphilis (via the Kahn and Hinton techniques), urine exams for bacterial infections, and excrement analyses to check for parasites. For inmates to be admitted to the penitentiary hospital, they had to have a hundred-degree fever or higher.[108] If the resources to diagnose and treat the infirm were unavailable in the prison, then medical staff sought answers beyond the walls.[109]

Physicians like Méndez Polo often decided that surgery was the best available treatment in general. In summer 1950, he discussed in *El Despertar* his experiences with a young prisoner who underwent two surgeries with him. The first surgery extracted construction nails from the inmate's intestine. The second surgery removed a piece of iron and a laboratory needle from the same site. The convict recovered quickly and received psychotherapy. During therapy sessions, he claimed that problems with other inmates had induced him to ingest hazardous objects. For Méndez Polo, physically salvaging inmates debilitated by anemia was a priority in itself, but even more so when the effort was linked to securing their labor power for the institution and state.[110] Psychotherapy complemented biomedical intervention after the fact to help incarcerated people obtain sound minds en route to their renewed bodies being channeled into a changing Puerto Rican political economy.

Medicine was not always objective or just about reviving deteriorating and infirm convict bodies, however. It could also be politicized and deployed in acrimonious ways that harmed incarcerated people. Heriberto Marín Torres, for instance, who participated in the nationalist insurrection of fall 1950 and served an extended sentence across Puerto Rican penitentiaries that decade, recalled persecutory medical experiments that were carried out in prisons. While he was imprisoned in Oso Blanco, two high-ranking US military officials accompanied by a local sergeant visited every day. They experimented on prisoners in the penitentiary laboratory in exchange for cartons of cigarettes.[111]

One such guinea pig was a convict named Héctor Gabriel Moreno, a Korean war veteran who worked in the prison hospital. Having been previously infected with bilharzia, army officials studied his body and gave him a pill-based treatment to determine his health status. While Moreno had no qualms about the treatment because he was ex-military and therefore trusted the institution, other prisoners were subjected to similar experiments and subsequently died—almost all of them with "swollen bellies" and having endured "excruciating pain."[112] Moreno was no exception. Although eventually transferred to a hospital, pardoned by governor Luis Muñoz Marín, and released from prison, Marín Torres could not help but notice Moreno's "cadaverous" appearance during the final visit he made to Oso Blanco.[113]

Oso Blanco's hospital was remodeled after the prison rebellions of late October 1950 and late January 1951. The journalist Benjamín Santana wrote a brief article about the restored, better-equipped, and more sterilized facilities that summer.[114] The photograph accompanying the article, of a surgery in motion, gave readers the impression that prison biomedicine had, again, turned over a new leaf in the march toward progress. In some ways, Puerto Rico's rehabilitative carceral project intersected with the pioneering work of Health Secretary Guillermo Arbona, who would institute a transnational public health model later in the 1950s that integrated preventive and curative care and oriented medical education to be supportive of such systems.[115] But the testimonies of Marín Torres and others invert the medical class's heroic self-image and shed light on how medicine could do violence to prisoners. Reinforcing or redirecting health facilities could not save and regenerate all convict bodies when that very infrastructure was used to harm them as well.[116] A bottom-up suspicion of medicine, its logics and practices, and its technologies circulated in midcentury Puerto Rican prisons, tempering but not entirely undoing the idealism that pervaded rehabilitative corrections.

Conclusion

Prison biomedicine in Puerto Rico evolved after US citizenship in 1917. In the 1920s through midcentury, it entailed tremendous scrutiny of convict bodies. The process of understanding and treating prisoners' physical bodies began outside of them. When fresh inmates first entered prisons like Oso Blanco, guards logged their arrival and christened their institutional case files. The task of photographing new arrivals was typically assigned to trusted convicts. By the 1930s, mug shots formed part of everyday criminal-legal practice. They were a central feature of incarceration and the broader taxonomic culture of information gathering and synthesis characteristic of modern penitentiaries. Criminal anthropology and phrenology still informed how prison authorities in Puerto Rico went about archiving punishment, but the eugenic rationales connected to them were muted considerably.

While mug shots continued to shape how the state archived punishment, their association with ascendant cultures of rehabilitative corrections signaled that they did not always have to lead back to pseudoscience. Physicals followed penitentiary central booking. After an extensive intake process, prison authorities escorted new inmates to Oso Blanco's hospital, where physicians examined their case files, photographs, and bodies. They completed a series of forms chronicling the condition in which they found prisoners, noting discernible symptoms, defects, overall health, and if necessary, the results of preliminary laboratory studies. Once this initial health screening was completed, inmates were sent to their cell blocks or other penitentiary health-care facilities, such as the tuberculosis ward. There, they awaited next steps in their treatment, which sometimes meant being delivered to nearby welfare institutions.[117]

The purpose of screening and documenting Puerto Rican convicts and their infirmities served multiple interrelated purposes. Physicians represented the first community of care that sick prisoners happened upon behind bars. They provided needed and even life-saving diagnostics and treatment at a time when these were not readily available in convicts' communities of origin. Doctors wanted to improve the health and lives of the incarcerated both for the person *and* to show the modernity of the prison while preserving and enhancing its reputation. In turn, this allowed for better control of the incarcerated and their social management. Finally, diagnosis and treatment determined the labor potential of inmates. Healthy bodies meant exploitable labor. This contributed to Oso Blanco's self-sustenance, the stability and expansion of its industries corporation division, and prepared inmates for societal reinsertion. Raising the living dead commenced with physically salvaging and regenerating their bodies, but medicine could also serve a range of nonrehabilitative purposes and do them harm. Penitentiary health care merged positivist science, eugenics, and tropical medicine in a single brew, laying a foundation for the robust prison social science of the 1940s.

To Classify and Treat:
Correctional Psychology and Psychiatry

On April 24, 1945, a twenty-four-year-old black former bartender and mechanic from Caguas named Marcial Hernández García entered the Insular Penitentiary. A week prior, the Caguas district court sentenced him to eight years for a bundle of offenses, including breaking and entering, multiple counts of theft, and a crime against nature. Hernández García claimed to have committed all these acts under the influence of drugs and alcohol. Behind bars, the convict was studied and interviewed by penitentiary health professionals, who were interested in his life before prison and his physical, mental, and social health while incarcerated. Many of these individuals participated in Oso Blanco's Classification and Treatment Board, an interdisciplinary and medico-legal entity founded in the mid-1940s on the heels of Frank Loveland's visit that imagined and implemented rehabilitation programs for prisoners, in effect advancing a kind of social medicine (fig. 2.1).[1] The psychiatrist José R. Maymí Nevares, for instance, learned that Hernández García suffered from mental maladjustment, or more specifically, episodes of bewilderment during which he observed "abnormal" and "undisciplined" conduct.[2] His erratic state of mind was confirmed by several individuals familiar with him in Caguas before he was imprisoned. These potential advisers had since distanced themselves from him, telling parole officials he was "half-crazy."[3]

To treat Hernández García's mental instability, he was isolated in a cell and observed on a regular basis. An intelligence exam (Wechsler-Bellevue Intelligence Scale) administered by the Columbia University Teachers College graduate and University of Puerto Rico–Río Piedras (UPR-RP) psychologist Juan B. Picart, on which the prisoner scored a 63 (indicative of mental deficiency), corroborated traces of "organic cerebral disease."[4] While the use of such an exam in a US settler colonial context suggests the gravity of a

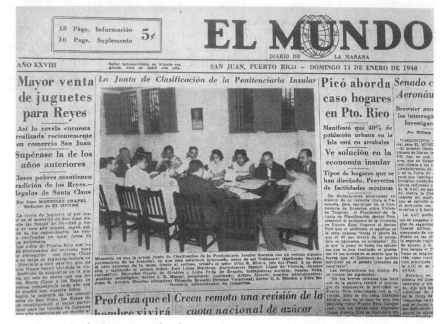

FIGURE 2.1 Insular Penitentiary Classification and Treatment Board in session. *El Mundo*, January 11, 1948. Biblioteca y Hemeroteca Puertorriqueña, Universidad de Puerto Rico–Río Piedras.

racialized dynamic—that is, a "civilized" white center imposing its technologies on a "savage" dark periphery—Picart, too, was of color.[5] His race-neutral clinical and vocational analysis confirmed Hernández García's cognitive and applied shortcomings, leading prison technocrats to believe that mental infirmity was why Hernández García neglected to study or learn a new craft while in Oso Blanco. This could become a problem, as reform and rehabilitation prevailed in the penitentiary *alongside* carceral capitalism.

When Hernández García was finally eligible for parole between late 1948 and early 1949, officials rejected the prospect given that his mental state and behavior had not improved much. Parole officer María Casasnovas cosigned their reservations, and in the end, Hernández García remained imprisoned. Still, penitentiary health professionals sensed the man was treatable and therefore salvageable. They insisted that solitary confinement, psychiatric observation, psychological examination, social work interviews, an appropriate labor assignment, and sports would achieve his rehabilitation. In fact, Oso Blanco Classification and Treatment officials continued to forecast Hernández García's rehabilitation as "regular," so they went about preparing him for parole reconsideration.[6] This meant that Classification and Treatment and parole agents viewed evidence of his impaired mind as surmountable, especially if addressed across rehabilitative techniques, and more importantly, as but a sliver of a panoramic whole that also included the body, social relationships, and the soul.

This brief foray into the penal experience of Hernández García, who was studied, interviewed, and ultimately deemed worthy of rehabilitation by an interdisciplinary group of penitentiary health professionals, reveals myriad overlapping encounters between different practitioners and convicts and the frequent exchanges and loops between them. In this case and many others, psychologists and psychiatrists played key roles in shaping mental health interventions and treatment programs. Psychometric tests spanning intelligence, ability, and personality enabled mental health experts and their social work collaborators to forge what they believed were objective assessments of prisoners.[7] In turn, these guided health professionals' decision-making about the vocational substance of rehabilitation on a case-by-case basis. The creole Puerto Rican project of socializing medicine in corrections helped mute and overturn long-standing colonial assumptions about the inevitability of tropical unfitness. The irony was that psychologists and psychiatrists aspired to rehabilitate inmates while reinforcing common tropes of their intellectual dysfunction.[8] Rehabilitation had a positive impact on many incarcerated people but also reified structures of criminalization and colonial subjugation.

Using parole records, historical periodicals, and other sources, this chapter traces the emergence of mind science in midcentury Puerto Rican prisons. Penitentiary psychologists and psychiatrists used psychometrics and the broader social sciences to measure the intelligence, skill sets, and personalities of prisoners, and to pin down how to best uplift them (usually via labor therapy). These diagnostic and descriptive tools revealed that convicts required discipline, tutelage, and treatment, but they also had redemptive potential regardless of social difference. This socioscientific double imperative troubled linear notions of human progress, tempered professional preferences for certain technologies of power over others, and formed and made visible the value commitments of prisoners and the experts charged with evaluating and shepherding them.[9] Mind science professionals catalyzed forward-looking treatment programs, illustrating how intersubjective exchanges and multiple agencies transformed Puerto Rican corrections, at least for a time.

Psychometric Testing

In the twentieth century, global psychometric instruments failed to universalize the human but nonetheless contributed to colonial expansion. In Puerto Rico, the competitive dust between Spanish and American colonial

frameworks had more or less settled by midcentury. The ensuing nationaliza-
tion of science and parallel pursuit of a comprehensive human science under
colonial populism subverted exclusively Spanish or American approaches to
rehabilitation. Spanish, American, and creole flows of scientific knowledge
production crashed into one another in the first half of the twentieth century,
with the latter becoming prominent between the 1940s and 1960s. Creole su-
premacy within Puerto Rico's borders circumvented conventional colonial
relations, reversed values, and upset predominant social structures and hi-
erarchies.[10] Settler colonial conceits that informed acceptable manifestations
of modern state formation remained visible in how psychometric tools reproduced certain standards and tropes during the era of the Partido Popular
Democrático but were also translated over.

Puerto Rican psychopathologists were involved in the application of psychological methods to criminology on the US mainland.[11] The development
and use of psychological tests and measures in the Western world and Puerto
Rico spans more than a century.[12] In 1920, adaptations of the Pintner tests of
nonverbal intelligence circulated on Puerto Rico's main island.[13] The Stanford Achievement Test appeared next, by 1925.[14] These were followed by other
exams administered to public school students and incarcerated youths.[15] In
1927, for example, the attorney general George C. Butte of Texas reported that
much attention had been granted in the previous year to the health of incarcerated young people in Puerto Rico:

> Examinations for syphilis, hookworm and malaria have been made, to ascer-
> tain the exact health conditions of the inmates, and proper treatments were
> given in an effort to eradicate the diseases. The [reform] school [for delin-
> quent boys in Mayagüez] also had the cooperation of Dr. [Fred C.] Walters
> and Professor [F. E.] Morse of the Department of Psychology of the University
> of Porto Rico, who made an educational and mental survey of the inmates,
> using, among other tests, the Stanford Test of Ability, which was used by the
> Commission from Columbia University in a study made of the children of the
> public schools of Porto Rico.[16]

While mental tests became a fixture of Puerto Rican psychology in the early
twentieth century, clinical services were not routinely offered in psychiatric
hospitals, facilities serving veterans and children, and prisons until the 1940s
and later.[17] This laggard expansion coincided with the maturation of the field
of psychology as an ascendant academic discipline that emphasized mental
processes, interpersonal relationships, introspection, and behavior.[18]

Psychologists trained in the United States and elsewhere aimed to perfect
mental tests attuned to the linguistic and cultural milieu of Puerto Rico.[19]

This was because mistranslation weakened the reliability of these diagnostic tools. Therefore, it was difficult for Puerto Ricans to obtain the expected mean intelligence quotient, or IQ, of 100, the prevailing standard in Anglo-America. Psychologists and educators recognized that a bias emerged when Spanish speakers were tested with instruments designed for English speakers.[20] Class bias also bedeviled the search for "culturally fair" mental tests.[21] In response, researchers tried to devise culture-free tests that could universally estimate the intellectual functioning and manual capabilities of different groups, in theory resulting in a more equitable assessment of Puerto Ricans.

Multiple tests were translated and adopted in Puerto Rico between the 1930s and 1950s. These included, among others, the Wechsler Adult Intelligence Scale, the Wechsler Intelligence Scale for Children, the Binet Intelligence Scale, and the Goodenough-Harris Draw-a-Man Test.[22] The use of mental tests in Oso Blanco aligned with the growth and application of psychology in Puerto Rico at large. Prison psychologists connected to UPR-RP measured the intelligence, cognitive and mechanical abilities, and personalities of convicts. Exam results reiterated to the Classification and Treatment Board that inmate minds harbored rich data that could and should be socio-scientifically excavated, explained, and deployed to rehabilitate incarcerated people. In mapping prisoners in this way, penitentiary social scientists laid bare their own moral and behavioral preferences.[23] For them the end of a rehabilitated Puerto Rico by and large "free" of colonial mismanagement and subjugation justified the means of utilizing psychometrics on prisoners to confirm their dysfunction and redemptive potential.

In its first decade of existence, Oso Blanco endured socioscientific growing pains. Shortly after officially opening in 1933, the penitentiary still lacked a psychopathological clinic to examine, diagnose, and treat convicts suffering from mental conditions.[24] The next year, in 1934, the attorney general Benjamin J. Horton of Kansas encouraged Puerto Rican legislators to carve mind science positions into the new fiscal year's budget. A psychiatrist and psychologist were "indispensable" for the study of prisoners' "defects" and treating the "mental disorders" either caused or instigated by the crime(s) they committed, Horton insisted.[25] As of 1935, the posts lingered as an idea.[26]

There is little to no mention of carceral mind science in Puerto Rican Justice Department publications between the mid-1930s and mid-1940s. By 1946, however, in the wake of Loveland's visit and the administrative schematics he introduced, psychiatric and psychological services were routine in Oso Blanco and overlapped with one another. Psychological testing fell under the umbrella of psychiatry in terms of government reporting. The attorney general Enrique Campos del Toro, for instance, observed: "The number of new cases taken care of during the fiscal year by the psychiatrist at the Penitentiary were 138, of which the majority were cases of mental deficiency, psychopathic personality and psychoneurosis. Fifty-seven did not reveal apparent mental disturbances."[27] In part, mental test results let prison authorities draw these conclusions. Governor Jesús T. Piñero relayed the following year, in 1947, that "medical care to the indigent and public welfare activities in general increased throughout the Island, and a modest educational program [and census] on mental hygiene, with special emphasis on the problem of the feebleminded, was undertaken."[28] The category "feebleminded" surfaced in the US in the mid-nineteenth century to describe people exhibiting a lack of productivity and other heterodox behaviors. To be feebleminded equated "mental deficiency" and denoted a level of functioning just above "idiocy."[29] Puerto Rican penitentiary health professionals imbued the category with similar opprobrium in their assessments of incarcerated rural people in the mid-twentieth century.[30]

The end of World War II boosted the progress of clinical psychology in Puerto Rico. Psychologists active on the UPR-RP campus, including Picart, administered intelligence tests and conducted psychodiagnostic studies through projective tests that evaluated personality and intrapsychic conflicts.[31] In 1945, "apolitical" educator Ismael Rodríguez Bou gauged the intelligence of 642 penitentiary inmates using the Interamerican General Intermediate Ability test (Form AS). He found that 97 percent of those examined had an eighth-grade education or lower. Rodríguez Bou's research indicated Oso Blanco had a serious illiteracy problem and that there was a correlation between criminality and educational level.[32] Mental health professionals charged a similar relationship existed between crime and degrees of oligophrenia.[33] Potential measures to manage young oligophrenics, for instance, required a register of all known cases, the founding of an agro-industrial colony where they could be isolated, the preparation of a trained socioscientific workforce to serve them, the establishment of special education curriculum, economic aid, social services, and clinical orientation.[34]

As for prisoners, they were evaluated in the penitentiary and on the UPR-RP campus. Importantly, performing well or poorly on intelligence tests did not preclude their rehabilitation. For example, in the January 1949 case of a thirty-one-year-old white "psychopathic" civil guard named Santiago Ocasio Soler who grew up between San Juan and New York, Picart secured numerical values for the inmate's verbal and manual skills by having him respond to arithmetic problems, order blocks, and finish drawings.[35] There was a discrepancy between Ocasio Soler's verbal and nonverbal scores because he took longer than expected to complete the former and was too sure of himself on the latter. Yet his "mental deterioration" was an "insignificant seven [percent]," and overall, he scored a 118 (in the normal-superior range).[36]

Ocasio Soler's performance on the Wechsler-Bellevue test suggested he was rehabilitable. He had a favorable attitude toward the test, performed all related tasks, and appeared to have control over his emotions. His responses were "clean, quick, and precise," Picart asserted.[37] Picart's findings with regard to Ocasio Soler contrast sharply with those he articulated several months earlier (in September 1948) for Enrique Carmona—a seventeen-year-old wheat-colored (*trigueño*) and "rebellious" errand runner from Toa Alta.[38] Carmona took the Wechsler-Bellevue test (Form I) on the UPR-RP campus and earned a total score of 56, which meant he was "mentally retarded" or a "high moron."[39] However, Carmona had "psychological potential" and would thrive "under favorable environmental conditions."[40] His petulance and firm independent streak aside, rehabilitation was not out of the question for him. In fact, his rehabilitative prognosis was "good."[41]

Mimicking developments in the United States to an extent, psychometric tools in Puerto Rico formed part of a culture of observation and evaluation that consolidated and expanded vertical forms of social control.[42] Notwithstanding the cultural and linguistic limits of many exams, psychologists like Picart deployed a variety of mental tests to determine on which minds different tests could be applied. Their work, in conjunction with the efforts and interpretations of the Classification and Treatment Board, tended to harden the otherness of "mentally deficient" prisoners. Convicts thus served as psychological specimens. However, many social scientists also valued the egalitarian, social reformist impulses animating rehabilitative corrections under colonial populism and wanted prisoners striving for rehabilitation to as well. As convicts showed signs of conforming progress, evidenced by their conduct during interviews and the testimonies of others, the liberatory effects of colonial-populist rehabilitation became more pronounced. The scientific tools of settler colonialism were translated over in the process.

Intelligence, Motor Skills, and Personality

The mental dimension of rehabilitative corrections in Puerto Rico commingled with its social dimension. The work of psychologists and psychiatrists represented but two components of classification and treatment. Oso Blanco's Classification and Treatment Board also dispersed social workers to investigate the lives of convicts and synthesize the health studies completed by their peers. In turn, they generated panoramic and voluminous profiles of inmates.[43] Social workers trained in socioscientific concepts and methods accumulated health and social science data they later transmitted to modifiable treatment programs. These covered the medical, psychological, psychiatric, social, educational, and vocational aspects of rehabilitation, and usually concluded with a bottom-line prognosis indicating whether individual prisoners could be rehabilitated period.

Classification and Treatment personnel utilized diction like "good," "bad," "regular," and "difficult," among other words, to convey inmate rehabilitative prospects. Proclaiming that prisoners were "rehabilitable" meant they were salvageable physically, mentally, socially, economically, and civically. Psychometric exams such as the already-mentioned Wechsler-Bellevue, as well as the Otis Mental Ability test and the Rorschach inkblot test, either set the interpretive tone for Classification and Treatment Board efforts or built on already available critical ethnographies of convicts.[44] In short shrift, however, the board rejected exclusively considering intelligence quotients on their own. Instead, they made a habit of contemplating exams intersectionally, meaning on the one hand that mental tests spanned intelligence, aptitude, and personality, and on the other that psychologists and their Classification and Treatment colleagues believed that multiple exams disclosed more together about individuals' rehabilitative prospects than they did apart.

Although mental tests pointed to the purported intellectual, interactive, and mechanical deficiencies of inspected incarcerated people, they also served as a compass for the prison technocrats charged with crafting treatment programs. Regardless of inmate identities (e.g., race, class, sexuality) or the nature of their crime(s), they were generally considered eligible for rehabilitation—even if getting there would be an uphill climb. Psychometric exam results were key pieces of the rehabilitative puzzle, not the first, last, or only relevant variable. Rarely, if ever, did such results dictate the rehabilitative prospects and outcomes of individual inmates. Bodily health, education, vices, and security status colored most inmates' situations and prognoses as well. Critical ethnography provided windows into these and other pertinent aspects and imparted further steps that penitentiary health professionals could take to achieve rehabilitative success.

The confluence of convict ethnographies, mental tests, and treatment programs repeatedly appear in the archival record. For example, in March 1950 prison authorities considered the case of Onofre Rodríguez López, a twenty-five-year-old white agriculturalist and chauffeur from Cayey serving time for mutilation. The Classification and Treatment official Gloria L. Umpierre reported that the convict was well educated and appeared to be a "trustworthy," "serious," and all-around "normal" person.[45] Moreover, he showed repentance for his crime, possessed an excellent attitude, and was willing to adapt to what authorities demanded of him. All of this made him a "good" case for rehabilitation.[46]

Rodríguez López underwent protracted psychological testing while incarcerated. The assistant psychologist Jesús Palmer reported that he earned a high average score of 118 on the Otis test. More impressive was the fact that he answered questions quickly and correctly. Rodríguez López scored 39 points on the Bell Adjustment Inventory, which measured domestic, health, social, and emotional adjustment. The result implied he was "relatively well-balanced" compared to his immediate peers.[47] Yet his social skills needed improvement, for he was an "isolated type."[48] The answers he gave to questions about interpersonal interactions exposed his social shortcomings. Psychologists also probed Rodríguez López's manual competence via the MacQuarrie Test for Mechanical Ability, an exam that measured spatial relations, speed of decision and movement, hand-eye coordination, muscular control, and visual activity.[49] He boasted average mechanical ability, performing well on the spatial, speed, and visual portions of the test but underperformed on others. Prison officials recommended that the convict be given vocational work assignments to take advantage of the skills he had and to cultivate those he lacked. Interviews and religious services could further enrich his rehabilitation process, Classification and Treatment experts believed.

As Rodríguez López's case suggests, midcentury Oso Blanco social scientists presumed that the accurate mathematical prediction of intelligence had to be complemented by the measurement of nonintellectual characteristics, such as personality traits and disorders.[50] For example, in April 1950, Oso Blanco's Classification and Treatment Board studied a twenty-seven-year-old mulatto agriculturalist and carpenter's assistant, Antonio Hernández Alamo, from Guaynabo who was serving time for homicide. The ebullient Hernández Alamo impressed board members as "humble" and "trustworthy" but also as "a bit ignorant" and emotionally volatile.[51] He earned a 77 on the Otis test, a borderline deficient score. If exposed to interviews, religious guidance, challenging recreational activities like reading, and agricultural labor therapy, however, Hernández Alamo was a good case for rehabilitation. The prisoner teemed with "plenty of rehabilitable material."[52]

Hernández Alamo's Otis test result was but a component of a rigorous psychology that also depended on a social worker's evaluation of his personality. In his case and scores of others, penitentiary social scientists bridged ethnography and psychometrics, two constitutive elements of Puerto Rican rehabilitative corrections. The experience of a thirty-eight-year-old black asthmatic inmate from Guayama serving time for homicide, Adolfo Ortiz Gutiérrez, who "feared the dark" and was plagued by nightmares about ghosts, is also instructive in this regard.[53] According to Classification and Treatment experts who evaluated the convict in July 1950, he seemed to have "emotional problems," found "lying satisfying," and earned a 74 on his Otis test (borderline intellectual deficiency).[54] These findings convinced psychologists that they needed to administer personality tests to better diagnose and treat Ortiz Gutiérrez. Still, all was not lost. They thought he had a regular chance to be rehabilitated, and they stressed that interviews, religion, reading, and films could help bring him back from the mental and social brink. When specific tests were not used, social workers read personalities through body language and facial expressions.[55]

Oso Blanco social scientists experimented with combinations of tests, oftentimes with an ethnography at their disposal, sometimes without an ethnography at all. The perceived mildness or vulgarity of prisoners' crimes, their racial backgrounds, upbringings, labor histories and infirmities, and their (un)favorable personality traits, vices, and test scores did not automatically qualify them for or disqualify them from rehabilitation. Education, vocational training, agricultural labor therapy, social orientation, religious services, mentorship, and so on could mark a turning point in *every* convict's life, although this was not guaranteed.[56] The triangulation of prisoners' socioeconomic histories, their psychometric test results, and their treatment plans defined the research output of Oso Blanco's Classification and Treatment Board well into the 1950s.

Classification and Treatment officials adjoined psychometrics with ethnographic research about the socioeconomic histories and health circumstances of convicts. Some prisoners recognized the importance of having psychologists and social workers "study, diagnose, and analyze" their personalities.[57] A holistic approach to rehabilitative corrections engendered layered portraits of individual prisoners, which in turn pervaded health professionals' thinking about who was (in)corrigible and why. The Classification and Treatment Board utilized social science tools and methods to identify rehabilitative routes for inmates. These routes included medical, labor, recreational, social, and religious options. While psychologists and social workers had occasion to trivialize convicts, implicit in their pursuit of understanding prisoners' affective worlds and articulating original rehabilitative programming for them was the belief that inmates could be raised from intellectual, social, and ultimately civic death. Raising the living dead affected the reformist, constituency-building project of Puerto Rico's colonial-populist state in the mid-twentieth century, even if colonial-populist branding was not splashed all over the project. Social scientists and incarcerated people together made

the human sciences more human in a place (the prison) where dehumanization was and remains the expected norm.

Psychiatry

Psychology and psychiatry in Puerto Rico were interrelated in the mid-
twentieth century. Hundreds of prisoners received psychological and psychiatric treatment.[58] Penitentiary psychiatrists often reviewed the results of
mental tests administered by psychologists before embarking on their own
studies of prisoners, although they just as frequently studied convicts prior
to their psychology colleagues. Puerto Rican psychiatry, for its part, emerged
in earnest between the mid-1940s and 1950s.[59] During World War II, it was
cast as relevant to local and broader US national security.[60] Preventive mental hygiene to discipline the mind, sedatives and antispasmodics to address
symptoms of anxiety, and treatments in the form of electroshock therapy,
psychotherapy, psychoanalysis, and surgical lobotomies were routinely refer-
enced in the medical literature of the period.[61]

A prisoner named Tomás G.D. recalled that, for him, psychiatry blended
military and private practice. This was because he was treated in the psychiatric
ward at Fort Clayton, Panama, during the war and the Juliá Clinic once back in
Puerto Rico.[62] A group of psychiatrists trained in the United States, who later
became known as the Circle of Psychoanalytic Studies—Luis M. Morales, Juan
E. Morales, Juan A. Rosselló, Fernando Canino Pont, and Ramón Fernández
Marina—especially accelerated the professional development of Puerto Rican
psychiatry.[63] Several others who received training in Iberia and later pursued
their craft in Oso Blanco contributed as well. Maymí Nevares and Rafael Troyano de los Ríos, a Spanish exile who practiced in the Dominican Republic
before traversing the Mona Passage, were two of the most prominent research
scholars working at the interface of punishment and psychiatry in the mid-
twentieth century.

Maymí Nevares focused on neuropsychiatry and the union of the body
and the mind. After graduating from the University of Paris in December
1936, he began practicing medicine in Puerto Rico in October 1937. He joined
the local Medical Association in July 1940. In short order, he cofounded the
Medical Association's Psychiatry and Neurology Section. He started working
at Oso Blanco sometime between 1941 and 1942. Before his untimely death in
1951, Maymí Nevares presented his work at academic and public welfare conferences. He also published widely in medical and social science journals. In
El Heraldo Médico, for example, he broached topics of specialized and general

medical interest, including mental health and the role of the medical expert in legal processes.

Although his publications in *El Heraldo Médico* did not explicitly refer to incarcerated people like many of his other writings, Maymí Nevares used them as an indirect point of reference in his analyses. In Oso Blanco, he interviewed and observed convicts and examined their case files to recommend treatment options. Classification and Treatment Board narratives instructed him about the different crises and traumas they had faced in life. Maymí Nevares ruminated that prolonged emotional crisis and trauma could, in the long term, affect organ function through the nervous system. Canvassing nerve tissue did not in itself reveal anything about mental patients. Rather, an examination of emotional causalities was required. These needed to be extracted from patients' psyches, analyzed, and related to tangible symptoms to determine the degree to which psychological and physiological mechanisms were at work in specific cases and scenarios. To treat emotionally engendered mental problems, patients would have to modify how they reacted to external and internal disturbances.[64]

According to Maymí Nevares, one's inability to react correctly to emotional and mental challenges distinguished normal people from abnormal people, as did the extent to which individuals were extroverted or introverted. He defined normality as relative and elastic. " 'Normal' is only a statistical term for practical use, which is to say [in relation to a notion of] an average man, and a social term, which is to say a mind that responds . . . to established social norms" regarding discipline, preference, and morality in specific geo-cultural contexts.[65] Norms in France, Turkey, and Mongolia played out differently than in Puerto Rico, he insisted. But regardless of geography and culture, abnormality could surface in the extremes of extroversion and introversion, particularly in the absence of balancing qualities or when an extrovert or introvert failed to adapt to their environments and even their own egos. A "normal mind," in contrast, enjoyed "a sufficient amount of energy flowing constantly, free of inhibitions and obstacles," "a sufficient amount of friendly and affectionate feelings" in human relations, and "felicity or serenity, or rather, sufficient capacity to feel pleasurable and satisfying emotions," above all "self-satisfaction."[66]

Echoing the Austrian neurologist Sigmund Freud, Maymí Nevares claimed that normal men were rare. Men hovering between average normality and abnormality abounded, however, and these were the men he regularly came across in Oso Blanco. Difficult circumstances and challenges frequently accosted such prisoners, feeding debilitating inferiority complexes and hypochondria in them. Maymí Nevares elaborated on the reassuring internal and social safety valves they invoked, such as spectacle role-playing, "the desire to overcome," and "day-dreaming."[67] The rhetoric of overcoming confinement, specifically, marked the carceral situations of many midcentury prisoners, who eagerly anticipated the respective days they would leave prison, return home, and lead better, successful lives. Maymí Nevares suggested that inferiority complexes were embedded within these seemingly harmless expressions. They manifested themselves in peculiarities of character, awkward social behavior, and in a chronic nervous tension approximating the delusions of the protagonist in "The Lawyer of Glass," a seventeenth-century short story by the Spanish novelist Miguel de Cervantes Saavedra.[68]

Convicts were also indirect strawmen for Maymí Nevares in his views on drinking. He made clear that, from his vantage point, there was a difference between those who consumed acceptable amounts of alcohol and neurotic or degenerative individuals who drank in excess for psychopathological reasons. Maymí Nevares argued that social drinking could spiral out of control over time, resulting in violent outbursts and criminal behavior. While limited alcohol consumption reduced mental friction and facilitated social exchange, dependency on alcohol was also a possibility in weaker personality types. For people with "abnormal or unstable personalities," Maymí Nevares wrote, drinking could lead to "chronic alcoholism with all its range of physical and mental pathology."[69] In other words, in the wrong hands drinking could be dangerous and destructive, as evidenced by the scores of inmates (more than 80 percent) serving time in Oso Blanco and other main island prisons whose crimes were (in)directly related to stimulant depressants like alcohol.[70] Some prisoners recognized group therapy–conduced mental sobriety as a treatment and the basis of their postrelease emotional stability. To function in society, such sobriety had to be achieved in prison first.[71]

Maymí Nevares unified American, Iberian, and broader European psychiatric currents. He classified which experts could best explain phenomena like the physical symptoms of mental illness, throwing shade at practical psychologists and Spiritist healers while stressing the superiority of neuropsychiatrists. For Maymí Nevares, the psychological and physical sides of emotion were concomitant and inseparable. Freud himself, who before becoming a psychiatrist was a physician and neurologist, always recognized the somatic foundation of psychology and regretted that many of his colleagues used psychoanalytic theory and methods to argue that the theory was exclusively psychological. Emotions acted on the body through the nervous system, as corroborated by the work of the French psychiatrist and neurologist Jean Delay, the American neurophysiologist and historian of science John Farquhar Fulton, and the American physiologist Walter Bradford Cannon, Maymí Nevares affirmed.[72]

To elaborate on the emotional causes of mental illness symptoms, Maymí Nevares discussed Cannon's and Philip Bard's studies of animal physiology, during which they performed lobotomies on mammals to highlight the role of the brain in generating physiological responses and feelings.[73] Cannon and Bard developed a theoretical model of emotion based on thalamic processes. The key component of this theory is that the thalamic region of the brain is the coordinating center for emotional reactions to stimuli. When the thalamic discharge occurs, bodily changes coincide with the emotional experience. However, these happen separately and independently of one another. Physiological incitement does not have to precede emotional expression or experience.[74] Maymí Nevares pointed to Cannon's lobotomy of a cat, whose cortex and hypothalamus were forcibly separated to show that the feline was "mindless" even though it could still respond somato-emotionally.[75] The bodily basis of a normal man's emotions and his nervous system, Maymí Nevares believed, could be extended to a nervous man or neurotic, the only differences being degree, intensity, and duration. In Oso Blanco, he came across his fair share of such men.

Inside Prisons

Oso Blanco's reform program included psychiatric treatment of the psychic lesions or disorders causing and influencing crime.[76] According to one prisoner, psychiatrists "performed a thorough analysis" of convicts' "mental processes to determine the presence of any mental anomaly. [They are] questioned and observed to see if [they show] signs of mental or emotional instability, phobias, abnormal attitudes, etc. When anomalies are discovered, [they are] submitted to psychiatric treatment."[77] Maymí Nevares treated epileptic inmates and tendered psychiatric reports of mentally infirm convicts to prison and state administrators when necessary or requested.[78] His reports chronicled the various mental symptoms and conditions of prisoners, as well as the pathological rationales and behaviors associated with their phrenic deficiencies. For instance, in October 1942, Maymí Nevares presented a diagnostic report to warden Saldaña concerning a twenty-nine-year-old mulatto day laborer from Carolina named Félix Calderón Parrilla who was serving ten years for second-degree murder. He determined that the prisoner suffered from paranoid schizophrenia, an "acute outbreak of arousal of the catatonic type" that arose from the depths of an "accentuated psychopathic personality."[79] Maymí Nevares examined Calderón Parrilla's mental history and learned that his "schizoid and paranoid traits" had gradually come to externalize themselves in the form of "isolation, suspicion, and strange behavior."[80] Authorities often found him in the restroom grimacing, gesticulating, caterwauling, talking to himself about persecution, hallucinating, and hearing voices. Because of this, they recommended that he be transferred to the nearby insane asylum.

Interviewing and observing convicts and studying their histories enabled Maymí Nevares to generate psychiatric knowledge about incarcerated people in abundance. In another case, he assessed a forty-four-year-old white entrepreneur from Aguas Buenas named Arcadio Vargas Pagán, who was serving five years in the penitentiary for incest. He reached out to warden Saldaña in January 1943 to discuss the prisoner, whom he called a "mentally deficient moron" with "intellectual deficit" and "impoverished affective tendencies."[81] Vargas Pagán was an emotional simpleton, and it showed in his "abnormal" and "asocial" conduct.[82] The environment also contributed, particularly his overcrowded and promiscuous lifestyle (his family of nine inhabited a single room). Cohabitation of this sort stirred unnatural sexual attraction with a teenage daughter and undermined spiritual order within his household. While Maymí Nevares confidently analyzed Vargas Pagán, he also acknowledged there were limits to what he could put forward in terms of findings. Evaluating the consciousness and subconsciousness of Vargas Pagán's daughter, who may have had an "Oedipus complex," for example, proved difficult, as she was beyond the immediate reach of penitentiary psychiatrists.[83]

Incest was just one of several sexualities documented and psychiatrically dissected by Maymí Nevares. The probation officer Tomás Rosario submitted a report in fall 1946 about a twenty-four-year-old white laundry worker from Jayuya named Armando Rivera Colón, who was serving two years for a crime against nature. Community members familiar with the convict and interviewed by Rosario signaled that Rivera Colón was a sexual invert, "a biological defect for which he is not at fault."[84] Maymí Nevares labeled him sexually abnormal and in the process identified such cases as soaring in the penitentiary.[85] He singled out four types of sexual abnormality: vicious, neurotic, psychopathic, and glandular.[86] In Oso Blanco, sexual abnormality rooted in vice predominated, although in Rivera Colón's specific case a glandular problem was to blame. To properly address the situation, Maymí Nevares proposed, the infrastructure for treating such prisoners had to be improved.[87]

At a social work convention held in 1947, Maymí Nevares confirmed the various mental health treatments for which Oso Blanco prisoners qualified. Drawing from more than five hundred penitentiary cases, he stressed the importance of preventive measures in the educational, economic, and social lives of convicts and collaborative clinical interventions (meaning treatment that blended psychiatry, psychology, and social work but under the auspices of a qualified psychiatrist). What he called "curative" measures, or rather, the diagnosis and prognosis of individual cases, were to be advanced in the court system and through reentry structures like the Parole Board. In these different settings, targeted psychiatric treatments could be pursued. Finally, he viewed incarceration itself as a treatment measure. It "cured" those feeling guilty about their transgressions, having the effect of resolving the principal emotional crisis that landed them in prison in the first place.[88] Psychoanalyzing every prisoner of this kind was not feasible, Maymí Nevares argued, but general patterns could be ascertained after a few interviews with them. He learned that crimes against persons, for example, were often anchored in "maternal fixation."[89] Indefinite confinement, meanwhile, gave prison mental health professionals the chance to "study, treat, and advise" convicts so long as such surveillance was rooted in empathetic understanding and humane treatment.[90] Inevitably, Maymí Nevares concluded, there would be those who could not be treated at all because of some underlying pathological feature.

Maymí Nevares's pessimism about extreme cases of psychopathology did not dissuade his administrative peers from entertaining the possibility of discovering other cutting-edge treatments, however. In August 1948, *El Mundo* reported that Puerto Rican correctional professionals were studying a months-long group psychotherapy model developed in New Jersey prisons by the penologists Frederick Lovell Bixby and Sanford Bates. Lovell Bixby and Bates based their model on a promising one used by the US Army in Fort Knox in 1943. Using techniques drawn from psychology and the broader social sciences, the New Jersey experiments sought to change the basic attitudes of prisoners by adjusting their disruptive personalities. Inmates learned about mental hygiene concepts before diving into hands-on work with therapists and, in the end, attempting to extirpate any antagonisms or hostilities that persisted in their psyches. Puerto Rican officials were eager to apply the model in Oso Blanco, although it is unclear if they did right away.[91]

While correctional mental health therapeutics were still in their infancy in midcentury Puerto Rico, diagnosis was another matter. According to Maymí Nevares, the symptomology of mental illness was expansive. Four types were apparent in the context of incarceration: mental deficients or oligophrenics, the criminally insane, neurotics, and psychopaths.[92] When a case escaped these categories, deeper psychiatric scrutiny became necessary. This happened to a twenty-two-year-old white prisoner serving time for theft, Modesto Matos Rodríguez, who manifested "affective indifference, mutism, obsessions, hypochondriacal delusions, and abnormal conduct (semi-stupor and catatonic positions interrupted by impulsive raptus during which, lately, he attacked other prisoners)."[93] Matos Rodríguez also went on hunger strike and had to be fed intravenously. These cumulative circumstances convinced

Maymí Nevares that the prisoner's schizophrenic reactions would be better addressed in the nearby insane asylum.

Aside from submitting institutional reports on the mental health of incarcerated people, Maymí Nevares published several articles about prisoners in the *Revista de Servicio Social*, an interdisciplinary academic journal focused on social work. He drew from prevailing psychiatric language and tropes (categories like "psychotics," "feebleminded," "psychopaths," "psychoneurosis," and "maladjustment") and the psychoanalytic contributions of the British American psychiatrist and criminologist William Healy to unpack his own approach to classification and treatment. Neuropsychiatry, as he put it, had a role to play in socially redeeming criminals by offering specialized technical knowledge and support to penal administration.[94] Psychosocial intervention was needed because a quarter of Oso Blanco inmates qualified as mental cases.[95] Assessing this population, Maymí Nevares maintained, meant being attentive to environmental and social factors. He established a protocol determining exactly who should be examined (the obviously insane, sexual deviants, elderly first-time offenders, murderers without motives, and those who committed creepy and horrendous crimes), and for what reasons (juridical, social, psychiatric).[96] The decade or so Maymí Nevares labored in Oso Blanco gave him access to the raw material he required to advance his investigations and problem solve carceral mental health. When he departed, the inmate Víctor F.F. wisecracked, "few crazy prisoners remained" in the penitentiary.[97]

After Maymí Nevares resigned and unexpectedly passed away in 1951, Troyano de los Ríos became Oso Blanco's resident psychiatrist and medical director. Before arriving at the penitentiary, Troyano ran the nearby insane asylum, where he would have interacted with infamous patients like David Luis Phillips of Saint Kitts.[98] He also published in Puerto Rico's flagship medical journal.[99] While based at the asylum, he ordered inmates to sanitize hospital grounds. His valiant efforts were trumpeted by some asylum patients. A few of them also reminded him of the colonial-populist politics he was supposed to represent and promulgate.[100] At Oso Blanco, Troyano equally had his work cut out for him. In the early 1950s alone, he interacted with several high-profile prisoners, including "paranoid" fugitive extraordinaire José Aníbal Gerena Lafontaine (known as "La Palomilla") and the radical nationalist Pedro Albizu Campos, whom he found to be suffering from persecutory hallucinations.[101]

Troyano spent most of his time engaging and studying common prisoners, however. The bulk of surviving psychiatric evaluations in penitentiary parole files concern ordinary inmates. These primarily date to the early 1950s.

Troyano interviewed, observed, and classified prisoners, and recommended treatment options, most prominently labor therapy.[102] Agriculture and skilled apprenticeships (e.g., carpentry, construction, electrical wiring, plumbing, shoemaking, tailoring) were among the labor assignments he designated. At the insane asylum, he had been a major proponent of hydrotherapy, physio-therapy, and calm-inducing injections.[103] As for drug regimens, penitentiary health professionals prescribed epamin tablets to inmates with epilepsy.[104] The use of psychotropic medications would not become mainstream in the Puerto Rican prison system until later in the 1950s and beyond.[105] There-fore, Troyano seldom referred to them in his evaluations of convicts. Other sources reveal alternative ways of delivering mental health treatment alto-gether. Joaquín R.B.V., for example, insisted in El Despertar that recreational activities like dominoes and sports like baseball and volleyball productively channeled mental energies, thereby curtailing violations of prison rules.[106]

Overall, Troyano's brand of psychiatry resembled Maymí Nevares's. Both men understood that crime in Puerto Rico, and elsewhere for that matter, could be traced, in part, to mental and especially sociological factors.[107] He emphasized the physical body and everything from disease and skin complex-ion to nourishment and corporeal type—such as acromegaloide, adenoide, athletic, eunucoide, feminoide, oligoide, and so on.[108] Troyano was also as attuned to stratified context as his deceased colleague. He underscored where convicts came from, the circumstances of their lives and crimes, their edu-cation, their vices and prison behavior, and the treatment options for their pathologies.[109] Troyano linked the pathologies he described to precise de-mographics, such as working-class or jíbaro men and homosexuals. Certain traits characterized jíbaros, including poor nourishment, reticence, coming from large families, working in agriculture, and mis- or undereducation.[110] Homosexuals exhibited personality tendencies that were behaviorally legible. Troyano recognized a twenty-two-year-old white pimp from Mayagüez serv-ing an extended sentence for crimes against nature, for example, as a "psycho-pathic homosexual" who gambled, attacked peers, raped younger prisoners, and caused scandals.[111]

Troyano and Maymí Nevares advanced psychiatry in Oso Blanco while distancing it from carceral psychology. By the late 1950s and into the 1960s, prison and health officials definitively turned toward providing forensic and penal psychiatric service with less recourse to psychology than ever before.[112] The growing distinction in practice between psychology and psychiatry did not mean the two fields became anathema to one another, however. Both fields influenced the penitentiary Classification and Treatment Board and often coalesced in swaying the board in a specific psychosocial direction when cases involved mentally dubious or infirm prisoners. What is more, some prisoners viewed psychology, psychiatry, and sociology as a penological trinity.[113] But clinical sociology in partnership with UPR-RP inside the penitentiary would not materialize until later in the 1950s.[114] Mental tests, interviews, observations, and labor-oriented treatment models proved to be psychologists' and psychiatrists' most reliable tools in their collective quest to mentally raise the living dead, thereby paving the way toward what they hoped would be effective education or vocational training and subsequent societal and labor market integration.

Conclusion

Correctional psychology and psychiatry evinced the second phase of carceral rehabilitation: the living dead needed to be raised intellectually and vocationally. From the vantage point of the state, refining prisoners' intellectual and vocational skills would activate their labor power and give them a taste of civic dignity. For this to occur, mental health professionals required a foundational catapult for launching their efforts, which intelligence testing provided. Penitentiary psychologists administered a variety of raw intelligence tests but later combined them with motor skill and personality exams.[115] After gauging convicts psychometrically, many of whom tested deficient or nearly deficient in all three facets, psychologists analyzed the data and shared the results with partnering psychiatrists who emotionally and sociologically contextualized prisoners, assessed whether they had glaring mental illnesses, and recommended labor therapies. Oso Blanco's Classification and Treatment Board incorporated these mental pieces of the carceral puzzle into their work, using them to decide what individual treatment programs would look like.

Prisoners—a "problem population" needing to be psychiatrically managed—were mentally dissected in Oso Blanco.[116] But just as significantly, social scientists also desired to civically redeem them, transforming the meanings of socioscientific knowledge production in a colonial-populist context. Psychometric instruments represented a step toward comprehending inmates and helping them plan for their postcarceral lives. Psychologists could take the rehabilitative process only so far by themselves. A layered understanding of prisoners was required if even a bare majority of them were really going to be rehabilitated. Therefore, the Classification and Treatment Board ordered and supervised ethnographic investigations into convict lives, their health, and their civic prospects. The resulting narratives about individual prisoners capacitated the board to establish parameters for mental and social interventions. Asymmetrical power relations and scientifically legitimated stereotypes are embedded in mental test results and Classification and Treatment ethnographies, but so is a comprehensive human science of rehabilitation. Within the colonial context of Puerto Rico, rehabilitation's professional adherents looked inward and sought to repair the incarcerated population for (re)incorporation into the local body politic and economy. They also gestured outward by conveying to the US that they were more than capable of redeeming their own people. Like physicians earlier in the twentieth century, who reclaimed a political space for themselves by contesting US colonialism, rehabilitating inmates became a mechanism for Puerto Rican mental health professionals to rehabilitate their own identities as colonial citizens as well.[117]

Whereas psychometric exams generated numerical results pertaining to the intelligence, motor skills, and personalities of prisoners, psychiatric evaluations could be more abstract. Psychiatrists contextualized the lives of incarcerated people before and during their exposure to state rehabilitation, uncovered how their minds functioned through observation and interviews, and clarified the symptoms of mental illness they endured to identify treatment paths. Compared to psychology, psychiatry seemed better equipped to guide convicts to social goals. In general, the two fields often reinforced each other. The contributions of psychiatrists and psychologists built on the work of physicians, who salvaged the bodies of inmates, and complemented the work of social health experts, who (re)socialized the living dead. Of all the health professionals involved in rehabilitating prisoners, social workers and parole officers perhaps carried the heaviest burden.

Interactional Care:
Social Workers, Parole Officers,
and Social Rehabilitation

In late November 1949, Oso Blanco's Classification and Treatment Board met with a 25-year-old white-wheat cane worker from Maunabo named Jorge Díaz Ruiz, who was serving time for having mutilated his drunken brother Clemente during a struggle over a firearm. Díaz Ruiz impressed Classification and Treatment officials as a sincere extrovert. He did not look like a violent fighter but in conversation revealed himself to be just that, as well as bitter and vindictive toward the person who was responsible for his having been previously imprisoned for theft. Díaz Ruiz boasted of having a bad temper and that, for years, he made a habit of carrying an unregistered revolver. When parole came up, in an instance of likely accismus, Díaz Ruiz showed little interest. He preferred to max out his sentence because, as he put it, he might slip up on the street by not tolerating anyone's shenanigans. His position was not definitive, for he also suggested to Classification and Treatment officials that he would discuss parole with an uncle. If he did get out earlier than expected, though, Díaz Ruiz expressed not wanting to go home to Maunabo. Otherwise, he would in all likelihood return to prison.[1]

Although Díaz Ruiz was pessimistic about his situation and parole, Oso Blanco's Classification and Treatment Board still thought he was a "regular" case for rehabilitation.[2] Board members believed that carefully developing a rehabilitation program for him might result in a desirable outcome. His social treatment consisted of religious services and interviews with social workers and psychologists. To tap into his preexisting skill set, the board assigned him to work on the penitentiary farm. Recreational activities such as games, sports, and movies also formed part of Díaz Ruiz's program. The key aspect of the prisoner's treatment plan, however, was helping him avoid the life of a troglodyte, which in his case meant figuring out how to repair his "family relationships."[3] This is why classification and treatment officials stressed pa-role in discussions with Díaz Ruiz. They understood how in cases like his treatment in the community represented the best course of action.

"Treatment in the community" was a core principle of rehabilitative cor-rections in midcentury Puerto Rico, beginning with reimagined probation and parole systems and temporary passes to visit family members.[4] Accord-ing to the National Council on Crime and Delinquency counsel Sol Rubin, who published a study about Puerto Rican corrections in 1951, parole and probation were cornerstones of community treatment. He wrote, "Since prac-tically every prisoner will sooner or later be released, and since the prison experience has not only interrupted community living but has created addi-tional problems of adjustment for the offender, almost every prisoner should be released on parole to provide him with the assistance of supervision, and to provide the community with the additional security of supervision."[5] For most Puerto Rican prisoners being committed at the time, Rubin asserted, community treatment was feasible. Despite Frank Loveland's previous call for the development of a parole system with supervision, however, few paroles were being granted.[6] Puerto Rican social workers and parole officers con-tributed to reversing this trend in the late 1940s but particularly in the 1950s.

A generation of social workers carved professional spaces for themselves in Puerto Rican corrections in the mid-twentieth century. Social workers and parole officers were on the carceral front lines and largely realized the project of prison reform and rehabilitation. As members of the Classifica-tion and Treatment Board, social workers served as designated factfinders. They researched prisoners' lives and crimes and mapped the contours of their health. Interviewing and observing convicts and engaging their families and wider communities provided social workers with data to construct ekphras-tic portraits (or socioeconomic histories) of inmates and drafts of treatment programs. Parole officials carried out similar duties for Puerto Rico's Parole Board, only they spent more time visiting convict communities (of origin and postcarceral residence) and talking to the people there. They interviewed the family members of prisoners, their neighbors, their employers, their cowork-ers, law enforcement, and many others who could speak to the rehabilitative progress or lack thereof of former inmates. Their research shaped the Parole Board's decision-making and divulged the successes and failures of social re-habilitation at a time when the rehabilitative ideal was at a fever pitch.

Using parole records, conference proceedings, and other sources, this chapter examines the contributions of social workers and parole officials to social rehabilitation efforts in midcentury Puerto Rico. After prisoners' bod-ies and minds were regenerated, the next facet of their improvement revolved around social life and relationships. A medico-religious ethic of uplift framed and guided the labor of social workers and parole officers, who exposed convicts to the etiquette and norms to which they needed to adapt, mimic, or perform if they wanted to secure freedom.[7] As Afro–Puerto Rican social worker Lydia Peña Beltrán notes, incarcerated people often complied with authorities' demands since securing parole depended on deference. Convicts went (and go) to great lengths to speak the language of the state and generate or preserve an image of repentance and moral conduct.[8] In midcentury Puerto Rican corrections, social workers promoted an interactional culture of care that aspired to raise the living dead socially. They and parole officials reconnected inmates to their kin both in narrative form and a literal sense, restoring the natal bonds and links to community that were ruptured by incarceration, while also celebrating prisoners for settling into prevailing social standards or denigrating them for not conforming.[9]

A Transnational Web of Social Work

In late 1930s and 1940s Puerto Rico, a major forum and outlet for social work knowledge production, debates, and activities was the *Revista de Servicio Social*. Throughout its life span this periodical showcased that a local and transnational politics of care determined the trajectory of Puerto Rican social work.[10] In the inaugural issue of the *Revista de Servicio Social*, Beatriz Lassalle linked the nascent discipline to charity and two salvific objectives: providing for the physical needs of the indigent and infirm, and pursuing social adjustment in others. She cited the child welfare leader Katherine F. Lenroot to convey her point that, to be successful, social workers had to possess certain characteristics: integrity, vision, enthusiasm, patience, faith, discernment, compassion, tolerance, and self-control. True social work, she added, "required knowledge obtained through conscientious study, experiential wisdom, emotional maturity, and spiritual strength acquired through faith."[11] For Lassalle, social work could uplift the lower classes, and in its ideal form sought to reconcile individual freedom and social security.[12] The collaborative nature of social work, its pedagogical utility, and its emphasis on solving social, economic, labor, and health problems made interaction, cohesion, and stability within social conglomerations possible.[13]

Social work education and practice in Puerto Rico can be traced to at least the 1920s.[14] Celia Núñez de Bunker acknowledged that it was by and large imported from the United States to address grinding poverty and its effects, such as Puerto Rico's low standard of living and the "deterioration of the mental and physical health of our people."[15] While the American Red Cross had a social work arm active in Puerto Rico at the time, the Health Department was the first local government agency to entrust social workers with creating an infrastructure for caring for vulnerable populations. This happened in tuberculosis and prenatal clinics, encampments, dispensaries, and community centers that in the long run served thousands of people. In the 1930s, the Puerto Rico Emergency Relief Administration, the Puerto Rico Reconstruction Administration, and Puerto Rico's Education Department brought social workers into their collective fold and deployed services with an eye on socially recomposing Puerto Ricans. The Education Department, specifically, trained visiting teachers (as social workers were originally known) to spur efforts in rural areas. Social workers understood that their labor could have communal impact, so they liaised with individual people and families.[16]

Puerto Rico's Justice Department commenced social services circa 1930 with the appointment of a probation official to the San Juan juvenile court. Oso Blanco was projected as a site of humanitarian social work as early as 1934.[17] By 1939, however, when an average of twenty new social workers joined the field every year and there existed more than two hundred overall, social work still was not a fixture of all the major courts or penal institutions of Puerto Rico.[18] The regulation of social work in 1934, the establishment of the university's School of Social Work and the government's Division of Public Welfare in the early 1940s, the implementation of penal reforms in the mid-1940s, and the creation of parole officer positions normalized social work in the criminal-legal system by midcentury.[19] The independent Insular Society of Social Workers identified the prison as a site where social rehabilitation could be realized. In 1939, the women's prison of Arecibo hosted the group's fifth conference. Educational, political, and social experts gathered there to discuss rehabilitative services, cultural, educational and recreation programs, and social problems like prostitution, mental hygiene, and juvenile delinquency.[20]

The 1940s marked a turning point for social work in Puerto Rican corrections. Social workers, justice officials, and others critically reflected on and debated crime and punishment issues in academic journals and conference settings throughout the decade.[21] Loveland's report, however, had established a precedent in terms of setting short- and long-range socioscientific goals for the penal and correctional program. He bemoaned the minimal use of probation and parole. Their "intelligent use," Loveland maintained, "is not only the best method of handling certain cases" but also "more economical."[22] Probation was preemptive while parole served two major purposes. "The first is to release the offender when he can be safely returned to the community, with full regard for the interest of the public welfare," Loveland pronounced, and the second "is to assist the released offender to make a satisfactory adjustment in the community and to return him to institution[al] custody if he has demonstrated that he cannot safely remain in the community."[23] Prioritizing probation and parole was linked to "intelligent classification and segregation," "specific programs," and dealing with offenders as individuals.[24] Puerto Rican social workers and parole officers helped propel these related ventures.

The intellectual currents shaping the social work stratum of rehabilitative corrections in Puerto Rico did not just trickle down from the United States. They also flowed from within the Spanish-speaking Greater Antilles. The Fourth Convention of Social Workers held in Río Piedras in 1947, for example, explored crime, its causes, and potential solutions not only in Puerto Rico but also in Cuba and the Dominican Republic. The Cuban delegation—Dr. Ada López Flammand, Ana María Perera, Lilandia Pividal, and Rafael Rodríguez Cuquerella—was sent by president Ramón Grau San Martín and conveyed advances in Cuban penitentiary science. Cuba's Presidio Modelo—an institution that could accommodate up to four thousand men, of all colors—in their view functioned as a school that realized agricultural and industrial activities like tailoring, shoemaking, carpentry, and marble masonry. The Cuban delegation stressed the need to establish social service departments in prisons to help prepare convicts for societal reintegration. This meant teaching them wage-earning skills and considering how personal, familial, and environmental factors shaped their lives and behaviors. They explained how such work was ongoing in their own youth facilities and bearing fruit.[25]

The Dominican delegation to the convention comprised of Consuelo de Prats Ramírez and Carmen Adolfina Henríquez Almanzar, the latter a social work official embedded in the Rafael Trujillo regime's Health and Public Assistance Department. Henríquez Almanzar zoomed in on juvenile delinquency in the Dominican Republic, drawing attention to how poverty, vagrancy, and parental neglect and abandonment combined to produce criminals. Alcoholism, prostitution, and sloth set terrible examples within individual homes and destroyed families. To combat these ills, Henríquez Almanzar discussed how the Trujillo government had initiated nonviolent social improvement projects. These focused on preventing crime and treating those affected by it. Home visits, providing families with a share of their subsistence, primary education, vocational training in multiple fields ranging from woodwork to bookbinding to mechanics, and even public shaming curtailed crime. Separating predelinquents and rigid criminals was under consideration, as was creating a contingent of technocrats that could attend to paroled youths both inside and outside the juvenile court system. The goal of Dominican reformatories was to mold the character and social sentiments of offenders, to transform their personalities.[26]

That social workers and other social health professionals active in carceral care fields from around the Caribbean traveled to Puerto Rico for this conference suggests that participants viewed rehabilitative knowledge production in integrated fashion. Those in attendance were mindful of US trends concerning the entanglement of social work and health enterprise but also Caribbean, Latin American, and Pan-American innovations.[27] Within the Caribbean, Puerto Rico would become a refinery of social work. There is evidence that Dominican functionaries, for example, later crossed the Mona Passage to complete multifaceted training in the field. The training exposed them to the latest developments in social work administration, legislation, concepts, and best practices.[28] The Insular Penitentiary served a similar function within Puerto Rico itself, providing social work professionals and students with a laboratory where they could carry out research studies and produce social knowledge about incarceration. No doubt, the penitentiary functioned as a "laboratory of deficiency," but it was much more than that.[29] Oso Blanco was also a place where intellectually and socially "deficient" people could be civically empowered and mold penal reform.

Prison Research and Social Services

The meanings of social rehabilitation in the Insular Penitentiary revolved around the Classification and Treatment Board and by extension social workers. Peña Beltrán, who worked in Puerto Rican corrections across institutions for several decades, complicates the conventional definition of rehabilitation in carceral settings. She suggests that rehabilitation is assumed to mean restoring a preexisting normal conduct in criminals so they can respect prevailing social norms and coexist with the majority population. However, rehabilitation can also mean returning someone to a previous state, which for offenders might mean reviving aspects of their deprived and sordid pasts. Social workers have turned to the concept of resocialization to discuss how they approach teaching and convincing people of their erring reasoning and ways.[30] But as Picó has noted, it is difficult to resocialize someone who has, presumably, never been socialized.[31]

In mid-twentieth-century Puerto Rico, rehabilitation and (re)socialization functioned as synonyms even if social workers did not explicitly use the latter vocabulary. They viewed their craft as a salvific "ministry" advanced and defended by "crusaders" whose collective example organically attracted clients.[32] A Christian framework animated social work during this period, but so did science.[33] Puerto Rican social workers looked to American proponent of absolute idealism, Josiah Royce (1855–1916), for instance, as someone who adeptly blended scientific and religious precepts and was therefore worthy of emulation.[34] "You must be a true naturalist to study that living creature [the social work client] as a biologist would study cell growth under the microscope, or as a pathologist who carefully examines diseased tissues," he wrote, "but in order to study, you must necessarily love."[35] For social workers, "that living creature" was a human social patient who had to be engaged in person. Social workers leaned scientific in practice but were guided by righteous virtues.

Because exposure to human clients occurred face-to-face, social workers believed that social science concepts and methods provided a firm intellectual foundation for what they would find in the field.[36] University social work students encountered clients and social science through applied training, which gave them opportunities to conduct research in places like Oso Blanco. In so doing, they raised convict consciousness about the caring nature of their profession while objectifying prisoners to produce socioscientific knowledge. The domestic sciences student Esther Pou González, for instance, interviewed one hundred Insular Penitentiary prisoners in 1945. She asked them questions about their crime(s) and lifestyle(s), and used the information to produce a demographic and statistical picture of inmates. Pou González uncovered patterns detailing how age, race, education, lineage, birth legitimacy, marital status, hereditary diseases, income, property, and other categories of analysis shaped carcerality.[37]

Most of the incarcerated men Pou González interviewed were young adults who had no more than a primary school education. They came from large families. The predominant occupation for a third of them was transient day laborer (bracero) followed by carpenters, those who were unemployed, and a variety of other blue- and white-collar positions. Half were convicted for attempted murder, and another third for crimes against property. More than half were recidivists, many of whom had returned to Oso Blanco for the same crime. Pou González concluded that most offenders "come from the lowest social and economic levels. This is so because it just is or because justice is maladministered in our country."[38] Her study straddled individual and structural analysis, confirming young men's inability to see a clear and promising future for themselves. Crime would diminish, however, if the economic well-being of young people was addressed, Pou González stressed, for all the evidence indicated that socioeconomic conditions had created psychological imbalances in the young men studied, resulting in their delinquency.

Pou González referred to alcohol abuse as well. A few years after she published her brief reflection, the social work student and future director of penitentiary social services, Jesús E. Palmer, published a short piece about alcoholism among Puerto Rico's penal population.[39] The first socioscientific alcoholism studies in Puerto Rico were issued in the late nineteenth century by the likes of the creole physician-anthropologist José Rodríguez Castro.[40] By the mid-twentieth century, the problem not only persisted but also spread, and aspiring correctional professionals dove into the topic. Palmer discussed the bodily and social effects of alcohol and how it awakened and unleashed morally dubious sentiments and actions in people. Understanding this, he claimed, it was "easy to see how it [liquor] contributes to social delinquency (crimes, robberies, sexual offenses, etc.)."[41]

According to studies completed in Puerto Rican prisons and reformatories, many incarcerated people perpetrated their crimes under the influence of alcohol. Palmer suggested that, for some, liquor gave them a sense of independence or helped them forget. Others believed it brought out their true personalities and identities. They felt that the euphoria triggered by alcohol diminished their difficulties, inferiority complexes, frustrations, and introversion. There was a price to pay for years of substance abuse, though— namely psychosis. The temporary reprieve and ego stroke afforded by liquor was not worth it, Palmer noted. Unrestrained alcohol consumption might be misconstrued as a pleasurable fantasy for a time, but it ultimately became a degenerative vice. Liquor consumption was thus a psychological problem that required urgent attention and resolution.[42] Prisoners themselves recognized the scourge of alcohol in their lives in the late 1940s.[43] By the mid-1950s and later, justice and prison officials lauded the emergence of self-aware groups like Alcoholics Anonymous that used the gospel of rehabilitation to make inroads against the sickness of alcoholism.[44]

Knowledge of the socioeconomic conditions, substance abuse, and concerns of prisoners was compiled by social workers through open-ended interviews (fig. 3.1). They carried out comprehensive interviews in an official capacity as members of the penitentiary Classification and Treatment Board.[45] Frank interaction between social workers and convicts uncovered inmate sensibilities to the degree that issues like prison sexuality and other rehabilitative options that beckoned, such as engagement with humanities disciplines and techniques, could be contemplated.[46] Classification and treatment were initially pursued only at Oso Blanco. By the mid-1950s, these services were also available at the women's prison in Vega Alta, the institution for youths in Mayagüez, and the minimum-custody agricultural camps.[47] "Treatment" entailed all the activities, influences, and actions applied to individual prisoners with the goal of rehabilitating them; it was a long-term project that encompassed living arrangements, diet, medical, psychiatric and social services, education, labor training, recreation, and discipline.[48] As of 1949, Gloria L.

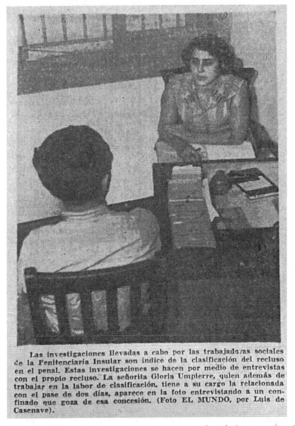

Las investigaciones llevadas a cabo por las trabajadoras sociales de la Penitenciaría Insular son índice de la clasificación del recluso en el penal. Estas investigaciones se hacen por medio de entrevistas con el propio recluso. La señorita Gloria Umpierre, quien además de trabajar en la labor de clasificación, tiene a su cargo la relacionada con el pase de dos días, aparece en la foto entrevistando a un confinado que goza de esa concesión. (Foto EL MUNDO, por Luis de Casenave).

FIGURE 3.1 Social worker Gloria Umpierre interviewing an unidentified prisoner in the penitentiary. *El Mundo*, August 23, 1952. Biblioteca y Hemeroteca Puertorriqueña, Universidad de Puerto Rico–Río Piedras.

Umpierre, Carmin Bravo Abreu, Luz Lladó, and Flor de María Monserrate, among others, served on the Classification and Treatment Board.[49] The total number of social workers active in the penitentiary administering rehabilitation grew thereafter. Broadly speaking, the board oversaw all technical matters in penal administration. In addition to social workers and wardens, a physician, a psychologist, a psychiatrist, a vocational counselor, and other technical personnel participated.[50] This team of professionals aimed to generate favorable rehabilitative conditions for prisoners and initiate treatment programs for them based on specialized knowledge.[51]

All penitentiary social services flowed through the Classification and Treatment Board. As the prisoner Luis M.C. noted in 1949, it was "the main axle" on which penal reform rested.[52] The assistant superintendent of prisons

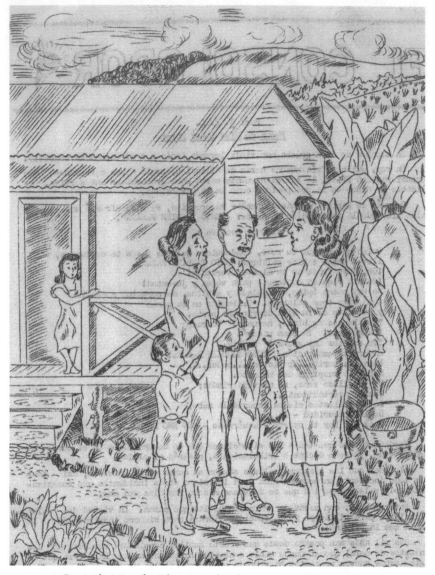

FIGURE 3.2 Convict depiction of social service work in the community. *El Despertar* 2, no. 2 (May 1950). Biblioteca y Hemeroteca Puertorriqueña, Universidad de Puerto Rico–Río Piedras.

Félix Rodríguez Higgins explained that same year that reform required the "decisive and voluntary cooperation" of everyone involved.[53] To ascertain which prisoners needed which services, the Classification and Treatment Board produced two key documents that health professionals utilized to manage convict rehabilitation: socioeconomic histories and treatment programs.

Socioeconomic histories narrated the lives of inmates from the womb (birth) to the living tomb (prison). They recounted the social situations of prisoners using (inter)personal, socioscientific, medical, and economic lenses, covering family and upbringing, personal information and references, observations about attitude and characteristics, treatment recommendations, occupation status, religion, physical condition, education, and recreational preferences.[54] Their compilation often required social service work in prisoners' communities of origin (fig. 3.2). Treatment programs paved the road ahead for convicts, and spoke to their rehabilitative prospects overall. They reiterated the finer points of classification and treatment histories but also underscored the factors impacting the conduct of prisoners, their weaknesses and potential, and what authorities assumed was the most important element of their treatment. Parole investigations became relevant if ex-prisoners violated the terms of their release. The interviews that were channeled into classification and treatment histories and treatment programs allowed prisoners to express themselves enough so that social workers could get a sense of how to best organize their rehabilitation regimen.

Convict Impressions

Convicts opined about how rehabilitation was structured, organized, and executed. Just as prisoners articulated their views on the bodily aspects of penitentiary health care, they also reflected on social work and classification and treatment. An Oso Blanco convict named Max P., for example, contemplated the "missionary labor of rehabilitation" in June 1949 and emphasized the involvement of social workers: "I personally have received great aid from the Honorable Classification [and Treatment] Board and have been able to digest the correct, scientific interpretations of [social worker] Mercedes Ossorio de Giráldez. She has guided me and to her I owe the adjusted and normal life I lead."[55] Max P. credited social work with pulling the wool from his eyes and teaching him that living on the margins of society was not a good life. Ossorio de Giráldez encouraged convicts to become useful to society. She conveyed to Max P. and others that beyond a religiously inspired sense of guilt, to be offended by one's transgressions and seek out productive alternatives encapsulated true rehabilitation. Ossorio de Giráldez taught Max P. about personal accountability, and as a result, he claimed a willingness to voluntarily shed his old mindset for a new, more righteous one. For every Max P., however, there was a Frank M.Q., who critiqued the overexertion characteristic of mid-century carceral social work and even questioned why reform proponents avoided seriously investing in and expanding it.[56] Others initially had an "acrid" attitude about Oso Blanco's classification and treatment program but remained hopeful.[57]

Throughout its short life span, *El Despertar* published a series of images and articles on what Max P. called the "praiseworthy" classification and treatment process.[58] In visual and narrative form, the series chronicled the different "situations" incarcerated people withstood, from prisoner intake and health evaluation to interviews with prison staff and release. The articles introduced how classification, treatment, and related advances in the midcentury present marked a major departure from what transpired behind bars before the era of penal reform. The cover page of the August 1949 edition of *El Despertar* captures this past-present dynamic. The drawing shows the transition from violent hard labor extraction to vocational training, productive labor, and righteous education (fig. 3.3). How prison conditions might be ameliorated further formed part of the conversation as well. For during these crucial years, inmates and prison professionals alike actively pondered the flagrant variance of punishment and rehabilitation.[59]

Meaningfully integrating families into prison rehabilitation represented one area of protracted struggle. Max P. reflected on the importance of family visits for incarcerated people and how they put rehabilitation into motion by "reviving" them and their "tribulated spirits" in an "instant."[60] "Archaic" realities, such as the lack of visitation space and disciplinary mistreatment in front of family members persisted, however.[61] Max P. mentioned how overcrowding and budgetary constraints linked to the supervision of visits were part of a structural problem and declared that a larger visitation room was therefore necessary. In fall 1945, the penitentiary population numbered some 1,600 prisoners. Between late 1949 and early 1950, that number swelled to more than 2,100 and then 2,300.[62] To meet the standards of modern penology, Max P. argued, family members had to interact with prisoners in "tranquil" spaces where they could learn about their incarcerated loved ones' problems and help them think through solutions.[63] The inmate Benigno D.R., in contrast, reflected on individual aspects of visitation, such as the shame endured by family members when they arrived at the penitentiary only to learn that their loved ones were being disciplined for some transgression. "With what face will they return next time they visit?" he asked rhetorically, in the direction of Max P.[64]

El Despertar put on full display the "multiple opportunities" at the heart of classification and treatment.[65] Convict Juan C.R. voiced in September 1949 that many Oso Blanco inmates embraced "their own reform" and that, in most cases, the socioscientific work carried out behind bars "gives good results."[66] In November 1949, Luis M.G. wrote an article about classification in Oso

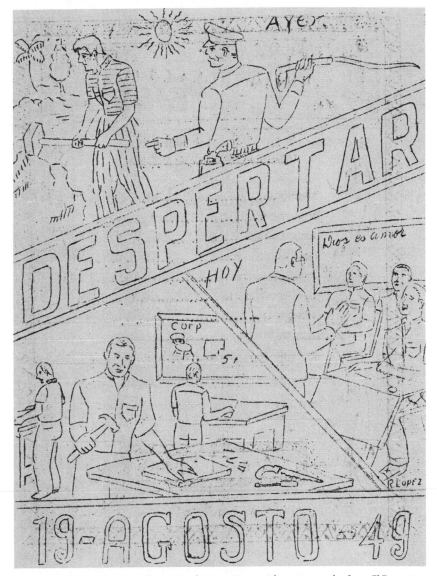

FIGURE 3.3 Convict depiction of transition from punitive punishment to penal reform. *El Despertar* 1, no. 4 (August 1949). Biblioteca y Hemeroteca Puertorriqueña, Universidad de Puerto Rico–Río Piedras.

Blanco and how it had served him well up to that point of his incarceration. He emphasized the impact of "orientation interviews," particularly the way they obligated him to scrutinize his past to understand his current predicament and to model a future for himself. Classification helped him identify his motivations, weaknesses, and treatment possibilities. Classification, Luis

M.G. expressed, taught him to work, "to earn my daily bread with my own sweat."[67] What really stood out to him was an interview session he had with the director of sociopenal services Susano Ortiz, who afforded him kindness, comprehension, and solidarity the likes of which he had never experienced before. After exiting Ortiz's office that day, Luis M.G. was a "completely different man, willing to struggle against all inconveniences to be worthy of the attention he is given" in prison.[68] The prisoner concluded his column saying that if *El Despertar* gave incarcerated people the opportunity to air grievances about penal reform and rehabilitation, then it was only fair that they convey what empowered them as well.

An authorless *El Despertar* article from April 1950 elaborates on the advantages associated with penitentiary classification and treatment. The institution dispensed health, vocational, educational, and social opportunities to convicts to help them deal with their problems and prepare them for their eventual return to society. They had to decide which components of programming to engage, however. Building and maintaining social bonds with prison professionals through rehabilitation could also keep inmates in the loop regarding developments at the communal, national, and global levels. Showing sincere interest, having a constructive attitude, and desiring to apply the knowledge obtained through classification and treatment foreshadowed good things to come for those who took the process seriously. The author of the April 1950 article encouraged his peers to value and seize the opportunities within their reach. Through it all, there had to be open communication between prison staff, professionals, and the incarcerated.[69]

While a subtext of the April 1950 article is that not *all* Oso Blanco prisoners were convinced that classification and treatment was for them, in general *El Despertar* remained a productive forum documenting the sharp turns of the reform moment. In the final editions of *El Despertar*, some authors decided that the upside of classification and treatment was still worth explaining. Joaquín R.B.V., for example, published a multipage article with illustrations in summer 1950 exposing peers to what was arguably the shining jewel of reform culture. He defined classification as "the total study of the individual prisoner," an effort that considered their needs and abilities in determining and recommending their "custodial status, work assignment, education, vocational training, medical treatment, etc."[70] A team of health professionals monitored the progress of convicts physically, mentally, and socially, leaving in their wake an extensive interdisciplinary paper trail. This team also adjusted individual programs on a case-by-case basis. All this work revolved around prisoners but was facilitated by the Classification and Treatment Board. Given that inmates were constantly entering and exiting Oso Blanco in the mid-twentieth century, information about classification and treatment perpetually circulated inside the prison to make newcomers and old-timers alike aware of their rehabilitative options.

In addition to classification and treatment, multiple articles in *El Despertar* reflected on developments in Puerto Rican and global prison reform more broadly. In August 1949, Joaquín R.B.V. identified 1946–47 as a crucial period for prison reform in Puerto Rico. These years coincided with the state's abandonment of corporal punishment and shift toward classification and treatment, reflecting the principle that all inmates are worlds in themselves. Joaquín R.B.V. distinguished between complete and partial rehabilitation, partial because "rehabilitation should continue as soon as prisoners are paroled or exhaust their sentences."[71] Oso Blanco's budding pedagogical orientation, Luis M.C. suggested, made it more of a "school" than a prison.[72] Precedents for this penological project could be traced to the work of the English activist Elizabeth Fry and the contemporary education efforts of the American Prison Association in the United States. Locally, it was advanced by the wardens Félix R. Rivera and J. Antonio Alvarado, the director of sociopenal services Susano Ortiz, and the assistant warden Arturo Alcover.[73]

Reform progress also played out on the terrain of clothing. The March 1950 edition of *El Despertar* recapped a recent visit by the attorney general Géigel Polanco to the Guavate penal encampment in Cayey, where he announced that the men there would be allowed to dress in civilian clothing. According to the authorless report, Géigel Polanco called the encampment a "prelude to freedom," a place where convicts could be reexposed to the routines, responsibilities, and privileges of citizenship.[74] Civilian clothing exercised a "psychological influence" on inmates by positioning them to cultivate self-confidence and to see themselves as "equal to others."[75] This erased the impression in them that they were mere objects without lives and personalities. *El Despertar* contributors appreciated the reform measure and hoped it would soon be introduced in Oso Blanco so that all prisoners could continue their march toward rectitude.[76] Prisoners recognized that penal encampments in Cayey and Río Grande afforded them "encouraging and stimulating" opportunities through the flexibilities built into how they were organized and operated. Permission to wear civilian clothing, in addition to two-day visits home and relative freedom of movement in a natural prison environment persuaded many minimum-security convicts that rehabilitation was not a ruse but a genuine exercise in "social prophylaxis."[77]

The Classification and Treatment Board worked with thousands of prisoners in the mid-twentieth century. In September 1949, Susano Ortiz disclosed statistics in this regard for the previous fiscal year. The board met fifty-seven times and reviewed 574 cases. Its members classified 477 convicts, debated twenty cases about transfers to the Guavate agricultural colony in Cayey, and eventually sent 56 inmates there and one to an institution for minors in Ponce. Ortiz reported that hundreds of prisoners were active in maintaining penitentiary grounds, in vocational workshops, and took advantage of access to libraries and recreation. A few years into the existence of the board, several benefits were apparent: segregation by crime, enhanced supervision, control and discipline, efficient productivity, and more organized, coordinated, and concinnated treatment regimens.[78] In November, Ortiz noted in *El Despertar* that more than 1,800 offenders had benefited from social orientation interviews.[79] High levels of inmate participation and their "trust" in the counsel of social workers and other social health experts denote that offenders embraced reforms and were receptive to Oso Blanco's culture of rehabilitation.[80]

Lives, Attitudes, and Characteristics

Classification and treatment reports reveal a great deal of information about the Classification and Treatment Board, social workers, and the rationales that went into framing and producing socioeconomic narratives of convicts. They are much more than this narrow assessment and critics of the "exclusionary" archival record would have us believe, however. Classification and treatment histories are one of the few documentary windows into the midcentury lives of convicts, their outlooks, and their wider social worlds.[81] There is no doubt that the histories are filtered and can come across as a long-winded megillah, but there is also no denying that convict raw material largely determines their form. In other words, the paper trail would not exist if incarcerated people had refrained from sharing their stories. Prisoners had less reason to subvert the data-gathering process that helped produce these histories than one might assume, especially if they had to max out their sentences or were serving extended or life sentences. This is not to suggest that inmates did not strategically present themselves to authorities, though. Rather, what I am proposing is that locking prisoners into strategy or even resistance for that matter obscures their internal diversity, as well as other equally or more important inspirations and factors that shaped how they decided to narrate themselves.

The Classification and Treatment Board and the histories they manufactured were the control center of rehabilitative corrections in midcentury Puerto Rico. Social treatment was broken down into four main areas: orientation interviews, the preservation of family bonds, observations of (mal)adjustment to prison routines and demands, and data verification.[82] Using convict stories, social workers generated a socioscientific perception of the dualistic natures of incarcerated people. Notwithstanding nuanced experience, this understanding tended to divide the convict body into a series of interlocked dyads: rural or urban, oligophrenic or intellectually capable, mild mannered or hot tempered, trustworthy or unreliable, and so on. Convict Joaquín R.B.V. commented in December 1949 that prisoners were viewed as moral or immoral, intelligent or dumb, hardworking or lazy. Keenly aware of the knowledge production around him that would determine his future, he intimated "[W]e are daily and greatly affected by what other people think of us" when the focus should be on "what we are [or were becoming] and not what we were" in the past.[83] Securing pearls required someone diving into the waters without preconceived notions, he concluded.

Rural convicts were further subdivided into several subgroups, including *jíbaros*, *jornaleros* (day laborers), *agregados* (those attached to someone's land in exchange for labor), and peons, among other categories.[84] Urban convicts were split into subgroups as well, such as townsmen, *barriada* (working-class neighborhood or shanty) residents, *arrabal* (slum) inhabitants, *caserío* (housing project) tenants, and so on.[85] Prison authorities deemed urban areas more complicated, if not depraved, than rural areas. They had more favorable views of inmates with roots closer to nature. However, rural people could move to urban areas and be corrupted by their new environments.[86] Journalist José A. Roméu validated this thinking in a May 1947 magazine article when he said that a portion of the *arrabal* population was full of rural peasants "in search of a better life" but "ill-prepared" to handle their new environments.[87] A passing glance at penitentiary inmate file cover pages reveals that many prisoners had rural roots but became offenders after moving to towns and cities. Yet it was not necessarily urban space itself that led people astray but what occurred in those spaces and the resulting self-destructive habits, such as drinking, fighting, promiscuity, and so on.[88] Through classification and treatment histories, social workers connected spatial location and behavioral and interactive pathologies. Socially pathologizing prisoners helped justify social work interventions on convict minds and behaviors. What prison officials and health professionals dubbed deviant, however, convicts often understood as survival or ordinary practice.[89]

The social duality of convicts emerged in classification and treatment narratives in at least two ways. On the one hand, social workers interviewed prisoners and critically evaluated their crimes, upbringings, economic statuses, attitudes, and characteristics. They approached incarcerated people from the outside in. On the other hand, inmates pointed to survival practices, power clashes at the local and interpersonal levels, and the minutiae of everyday life.

Classification and Treatment Board narratives, then, blend the interpretations of social workers and the voices of incarcerated people. For example, in 1951 Ligia I. Dávila compiled the history of a twenty-seven-year-old *trigueño* inmate from Guaynabo named Carlos Orizal Félix, who was serving time for robbery. Suffering from mental disequilibrium, he spent his teenage years in the madhouse near Oso Blanco (between the ages of fourteen and twenty). Although he would get excitable and attack employees, while in the asylum he benefited from labor therapy. Orizal Félix learned how to weave and started a small workshop when released, which partially earned him a living. The day he robbed someone for their cash and jewelry, police restrained him with a blackjack, injuring him. Orizal Félix entered the penitentiary a drug addict and sick with venereal disease. Dávila remarked that he was cooperative during the interview and "liked to give details. He is chatty. He recognizes that liquor, drugs, and the disorderly life he led are factors that have adversely influenced his life."[90] Regardless, he possessed the right attitude for rehabilitation and even believed that adopting Evangelical Christianity could help him defeat the vices contaminating him. The Classification and Treatment Board viewed his chances for rehabilitation as "regular."[91]

After establishing the contextual and interactive facts of cases, social workers proceeded to lay out salubrious recommendations. These covered custody, labor, social work, education, professional references and familial contacts, medical treatment, religion, and recreation. Sometimes social workers touched on all these aspects; more often they expanded on only those pertinent to specific individuals. Regarding Orizal Félix, he required minimal custody, was anxious to work, would benefit from orientation interviews, and should continue primary schooling. Dávila also solicited responses from the police officers and advisers closest to Orizal Félix where he grew up in Trujillo Alto, as well as the testimonies of living relatives. The Classification and Treatment Board concluded that he was "rehabilitable" but needed substantial social, vocational, religious, and moral guidance to help him achieve rehabilitation.[92]

As this brief examination of Orizal Félix's classification and treatment history shows, the priorities of social workers and agency of prisoners were inextricably linked. Classification and Treatment Board narratives presented critical accounts of convicts, their lives behind and beyond bars, and their decision-making but also suggested pathways toward interactional care and social rehabilitation. A thirty-six-year-old *trigueño* cane worker named Félix Enrique Soto Vélez, for example, entered Oso Blanco in September 1951. He was serving a few years for breaking into a store and seizing goods and eighty dollars in cash, which he used to buy clothing and other things he needed. Initially reserved, when Carmin Bravo Abreu earned his trust, "he narrated the facts of his life with apparent sincerity."[93] Soto Vélez had a long history of labor instability dating to his adolescent years, when he lost his mother. He did not get along with his father and therefore missed out on the supervision and orientation that, ideally, accompanied having a parent around. Over the years, he was unemployed most of the time, so he resorted to theft "to resolve his economic problems."[94] Bravo Abreu signaled that Soto Vélez's case demanded a program of vocational training, preferably as an electrician, given that he had some experience in the field. His eventual social treatment included orientation interviews and religious instruction.

The domestic instability that sabotaged Soto Vélez's social development surfaces in many classification and treatment histories. In another case, Gloria L. Umpierre reported in October 1953 that a fifty-year-old mulatto inmate from Coamo named Sandalio Mateo Vázquez required "an intense program of social orientation in order to reintegrate his deteriorating personality."[95] Growing up, he did not get enough personalized adult attention or affection. His mother died when he was young, leaving his father with the responsibility of raising nine children alone. The low moral standards Vázquez acquired over the years were to blame for him eventually abusing a child, which landed him in prison. Social and religious guidance, however, Umpierre insisted, could rehabilitate him. Although Vázquez and many other prisoners endured torturous upbringings, there were also convicts who enjoyed more tranquil domestic situations yet still ended up incarcerated. From the points of view of social workers, rehabilitation was a real possibility in either scenario.

Penitentiary social workers pushed a social diagnosis and treatment model that transcended national identities. In the late spring of 1951, for instance, Bravo Abreu filed a report about a twenty-two-year-old black Cuban prisoner with hearing problems, Carlos Osorio Acevedo, who was serving time for multiple counts of breaking and entering. As a child, the convict bore witness to and experienced physical abuse in his household. The same violence was replicated in his schooling through tense exchanges with teachers. During his adolescence, he picked up the regrettable habits of gambling and drinking, which flooded the calumnious and combative Santurce neighborhood in which he lived (Stop No. 25). The chaos appears to have affected Osorio Acevedo socially and in terms of his labor output, Bravo Abreu lamented, for he came across as "imprecise," "insecure," and "mentally retarded."[96] His treatment program included orientation interviews, library access, religious services, and exposure to a craft familiar to him—carpentry and sanding. Bravo Abreu deemed Osorio Acevedo's rehabilitative prospects as "difficult."[97] Only further surveillance and study of the inmate could shed more light on the matter.

The observational prowess of social workers is embedded in their classification and treatment insights. They had to fuse the disparate statements
of convicts into coherent narratives while being mindful of lapses that could
make or break rehabilitative programs. If classification and treatment ma-
chinery was operating as intended, other members of the board would catch
wind of the lapses and address them in later rounds of health professional–
convict exchange. Teodosia Boneta asserted in 1954 that a fifty-eight-year-
old white prisoner from Río Piedras serving a short sentence for mutilation
named Enrique Astacio Cruz assumed a respectful attitude during his interview but was a nervous wreck. He had an extensive criminal record for
alcohol-inspired fights and aggravated assaults, which made her suspicious
of him. The nature of his job—he was a fisherman that traveled to nearby
Caribbean islands and was therefore away from home for extended periods—
reflected the instability of his life. The lawlessness of life at sea manifested
in his having lashed out on someone for disrespecting him verbally. Astacio
Cruz's inconsistent self-presentation led Boneta to believe he was insincere.[98]

Given Boneta's and other social workers' heavy caseloads, there was no
way for them to determine classification and treatment on their own. Oso
Blanco mental health and educational professionals enriched and layered the
original canvassing performed by social workers. In Astacio Cruz's case, the
psychologist reported a Rorschach score of 26 percent, immaturity, and introversion. The psychiatrist noted his corybantic irritability and carelessness
about being incarcerated. Pedagogically, the convict demanded an "intense
social orientation program to readjust his personality."[99] His rural outlook
and tendencies and lack of penitence complicated social treatment, however.
Still, the director of prison social services Jesús E. Palmer, the final arbiter
of classification and treatment by the mid-1950s, decided that Astacio Cruz
would be best served in an agricultural penal encampment, so he authorized
transferring him to Zarzal, Río Grande.

Not only did social workers piece together the lives, attitudes, and characteristics of prisoners in narrative form, but they also studied them ethnographically to cull data. During interviews, they were attentive to manner-
isms, gaze, body language, and other corporeal expressions, mindful of any
sign that could help them decipher the behavioral and social pathologies
afflicting incarcerated people. Iván Graciano Núñez, a twenty-two-year-old
white convict from Arecibo serving eight years for a crime against nature,
was described in the following way: "He speaks with the simplicity of a child
and gives the impression that he cannot kill a fly. As he speaks, he lowers his
eyes and has a humble tone that makes a very favorable impression on the
listener."[100] Despite being an excessive drinker, Graciano Núñez intended to

rehabilitate himself. If his "external appearance is not *camouflage*, the man can receive treatment here to help him."[101] This final statement encapsulates the interpretive dilemma faced by midcentury correctional social workers. They had to be cautiously optimistic about socially raising the living dead.

Responding to Rehabilitative Failure

Conditional parole by executive decree in Puerto Rico dates to the early twentieth century. Modern parole emerged in 1946 via Law 266.[102] Loveland laid out the parameters for modernized parole in his report. These revolved around adjusting to community life, obtaining and retaining employment, and exercising responsible citizenship. "Careful planning for release and supervision by qualified parole officers following release," he noted, would result in "a minimum number of violations of parole and law."[103] The philosophical roots of parole in Puerto Rico ran much deeper, however. Puerto Rico's Penal Code was modeled after that of the US state of California, but in the early 1950s, José S. Alegría, president of the Parole Board, traced the Puerto Rican parole system to nineteenth-century Mexican and Swiss penologists (Antonio Martínez de Castro and Carl Stooss, respectively). These thinkers posed treating prisoners as recovering patients and using fear and hope to manage their behavior.[104] Because punishment itself did not reform and could strengthen criminal tendencies, prison sentences had to be complemented by sound preventive and reentry systems. The rough equivalent of parole in the British Caribbean, for its part, was known as "after-care."[105]

Proponents of midcentury rehabilitative corrections realized that punitive punishment no longer, if it ever, served any meaningful social function and therefore could be considered a failure. Puerto Rican justice officials and collaborating health professionals had to improve or, if necessary, altogether change the social "medicine" convicts received in response to their criminal behavior.[106] Parole humanized punishment by providing judges and other correctional stakeholders with portraits of prisoners, not just their rap sheets. Narrating inmate family circumstances and relations, their physical and mental conditions, education, labor history, and socioeconomic status gave parole officers windows into the variables influencing individual parolees. This information allowed them to socially diagnose convicts and their situations before approaching the courts with recommendations. The key decision parole officers had to make revolved around where prisoners could receive premier social treatment: inside prisons or elsewhere, such as another institution or in their home or host communities. If beyond prison walls, then ongoing, periodic supervision was required until determined otherwise.[107]

Realizing the most utopic version of parole necessitated personnel, however, which as of late 1948 was still lacking. In response to high demand, Puerto Rico's Parole Board contracted the services of eighteen new officers. These officers were assigned the task of investigating unclassified penitentiary prisoners to see if they qualified or were primed for parole. Their studies on those deemed unprepared were distributed to the Classification and Treatment Board.[108] Parole officers performed this preemptive work, but also investigations after the fact. Parole violation investigations were as deep as those that went into producing classification and treatment histories, if not more so. Given all the idealism permeating penitentiary science and parole, failure was a bitter pill to swallow for the social workers involved with prisoner release and committed to seeing the rehabilitative process through to the end. Like classification and treatment officials, parole officers interviewed prisoners and people in their immediate communities who could elaborate on their life trajectories. Engagement with the wider communities of parolees was even greater for obvious reasons, for parole officers had to decide whether to recommend revocation of their clients' freedom.

Classification and treatment officials provided the board with initial, rigorous snapshots of the physical, mental, and interactive needs of individual prisoners. Parole officers added new layers to these snapshots by contributing accounts of how inmates responded to accusatory fingers being waved at them. For example, a twenty-three-year-old white root crop and vegetable salesman with kidney problems from Sabana Grande named Pedro Ortiz Figueroa arrived at Oso Blanco in October 1949 to serve up to three years for a crime against nature. During his interview with Carmen Sylvia García in early 1950, the social worker was attentive to his body language and observed that, when discussing his crime, he grew restrained and lowered his head. These and other factors, such as his alcoholism, led her to believe that he needed "moral, religious, and recreational orientation to help him get better."[109]

It took two years for Ortiz Figueroa to finally earn parole, which he achieved in May 1952. He lasted one year beyond the walls before violating the terms of his early release. Parole officer Jorge Enrique Arroyo submitted a report to the Parole Board in summer 1953 detailing the circumstances of the ex-convict's most recent run-ins with the law. Ortiz Figueroa's mentor and the broader Sabana Grande community expressed disappointment in him and blamed alcohol abuse for his inability to turn his life around. Arroyo, who visited Ortiz Figueroa at least six times before he was arrested, never noticed there was something amiss. Instead, the former prisoner "gave the impression that he was advancing his rehabilitative process."[110] It turned out, though, that

Ortiz Figueroa and his brother Daniel frequently pursued illegal gambling and disturbed the peace.

Ortiz Figueroa denied the allegations and insisted that although he enjoyed an occasional drink, he never reached the point of drunken stupor. "Every time something happens in this town and the culprit is not discovered, I get blamed for it. The police do not leave me alone for a second. I am always getting threatened with being sent back to prison," he declared.[111] Before recommending that Ortiz Figueroa's parole be revoked, Arroyo advised him to exchange Sabana Grande for Mayagüez, where he had an uncle and a chance for a fresh start. Ortiz Figueroa stayed in Sabana Grande. This resulted in further tensions with locals, who increasingly found him and his brother aloof and repugnant. Townspeople even started calling the brothers *llaneros* (plainsmen), a way of communicating their preference for an existence on the margins of society and the law. All this frustrated Arroyo. He felt that Ortiz Figueroa had slighted the Parole Board and every convict working hard to truly be rehabilitated. After a hearing before the board, Ortiz Figueroa's parole was revoked, and he reentered the penitentiary to serve the rest of his sentence.

After each visit made to a parolee, social workers filed supervision reports. These reports diagnosed the evolving social situations of formerly incarcerated people: their residence, attitude, health, and employment. They also detailed whether ex-convicts had new problems requiring a treatment plan. General observations concluded the reports. The parole officer Elisama Morales Torres (de Irizarry), for example, visited a thirty-seven-year-old mulatto man from Ponce named Ismael Barnés Figueroa at least twice in the spring of 1952. He had been on parole for about six months. The ex-prisoner's older sister Luisa was advising him soundly and, aside from having recently moved in with a new female partner, which he needed to report to the Parole Board as soon as possible, Morales Torres found his situation to be normal. Barnés Figueroa earned wages at the Ponce beach docks and conducted himself "as a good citizen," Morales Torres noted.[112] "Complete rehabilitation" was on the horizon for him.[113]

By 1954, however, the recently married Barnés Figueroa was under renewed scrutiny. A teenage girl with whom he had been pursuing a parallel relationship accused him of rape. Morales Torres immediately launched an investigation and uncovered that the teenager had a dubious reputation and incited Barnés Figueroa's lustful passion. Regardless of the girl's role, it could not be denied that, when it came to women, the former inmate "lacked self-control."[114] The rape allegation derailed his rehabilitation not simply because of the nature of the alleged crime but also because, "being married, he partially violated the terms of his release, for the purpose of the system is to rehabilitate criminals" and their character.[115] This situation assailed several key moral principles informally undergirding the parole system, including living to please God by being sanctified and avoiding sexual immorality. Morales Torres recommended that the Parole Board delay its own action until the case worked its way through the courts. Should Barnés Figueroa be vindicated, then the board would have to address his weakness for women through social programming so that he could avoid such illicit behavior in the future.

Female prisoners similarly navigated the gendered dimensions of parole and rehabilitation. In October 1953, the parole officer Virginia Otero de Rodríguez filed a report about a thirty-four-year-old black prisoner from Coamo named Nieves Torres Santiago, who authorities released from Arecibo prison in March 1952. Shortly after exiting prison, her former partner (a married man with children named Julio Juan Torres Tapia), whom she had previously attacked with a weapon and mutilated (this was what landed her prison), began visiting her at home and work. Their relationship was toxic. Torres Tapia wanted Torres Santiago to be his exclusive concubine; she rejected this in principle but not in practice and continued to seek him out. Several onlookers, including police officers, overheard them arguing on several occasions. Many of their scandals revolved around Torres Tapia's jealousy and him catching Torres Santiago interacting with other men.[116]

Coamo police officers accused both parties of disturbing the peace in August 1953. After leaving a baptismal afterparty, where Otero de Rodríguez believed the couple drank alcohol, the two had an altercation because Torres Tapia disagreed with Torres Santiago's ungraciously taking off her shoes to sit and rest on a curbside. The result was they squared up and got into a fist fight in public. Otero de Rodríguez noted that, besides her relationship with Torres Tapia, Torres Santiago's rehabilitation was going well. She received sufficient advising and either sewed or painted portraits to earn a living. The problem was Torres Tapia, so the parole officer recommended that Torres Santiago move to Guayama to live with an aunt. Only there was her complete "moral and social rehabilitation possible."[117] Otherwise, it was best to revoke her parole to separate the two. In this case, rehabilitation did not revolve around the technical outcomes of corrections, for Torres Santiago complied with what social workers and the board asked of her in terms of advising and employment. Rather, here rehabilitation was cast as an ongoing process. For it to conclude, the ex-prisoner had to unlearn concubinage, respectfully interact with male suitors, and ultimately get married.

While they were often supportive of their incarcerated loved ones (exemplified by letters and visits, for instance), family members and broader communities could be indifferent toward ex-prisoners. One inmate explicitly claimed that recidivism could be traced to ordinary citizens and their "rejection" of those exiting prisons.[118] Mothers, usually steadfast in backing their imprisoned offspring, could also cast doubt over the rehabilitation of their children. When an eighteen-year-old white inmate named Esteban Méndez Jiménez, who was serving a short sentence for breaking and entering, was about to exit the penitentiary in summer 1955, the social worker Pura Jackson visited his family, neighbors, and coworkers in barrios Salto and Guatemala in San Sebastián to get a sense of his rehabilitative prospects and socioeconomic stability once beyond the walls.[119] Guillermina Méndez explained to Jackson her son's incorrigibility and the shame his misdeeds brought upon the family. She feared he would fall into his usual bad habits, such as drinking and sloth, especially given that he would not be pursuing gainful employment. The sugar harvest, the only kind of work available to him, was still far off. Neither familial counsel nor prison time restored decency and honor in Méndez Jiménez, so Guillermina expected the worst. Furthermore, coworkers and other members of the community avoided him like the plague because of his short temper and confrontational tendencies. He did not respond well to jokes but enjoyed dishing out the most vulgar ones himself. These testimonies—indeed, the lack of acceptance and familial and communal opprobrium—convinced Jackson that it was best to preempt any trouble by having Méndez Jiménez complete the remainder of his sentence.[120]

Episodes of rehabilitative failure such as these destabilize the view that rehabilitation was an exclusively successful enterprise celebrated by everyone in an ex-convict's social circle. As the work of the Classification and Treatment and Parole Boards proliferated in the late 1940s and into the 1950s, cracks in the system developed. And this notwithstanding that by 1951–52, for example, there were more than 1,600 people on the bookends of the carceral pipeline (either on probation or parole) and some 2,000 on parole specifically by the mid-1950s.[121] Ex-prisoners left one social fray in the prison to enter another in their home or host communities. Socioeconomic exclusion and friction with kin, neighbors, police, and other members of the community could thwart the rehabilitation of parolees and return them to prison. This defeated the purpose of releasing them. Thus, recouping freedom required psychological preparation.[122] Since 1947, this included incarcerated people briefly returning home before release to have their rehabilitation tested and to build up self-confidence for the challenges that awaited.[123]

Mutual aid and community building were also possibilities.[124] The establishment of a parole school with clear criteria for release, postcarceral curriculum, and a job placement program could help ensure societal reintegration and reduce recidivism.[125] One inmate even called for replacing all prisons with regenerative "schools."[126] Not everyone incarcerated agreed with these steps, however, for certain peers would be selected to lead these efforts, leaving minimal room for others to contribute.[127] Another convict doubted the penitentiary could rehabilitate *all* prisoners. He instead stressed how Oso Blanco could easily become "a source of contagion" that diffused "innumerable ills" to its inhabitants.[128] The focus had to be on education, he argued, because most inmates came from circumstances that left them with little choice but to resort to violence and crime to survive. Compared to physical and mental rehabilitation, then, social repair could be the most challenging facet of rehabilitative corrections since the body under scrutiny was not just inward looking (individual) but outward looking (social and communal).

Conclusion

In midcentury Puerto Rico, social workers and parole officers played important roles in materializing rehabilitative corrections. They were indispensable to the work of the Classification and Treatment and Parole Boards, interviewed and observed the conduct of convicts, and produced socioeconomic histories of prisoners that integrated the different aspects of the rehabilitation process. Their accounts revealed the tragedies and traumas at the core of inmate social pathologies, but also the promise of moving forward. Despite the optimism surrounding rehabilitative corrections at the time, the line between success and failure was porous and contingent.

Social work added a distinct flavor to and complemented Puerto Rico's culture of rehabilitative corrections. Once convict bodies and minds were diagnosed, treated, and salvaged, they required interactional care and social rehabilitation. This meant the living dead had to be prepared to reenter society on society's terms and play by society's rules, both of which were being forged again by colonial populism. Their livelihoods and those of their families depended on the degree to which they conformed to long-standing and reconfigured social norms. To achieve social redemption, prisoners needed to maintain bonds with kin and community, which was not always a given, and to acquire or improve the skill sets that would enable them to thrive once finally beyond the walls. This was easier said than done.

Riding the coattails of the penal reforms of the mid-1940s, Puerto Rico's classification and treatment and parole systems were refined and strengthened. Within a few years, prisoners were being screened more holistically and their rehabilitative programming reflected a messy but humanistic turn in corrections. Yet even if they succeeded in meeting the criteria for rehabilitation in prison, when ex-convicts reentered society other people might be hostile toward them, which threatened their meeting the minimum standards of staying free. This meant they had to go back into the world ready to endure affliction and tribulation. Religious and spiritual logics and practices, among other humanities tools, positioned incarcerated people to cope with and confront living death on their own terms, however.

More Than Flesh:
Sacred Knowledge and Experiential Healing

On September 9, 1957, a young inmate of Puerto Rico's Industrial School for Women in Vega Alta named Nereida Ribot composed a love letter.[1] The letter was addressed to someone named Rabi or Rafi.[2] Although it is not entirely clear who Rabi was, Ribot provided several clues. She expressed being upset about his not attending a recent prison dance in a labor capacity. Ribot also referred to a letter Rabi wrote in which he urged her to wait for him when she left prison since he, too, was imprisoned and "when a woman loves she has to respect the man."[3] She identified Rabi as a good person, asked him for his address, hoped for his early release, and insisted she would not forget him. Aside from conveying her emotions and mindset in the letter, Ribot attached a "song" and "some saints," which she deposited in a separate envelope and sealed.[4]

Prison officials seized the love letter and sealed envelope before Ribot had a chance to mail them. When I first came across the sealed envelope, I hesitated to open it. I eventually did and a potent, bittersweet smell that had been trapped for more than fifty years finally made its way into the world. The sealed envelope's contents included a song, some saints (including an image of a Greco-Roman Jesus Christ), and a small, crimsoned figurine of the Virgin Mary. Given how I was positioned at the archive, these items fell into my lap. As all this exploration unfolded, it occurred to me that the letter and objects formed part of an elaborate ritual. Ribot blended religious iconography with a perfume smell designed to elicit romantic meanings in a context of unfreedom.[5]

Ribot's song was based on the Mexican composer Wello Rivas's bolero "Cenizas." The song's emotional lyrics warned of unrequited and dead love that turned into ashes the moment the once-beloved party became aware of a former admirer's strong romantic affection.[6] Ribot did not quote "Cenizas" word for word, however. She interpreted the song in conjunction with her sacred knowledge and made it the center of a fortune-making seduction ritual. Ribot recorded her lyrics on a separate sheet of paper and kissed the sheet twice, leaving traces of lipstick behind. She subsequently pressed an image of the Virgin Mary to the page with a waxy substance.

Clearly, Ribot meant for Rabi to read the love letter and open the sealed envelope. She expected him to inhale the smell, open the song, bear witness to the religious artifacts falling into his hands or lap, and read the song lyrics. Ribot sought to caress Rabi through the letter, song, and saints. Her intricate ritual showcases how far she was willing to go to shape her fortune and future. Living death (incarceration) could not detain her. She soothed her grievance and empowered herself by making a rite of writing a letter to Rabi, one that invoked the living dead of the spirit world and the conqueror of death himself, Jesus Christ. The love letter and contents of the sealed envelope encapsulated a powerful subjective performance. Smell and sensory experience allowed Ribot to narrate her story and well-being on her own terms.

Incarcerated people like Ribot understood the body and physical senses as central to performing beliefs. As several scholars have suggested, tracing the materiality of the experiential makes it possible to capture the complexity of medico-religious epistemologies and ontologies without reducing them to folly because they are not scientifically verifiable.[7] Religious and spiritual logics and practices offer windows into how inmates, through sacred knowledge and ritual, confronted and transcended living death, which in many ways meant living in a time out of time. Additionally, religiosities and spiritualities represented a collective rite of passage that convicts went through together, one that (in)formally intensified their solidarity while also revealing the sociocultural fault lines between them.

This chapter examines religious and spiritual activities and experiences in Puerto Rican and other Caribbean prisons in the mid-twentieth century. Denominational publications, prisoner reflections on the sacred, and other sources show that inmates used belief systems to rationalize their incarceration, build community, and recast those very systems as their own to tap into their healing power. While Oso Blanco's rehabilitative regime officially treated convict bodies, minds, and souls, the hegemony of scientific approaches meant that religion and spirituality played a peripheral role even as some medical professionals acknowledged the health benefits of faith.[8] When wholeheartedly exercised, however, beliefs expanded convicts' therapeutic options. Religiosities and spiritualities stimulated the senses of prisoners in ways that medicine, social science, and the broader humanities could not, although incarcerated people often fused all these forms of knowledge to re-sculpt their consciousness and heal themselves. There also were prisoners who doubted the sacred or otherwise had indecipherable beliefs, but the pages that follow primarily emphasize those who embraced the sacred.

Catholicism

Ribot's diasporic or vernacular Catholicism represented one of many reli-gious options in midcentury Puerto Rican prisons.[9] Unsurprisingly, Catholi-cism dominated the prison system's religious landscape. For centuries, the Catholic Church managed religious policy in Puerto Rico. As imprisonment was linked to Spanish colonial governance, Catholic clergy contributed to meeting the religious and spiritual needs of incarcerated people. In the nine-teenth century, while participating in the persecution of heterodox think-ers, priests performed last rites for sick inmates on the cusp of death and arranged for their remains to be interred.[10] By the mid-twentieth century, the roles of priests and nuns evolved. They became more involved in human-izing inmates. In district prisons and penitentiaries, for instance, Catholic chaplains and societies presided over conferences and feasts and organized libraries, and nuns sang for prisoners, offered classes, and delivered small gifts to them.[11]

Catholic priests advanced their Oso Blanco operation in the 1930s. Re-demptorist missionaries were particularly active in the Río Piedras tri-institutional complex and beyond, spiritually and materially edifying not only prisoners but also leprosy, mental, and tuberculosis patients. In the differ-ent insular institutions, these priests led mass (the main act of worship in the Catholic Church), administered communion, and piloted other cultural and recreational activities.[12] With regard to religious affiliation, in the 1930s and 1940s about two-thirds of Oso Blanco convicts consistently identified as Catholics.[13] Many of them attended mass every Sunday; others less frequently, if at all. Some inmates activated their Catholicism only during holidays such as Passover (*Pascua*) and Christmas.[14] A few insisted they had deep histories with the faith both inside and outside of Oso Blanco.[15] There were "specu-lative" Catholics, "superstitious" Catholics who believed in the deleterious health impacts of "witchcraft," and those who consulted "infernal books" and other demonological and occult texts.[16]

Several prisoners simply highlighted the ritual base of their devotion, for example the fact that they participated in communion or habitually prayed.[17] In one case, an inmate described the mental alleviation yielded by and the liberatory effects of prayer; that praying at night made him "feel so good" that he forgot he was in prison.[18] What prayer entailed for incarcerated people was further clarified in the April 1950 edition of *El Despertar*. The activist Carmelina G. Freyre, who regularly submitted book excerpts to be published in the magazine, suggested that it was not about "letting God know your desires," for "material things," or to "satisfy the ego."[19] Rather, it was about "finding harmony with God," serving God with "thanksgiving," and securing God's "guidance and protection," which in turn preserved and enriched one's well-being.[20]

Catholic mass could be small and intimate or large scale. In late July 1946 at the penitentiary, for example, Catholics organized a spectacle mass performed on the penitentiary's patio. *El Imparcial* reported that Father Juan Díaz Mesón (of Sacred Heart Church), Father José (of the Redemptorist Fathers and chaplain of the Catholic mission in Oso Blanco), and Father J. Ortiz del Rivero (of the Carmelite Sisters) met in the Santurce residence of a musical couple involved in prisoners' affairs to plan the event. The singers Delia Quiñones de Meyner and Alfonso Álvarez Torres, who hosted the clergymen, were to direct the vocal portion of the program. The violinist Jaime Pedró and the organist Francisco Vidal Tarraza would contribute instrumentation.[21] Everyone involved wanted to offer attendees a total sensory experience, for experiencing religiosity in this way was not only instructional and entertaining but also could be therapeutic. Singing in groups synchronizes heartbeats and triggers the release of endorphins, serotonin, and oxytocin, hormones that relieve anxiety and stress and are linked to feelings of trust and bonding.[22]

El Mundo reported on the mass organized by Díaz Mesón and company in mid-August 1946. A series of photographs told the story of this Catholic campaign. The images say more than words can about the mundane, communal, and experiential aspects of Catholicism in Oso Blanco. Speaking from an elevated position, Díaz Mesón led the religious ceremony. A microphone amplified his sermon to a large, multiracial crowd of visibly thin prisoners. Prisoners eagerly listened, and when the time came to pray and reflect, they did so.[23] At some point during the mass, presumably before it began or after it ended, inmates received religious materials, including Bibles and catechism booklets.

Figure 4.1 is from the August 1946 *El Mundo* press release on the Catholic mission. It captures when mission representatives and their institutional collaborators distributed Bibles and catechisms to a throng of Oso Blanco inmates. At the bottom-right corner of the image, a man dressed like a prisoner distributes religious texts. A woman shielding herself from the sun with a hand fan stands behind him. The presumed convict distributing texts exchanges words with another prisoner. The middle-aged, balding, light-skinned text

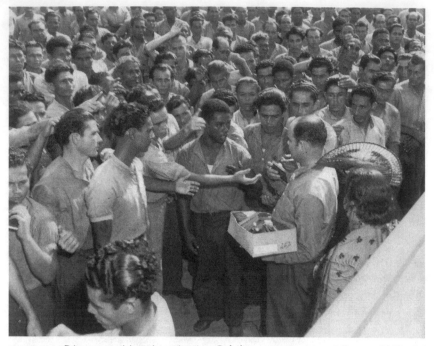

FIGURE 4.1 Prisoners participate in penitentiary Catholic service. August 1946. Proyecto El Mundo/ Biblioteca Digital Puertorriqueña, Universidad de Puerto Rico–Río Piedras.

distributor has a book in his right hand, but it is hard to tell whether he is withholding or about to extend it. The young inmate of color hoping to receive the text, on the other hand, lightly touches his chest as if to infer that he sincerely wants a text or should not be denied one. In the bottom-left corner of the image, another prisoner appears to be distributing texts as well. Meanwhile, other convicts are affixed to the unraveling situation. A few directly look at the camera. Several of them reach for the spiritual bread being apportioned.

Catholic priests and nuns carried out multiple large-scale masses and other activities in Oso Blanco around midcentury.[24] These were often linked to milestone rituals like communion. In September 1949, *El Despertar* announced a Catholic mission scheduled for that October 16–23. The Redemptorist Fathers advertised the event, which would focus on those inmates receiving the Eucharist for the first time. Each morning of the campaign, prisoners had the option of attending mass and Bible study. The Sisters of the Good Shepherd agreed to give doctrine classes in the afternoon. Convicts had access to confessionals, rosary prayers, sermons by the Jesuit reverend Gregorio S. Céspedes, and blessings every night. The mission concluded with a mass officiated by Bishop Jaime P. Davis of the archdiocese of San Juan. The Catholic mission was "a special time to receive God's grace" and understand "eternal salvation."[25] Comprehending the undeserved gift of grace allowed, in this case, incarcerated men to experience spiritual healing and turn a leaf in their lives. No longer tormented by who they were in the past or what landed them in prison, they could now strive to live according to the new creature principle elaborated by Paul in 2 Corinthians 5:17.

Prisoners later reflected on the Catholic mission in another edition of *El Despertar*. The text of the first page of this article was organized in the form of a cross, the symbolic source of new life for many of the men who attended the campaign. The highlight of the mission, writers agreed, was Friday, October 21, when prisoners performed the Via Crucis (Stations of the Cross) ritual. This rite pays homage to Jesus Christ through a series of stations, images or scenes that depict the story of his crucifixion.[26] Almost the entire inmate population either participated in or bore witness to this "solemn act bursting with religious fervor."[27] The procession was unlike anything *El Despertar* contributors had ever seen. Prisoners demonstrated "true spiritual retreat" during this part of the mission, as they clustered around several outposts that were representative of scenes of the Passion and awaited their turn to participate.[28]

The Via Crucis ritual in question put incarcerated people and Puerto Rico's cultural and political elites into close contact by having them share the same space and breath the same air. On Sunday, October 23, distinguished personalities of both genders attended mass, including philanthropists and social workers, prominent attorneys, civic club leaders, Parole Board and justice officials, university intellectuals, secular and church choir members, and so on. Several priests and government officials delivered speeches. Bishop Davis's solemn mass emphasized the "great spiritual significance" of the mission and exhorted prisoners "to maintain the spark" the mission had lit in their hearts and souls.[29] During the mission, some eight hundred inmates received communion, a ritual during which the bishop of San Juan fed convicts the symbolic body of Jesus Christ. Inmates knelt near one another in anticipation of their turn.[30] Furthermore, some seven hundred convicts enrolled in the Oso Blanco chapter of the Society of the Holy Name, which in the 1950s was led by a Cuban prisoner named Miguel Batalla.[31] In the aftermath of the fall 1949 campaign, inmates in Cell Block 15 agreed to make the time to pray the Holy Rosary. In subsequent weeks, five additional cell blocks joined. All of them chanted aloud in unison every night thereafter and expected others would enlist.[32]

Priests interacted with prisoners for nonritual purposes as well. In the San Juan district jail, Father Juan Vicente Rafael Rivera delivered a lecture in

October 1952 about the "restorative" power of religiosity.[33] Rivera met with convicts in rooms adorned with religious imagery, where they learned what a spiritual lifestyle entailed. He also let inmates vent, provided them with individual counsel, and had them reflect on the poetry of the Spanish philosopher Ramón de Campoamor.[34] Talking to priests like Rivera about the health benefits of religion in spaces decorated for the occasion afforded prisoners with opportunities for spiritual uplift and community building. Performing faith mattered to inmates not only because they could materialize what they believed in but also because doing so was fulfilling and even curative.[35] Harvesting feelings of certainty through religious instruction and ritual could raise convicts from living death.

Catholic work behind bars was not always amicable and orderly, however. In January 1958 in Vega Alta prison, for example, the assistant director Crucita Arzuaga Algarín wrote to her superior Lydia Peña (Beltrán) de Planas complaining about a Sister Imelda's intervention in bureaucratic affairs. This confused inmates about norms, procedures, and who really exercised power in carceral settings. Instead of sticking to a religious message, Imelda usurped the duties of classification and treatment officials and other administrators. She mistakenly trusted information collected from prisoners, many of whom were mentally infirm. One time, she even sought authorization to transfer inmate Lucía Ortiz's daughters from a welfare institution in Santurce to another in Ponce, where the girls would, in her view, receive better care. This conflicted with Ortiz's desires, who wanted the girls close so that she could see them under the supervision of a social worker.[36] Imelda neglected to recognize that religious authority did not trump secular authority within the logic and practice of rehabilitation. Nevertheless, as this case illustrates, holistic health issues were at the center of interactions and exchanges about prisoners' futures and the futures of their families.

Catholic services in Oso Blanco thrived well into the 1950s and 1960s. The Holy Name Catholic Knights Association did "outstanding" work there in 1957.[37] The church offered more than three thousand activities attended by thousands of prisoners by the mid-1960s.[38] Although in Puerto Rico Catholicism predominated behind bars, prisons were not the exclusive terrain of the Catholic Church. The Puerto Rican reality contrasts sharply with developments in the Dominican Republic, where Catholic priests largely monopolized prison religious life and limited the activity of Evangelicals.[39] Throughout the 1920s, priests delivered sermons in Nigua penitentiary and President Horacio Vásquez occasionally visited the facility to observe mass and other rites with convicts.[40] High-ranking clergy led mass in prisons in the 1930s.

The political prisoner Juan Isidro Jimenes Grullón, for instance, recalled the presence of the Italian archbishop Ricardo Pittini, whose holiday and Sunday cell visits he deemed "hypocritical" because of the priest's acquiescence to the political violence of the Rafael Trujillo regime.[41]

Despite constant exposure to Catholicism, Dominican convicts had limited access to the iconography and broader material culture of the church behind bars. An inmate named Diógenes, a healer who performed injections, improvised an altar.[42] One Catholic official petitioned Trujillo in the mid-1940s, asking that he order the placement of "comforting" crosses and images of the Virgin of Altagracia in Nigua and other prisons across the country.[43] A priest active in the mid-1940s in Puerto Plata prison, José Molné, reiterated the values of the dictatorship in his sermons. He exhorted prisoners to "regenerate" and dignify themselves by working hard and changing their lives.[44] This would benefit their well-being, that of their families, and that of the Dominican nation-state.

Catholicism prevailed in many midcentury Caribbean prisons. This was a consequence of cross-generational custom and habit but also the activism of people on the ground. Prisoners were receptive to the messages and rites overseen by priests, nuns, and other surrogates of the Catholic faith. They participated in Catholicism knowing there were spiritual and tangible health benefits to be obtained. However, the therapeutic uplift embedded in religious logics and practices was not exclusive to a single tradition. Several other creeds proliferated in prisons at the time.

Interdenominational Christianity

Throughout the first half of the twentieth century, interdenominational Christians buttressed United States empire and used laboratory medicine to raise Puerto Ricans and other Caribbean people from spiritual death and bodily infirmities. They helped build an expansive church and health-care infrastructure in the circum-Caribbean and beyond.[45] The president of the Adventist Inter-American Division put it best when he stated in 1947 that "medical work is the right arm of the [Gospel] and actually the 'entering wedge' to missionary activity."[46] Other key sites of Evangelical missionary activity during this period were jails, prisons, and penitentiaries. Across the Caribbean world—Medellín, Colombia; Isle of Pines, Cuba; Basse Terre, Guadeloupe; Río Piedras, Puerto Rico—pursuing the sacred behind bars could liberate the souls of men entombed in darkness, idleness, and living death and turn their hearts from sin unto righteousness.[47] Local and transnational believers

visited prisons, sang for guards and prisoners, preached to them, received letters from convicts, sent inmates copies of Christian literature, directed Bible
study, performed baptisms, and prayed for and healed prisoners.

While Catholics numerically predominated in Oso Blanco, the ranks of
Evangelical or Protestant-leaning Christians hovered around one-tenth of the
total penitentiary population in the 1930s and most of the 1940s.[48] Just about
all major denominations were represented: Adventist, Baptist, Disciples of
Christ, Lutheran, Methodist, Pentecostal, Presbyterian. Some prisoners fer-
vently identified with their denominations and read the Bible, attended services regularly, and tapped into the corresponding networks afforded by affiliation.[49] Others fused their faith to occult practices, such as "witchcraft."[50]
There were converted Catholics among the ranks of incarcerated interdenominational Christians who held that their new belief systems improved their
chances of subduing social diseases like vice and procuring better, healthier
lives.[51] Following the nationalist uprising of October 1950, which spilled into
Oso Blanco, a number of Catholic nationalists, one of whom previously practiced black magic, became Evangelical Christians. According to some of the
incarcerated nationalists themselves, several of these conversions occurred
because of the empathy and persuasive preaching of the New Zealand–born
British missionary Gladys B. Harrow.[52] The nationalist Catholic Heriberto
Marín Torres, for his part, draws attention to the dubious motivations of midcentury colonial missionaries, perceiving them as wolves in sheep's clothing.[53]

Interdenominational Christian activists in Oso Blanco were just as indus-
trious and resolute as their Catholics counterparts. Administratively, the Baptists led the pack. This was not by coincidence. By 1915 Baptists had spiritual
jurisdiction over the San Juan metropolitan area, where the penitentiary was
located.[54] Urban entrenchment positioned them to implement many projects
as soon as Oso Blanco opened in 1933, like organizing plays and other activities during the holiday season.[55] Baptists also held annual conferences with
other Christian denominations. Conferences advanced a preliminary agenda
for collaborative prison work, assigned a chaplain to the penitentiary and set
his salary, and documented spiritual uplift efforts in all major insular institutions. Conference minutes for some years even briefly refer to former prisoners who attended annual meetings and shared their testimonies about the
saving and healing power of Christ behind bars.[56] By midcentury, the interdenominational chaplain serving Oso Blanco, Juan Sánchez Padilla, published
articles, attended conferences, collected funds, and discussed the evangeliza-
tion of the Río Piedras scientific corridor. He fed incarcerated people spiritual
bread, exposed them to the cure for sin (genuine repentance leading to Jesus
Christ himself), and booked preachers and choirs for holiday services.[57]

Other denominations in Oso Blanco were just as effective despite their not having spiritual jurisdiction over San Juan and Río Piedras. Adventist work in Puerto Rican prisons, for instance, dates to at least the mid-1920s, when missionaries started visiting La Princesa.[58] They began putting down roots in Oso Blanco in 1934.[59] Rufus W. Prince, an Afro–Puerto Rican pastor with missionary experience in Santo Domingo, was among the most persistent Adventists active in the penitentiary in the 1930s. Prince secured permission from the Puerto Rican government to conduct a Branch Sabbath School—an evangelistic type of service for non-Adventists that includes worship songs and Bible study—there shortly after the prison opened.[60] He built and sustained a congregation in Río Piedras while collaborating with justice officials to offer religious programming at the penitentiary and over the radio.[61]

Although Prince helped plant the seed of Adventist radio in Puerto Rico, *The Voice of Prophecy* broadcast was not established in San Juan until 1943 (via WKAQ).[62] Missionaries began offering the program's Bible correspondence course in Oso Blanco soon thereafter.[63] A few years later, in 1946, Glenn Calkins reported that a culture of "preaching the message by radio" bloomed in the penitentiary, where convicts "are systematically studying the Bible under the direction of competent teachers, with many of the students asking for baptism."[64] Enrollment in Oso Blanco's *The Voice of Prophecy* Bible correspondence course grew exponentially, from a handful to several hundred. Prisoners completed the course in strong numbers. A Puerto Rican woman named Blanca Santiago cosupervised the radio Bible school alongside the missionary S. L. Folkenberg.[65]

Santiago and her husband, a police detective named Justino, spent most Sabbaths with prisoners, sharing the message of Christ's saving and healing power with them. During a typical Sabbath, Santiago mingled with inmates, helping them find Bible verses and with the pronunciation and comprehension of any difficult vocabulary they came across. She also collected modest tithes and administered the penitentiary baptismal class.[66] Baptism was and is among the most important rites of a Christian. As noted in 1 Peter 3:21, baptism does not remove the filth of the flesh but engenders a clean conscience toward God. Ideally, it marks a complete transition in the lifestyle and consciousness of the believer. The old self is buried with Christ, and a new person rises from the tomb with Jesus.

Santiago led Bible and baptism classes and utilized radio effectively. She understood the relationship between testimony and spiritual uplift in a context of unfreedom. In December 1945, she shared a convict's letter with Calkins that touched on these aspects. In the letter, the prisoner underscored the themes of spiritual rebirth, renewed history, and the battle between light and darkness, right and wrong, good and evil. In Oso Blanco, he had experienced several confusing trials. However, Christ "has extended His arms toward me, accepting me as a humble sinner."[67] The prisoner credited Christ for changing his thoughts and for bringing Santiago and *The Voice of Prophecy* Bible course to the penitentiary. Through them, he learned that the "things of the Lord" were about spiritual warfare (Ephesians 6:12) and therefore required spiritual medicine.[68] The penitentiary warden and his wife, who happened to be trained social workers, echoed this line of analysis, particularly the mental amelioration afforded by repentance.

While radio exposed convicts to religious healing through a new sensorial register, traditional experiential approaches persisted. Some of these coincided with the work of Oso Blanco's Classification and Treatment Board, which permitted well-behaved prisoners to visit their homes for days at a time in anticipation of release. An Evangelical convict was granted permission to go home for two days in December 1945, for example. The first place he visited was the Adventist church in Río Piedras. There, he "drank in every word of truth that was given."[69] The convict proceeded to give ringing testimony about his walk with Christ. He then went home to Juncos but did not feel comfortable there because of the irreconcilability of his new faith and old religion, which his family still embraced. At a small Pentecostal church, he again shared his testimony, above all what the Lord had done for him:

> How he had begun to study the Bible, the conviction that came to him that there is a higher law, and the necessity that we all have to obey. He then told them how hard it is to obey in our own strength, and how only through the assistance of our Lord can we live in harmony with His divine law. The point was then brought even closer home, that it is only through obedience to all the commandments that we shall be saved. He told them that we are going to have to serve our sentence for our transgression of God's law just as surely as he himself was even now serving his sentence for breaking the law of Puerto Rico.[70]

The convict subsequently returned to Oso Blanco, where he stood firm in his faith and continued to shine. He was living proof of the healing, stabilizing power of God himself.

Aside from Baptists and Adventists, Pentecostals also won over Puerto Rican prisoners. In the 1950s, charismatic transnational evangelists carrying a message of divine healing began visiting places like Peru, Chile, Cuba, and Puerto Rico. The Oklahoman Tommy Lee Osborn went to Puerto Rico several times in 1950 and 1951, drawing thousands to events around the main island.[71] Supernatural healing permeated these events. In June 1951, *The Voice of Healing* magazine reported that hundreds of Puerto Ricans "testified of having been completely healed of all manner of diseases [such as blindness and cancer] during last year's campaign and are still well today."[72] Osborn's exploits were confirmed by the testimonies of local medical experts and those he healed.[73]

During these revival campaigns, Osborn encountered and healed prisoners. At a Ponce crusade, for example, a physically disabled convict briefly escaped custody. The unnamed inmate had convinced district jail officials to let him attend the gathering. At the event, Osborn's message captivated the prisoner and the guards accompanying him. While the guards prayed, the inmate was healed, dropped his crutches, and ran through the crowd. The man then reappeared near the stage in tears. He had been miraculously healed and sprinting was the only way he could respond. Osborn cited Luke 5:17 during this episode, a story about Jesus Christ healing a paralytic whose relations went to great lengths to present him to the Lord.[74] He underscored not only the saving, but the healing power of Jesus, that Jesus was the world's preeminent physician, and that faith in Jesus was the best medicine.[75]

Pentecostals and Adventists remained at the forefront of Evangelical efforts in Oso Blanco through the 1950s and early 1960s. The Philadelphia Church of Chicago, Chicago Bible College, and Full Gospel Fellowship International, among other parishioner groups visited as well.[76] Evangelicals served nearly 8,500 inmates in 1963–64 alone.[77] Puerto Rican justice officials and their interdenominational collaborators held that Evangelical interpretations of doctrine and divine healing could teach prisoners about the limits of what they could control. Ministers like Gerardo López Rodríguez indicated this much regarding his efforts in La Princesa, suggesting that the result—spiritual uplift—was worth the time, energy, and sacrifice. However, prisoners had to do their part and determine what uplift would entail.[78] Interdenominational Christianities helixed one another and reinforced epistemologies and routines designed to foment certain mindsets, lifestyles, and emotional responses, all of which granted convicts access to holistic well-being.

Therapeutic religiosities and spiritualities could be found in other Caribbean penitentiaries as well. In 1940s Cuba, the Gospel reached prisoners through kin networks and *The Voice of Prophecy* radio programming. For example, an inmate named Manuel Suárez awakened interest in the Adventist message in the Presidio Modelo. Brief articles about Suárez were published in Adventist literature in late 1945 and early 1946. These were based on a report by Pastor G. C. Nickle, president of the West Cuba Conference, and the missionary Alvin J. Stewart, both of whom compared Suárez's incarceration to the biblical Joseph's experience in Pharaoh's Egyptian court (Genesis 39–41).

Stewart noted the various Adventist texts Suárez collected while incarcerated, including several books by Elder R. L. Odom, a copy of *Steps to Christ*, some old *Centinelas* and *Inter-American Division Messengers*, and some old *Missions Quarterlies* mailed to him by relatives. Further, Suárez led meetings every Sunday in the prison hospital or bakery, during which a cross-class assemblage of dozens of participants praised God and studied the Bible. Prison officials permitted Suárez to use a piano and two songbooks during the meetings. All who went enjoyed rousing services. Aside from a Methodist minister who used to visit the Presidio Modelo at the time, outside help was sparse. Adventist missionaries hoped the small Sunday school conducted by Suárez would become a full-fledged Sabbath school soon.[79]

Alongside Catholicism, interdenominational Christianity fashioned the religious and spiritual landscapes of Caribbean prisons between the 1930s and midcentury. Missionaries of different Christian persuasions dedicated themselves to teaching convicts scripture and preparing them for baptism, and more broadly to community building and serving those in need. Singing, praying, searching for God in the Bible, converting, baptism, and sharing testimony were but a few of the assorted practices through which convicts performed their beliefs in and beyond Oso Blanco. Through these activities, convicts experienced—indeed felt—their faith and secured salvation and noncorporeal healing.

Spiritism

In addition to multiple forms of Christianity, Spiritism was also practiced in Oso Blanco in the mid-twentieth century. According to the belief system's founder, the Frenchman Allan Kardec, Spiritism is a science that studies the origins, nature, and destiny of spirits, as well as their interactions with the corporeal world. But even this definition is narrow and does not fully account for all the varieties of Spiritism, including more vernacular manifestations. Many lower-class, racially mixed, and culturally syncretic Puerto Ricans, for instance, view Spiritism as a framework for understanding health and healing. They blend Spiritism with popular Catholicism, ethnobotany, and other logics and practices derived from indigenous, African, and creole heritage (à la Ribot, who blended sacred knowledges, deployed power objects, and ritually invoked spirit intermediaries whom she believed could make her fortune).[80]

While the Spanish colonial state in Puerto Rico perceived of Spiritists and other heterodox religious groups as threats, with US rule and religious freedom they assumed civic roles.[81] Following the establishment of an islandwide federation, Spiritists mobilized to transform education, end capital punishment, and reform prisons in the first decades of the twentieth century.[82] Spiritist activism in the criminal-legal sphere dates to at least 1905, when a government circular outlined how Spiritist meetings in prisons should be organized and executed.[83] By the 1940s and 1950s, Spiritists frequented Puerto Rico's district jails and penitentiaries.

In 1949, for example, a delegation of Spiritists and music students visited the Ponce district jail. The group was convinced that teaching incarcerated people the truth about intentionality and good works could save souls and "heal the existence of bad men."[84] The Spiritists counseled the inmates, explained to them the meaning of love thy neighbor, encouraged them to help the despondent, afflicted, and those in need of affection, and demonstrated that moral charity had not yet gone extinct. Music, poetry, and literature readings marked the session. Confirming the Spanish Caribbean circulation and consumption of Spiritist beliefs, the Puerto Rican Spiritist leader Adela Collazo read from the Cuban Spiritist Ofelia León Bravo's "Social Projection of Spiritism," a piece about how Spiritism could and must be amplified in society at large.[85] Moreover, "spiritual beings" (the dead) cooperated through "mediumistic dictations" to "awaken those souls dejected by their own negligence."[86] The prison warden approved of the sociofraternal therapeutics on display during the meeting and expected efforts to continue. "Lyrical-musical-literary" programs meant to undo "manual and mental idleness" and cleanse the body of the "impure effluvia" potentially responsible for inclining men to commit crimes in the first place were still being offered at Ponce district jail as of 1954.[87]

Spiritist gatherings in prisons enabled inmates to engage with people from beyond the walls, which positively affected their social health. When the Legion of Spiritist Women visited the Arecibo prison in late 1951, they threw a Christmas party for the women incarcerated there. The event revolved around poetry readings, speeches, and a Spiritist prayer because of the recent death of the facility's warden, Señor González Lebrón. Incarcerated women recited poems like "God Is Love," "Christmas Eve," and "December," the latter a humorous "jíbaro poem" that lifted the moods of everyone present.[88] Spiritists read selections like "The Whore" and "The Source of Life." The president of the Legion, Petra C. Aybar, used the occasion of González Lebrón's passing to discuss the immortality of the soul and the eternal life of the spirit. The festivities concluded with gifts, refreshments, and candy. Humanizing the incarcerated women in these ways illustrated to them that there were still communities of care invested in their health and rehabilitation.

Like Catholicism and interdenominational Christianity, Spiritism also formed part of Oso Blanco's complex religious landscape. Spiritists visited and lectured in the penitentiary on a regular basis. Spiritism itself allowed inmates to pursue intellectual and moral refinement. The ranks of Spiritists in Oso Blanco were steady in the 1930s and 1940s. Their numbers fluctuated between 3 percent and 6 percent of the total penitentiary population during this period.[89] Convicts who identified with Spiritism grew up around "centers," including the famed House of Spirits in Santurce.[90] In some cases, however, self-proclaimed Spiritists came of age far away from the urban areas where most centers were located, for example in forests.[91] Similar to certain Christians, incarcerated Spiritists could be disconnected from their belief system or sympathize with alternative beliefs.[92] Several prisoners recounted the healing power of Spiritist physicians and the conditions they treated, such as epilepsy.[93]

Classification and Treatment Board histories disclose fragments of what Spiritist healing practices entailed. A center-frequenting, thirty-one-year-old white Spiritist from Carolina named Ramón Molina Avilés, for example, realized income-generating spiritual works in the countryside by contacting ghosts. Elías de Jesús, the father of his eventual victim, recalled that he first crossed paths with Molina Avilés in Trujillo Bajo, where the man was "impersonating" an unnamed "great Spiritist."[94] Molina Avilés charged De Jesús $6.75 for the "medicines and baths" required to banish malignant spirits and treat his daughter's "rose sickness" (perhaps a severe case of pityriasis rosea, a skin condition, or a fungal infection).[95] He also claimed he could cure her with hand passes directed by a spiritual guide.

Compared to their Catholic and Christian counterparts, Spiritists played unglamorous roles in convict rehabilitation. Yet prisoners eagerly anticipated their visits. In the June 1949 edition of El Despertar, the magazine's director interviewed Don Eduardo Rivera, then president of the House of Spirits. The interview transcript reveals that Spiritists offered orientation programs and lectures in Oso Blanco. Many prisoners embraced these activities. Rivera also underscored the regenerative purpose of Spiritist work behind bars. He suggested that everyone, including prisoners, carried a divine spark. This "Creator-supplied faculty" needed only to be discovered and stimulated internally to produce intellectual, moral, and social fruit.[96] Spiritists remained active in Puerto Rican prisons through the 1950s, as was the case with the Spiritualist Society "Surcos."[97] Incarcerated people at the Guavate penal encampment founded a Spiritist center entering the 1960s, expanding the reach of Spiritism.[98]

Shaking the stereotypes associated with talking to and being guided by the dead proved difficult for Spiritists. Still, they carved civic roles for themselves in midcentury Puerto Rico's carceral archipelago. They mentored prisoners

like Catholics and Christians did but without the same levels of prestige, resources, and transnational support. Spiritist inmates took advantage of interacting with brethren from beyond the walls, and shared pieces of their lives
with prison social health professionals. Similar to Catholics and Christians,
Spiritists contributed to raising the living dead.

Other Ways of Believing

Christianity and Spiritism were the most cited and exercised belief systems in
Puerto Rican prisons in the mid-twentieth century. However, ample evidence
suggests that other ways of knowing and believing circulated as well. "Creed-
less" was consistently the second most common category overall in the 1930s
and 1940s, a significant feat in a historically Christian colony.[99] This category
was a catchall term, one that likely included everything from marginal Christianities and folk Catholicisms to Freemasonry, friends of all religions, and
the beliefs of foreign prisoners from Haiti, Hawai'i, the Philippines, China,
Turkey, the Arab world, and elsewhere. The new age and pantheistic Unity
School of Christianity, for instance, won converts in Oso Blanco, prompting
a Lazarus-like rekindling in believers.[100] According to annual justice reports
and other sources, there were other exceptions to these categorizations and
numbers; a theosophist served time in the penitentiary in 1933, nine did in
1934, and a convict waxed poetic about theosophy texts in 1949.[101] There is
also evidence that Islam and Buddhism circulated in Puerto Rican prisons,
but it is unclear if they did so experientially.[102]

Perhaps most revealing in terms of other ways of believing, Hindu philosophy was disseminated by the director of the Industrial School for Youths
in Mayagüez, Susano Ortiz, in the 1950s and early 1960s. "Hinduism" in the
Caribbean did not start as an organic religious category. Rather, Hinduism
was fashioned into a religion during the era of indentured servitude in the
nineteenth century and became a tool in the regulation of East Indian laborers struggling for autonomy.[103] While scholars of the Caribbean geographically locate the Indian diaspora in Trinidad and Tobago, Guyana, Suriname,
and Jamaica, where a plurality of the population resided in the mid-twentieth
century and still does, Hindu ideas crisscrossed the ethno-racial boundaries and colonial spheres of influence prevailing in the Caribbean region at
the time.

In the mid-1950s, Ortiz published short columns about Hinduism that
appeared in the mimeographed Industrial School magazine *Horizontes*. These
were Spanish translations of Hindu teachings accompanied by brief reflections. A September 1956 column explored the Bhagavad Gita (The Song of

God), a seven-hundred-verse Hindu scripture that is part of the second-century BCE Sanskrit epic Mahabharata, which narrates the struggle between cousins in the Kurukshetra War and the fates of the Kaurava and Pandava princes and their successors.[104] The Mahabharata also contains philosophical and devotional material. The Gita recounts a dialogue between Pandava prince Arjuna and Krishna, an avatar or divine incarnation of the Lord Vishnu. The context for the dialogue is that Arjuna is at a moral impasse, despairing about the violence and death that war will bring upon his kin. He considers renouncing the campaign altogether and seeks Krishna's counsel, whose answers in turn form the Gita. Krishna ultimately advises Arjuna to fulfill his duty and uphold the order of the universe.

The exchanges between Krishna and Arjuna cover a range of spiritual topics and broach dilemmas and philosophical issues that transcend the war Arjuna faces. The conflictual setting of the Gita is an allegory for the ethical and moral challenges and struggles human beings endure in life. Such a view of the Gita would have certainly resonated with Industrial School administrators, health professionals, and inmates, all of whom had to sit with their choices in different ways. Ortiz was adamant that the Gita had to be read with reverence so that it could answer questions, dissipate doubts, and materialize ideals. He extracted Gita fragments that applied to the circumstances of his audience, and transmitted lessons about "duty and reward" and "the secret of action," anticipating the seeds would fall into "fertile furrows, germinate, and produce fruit."[105] The next month, in October, Ortiz continued down the path of the Spirit with Gita extracts about "peace and serenity," again hoping they "find fertile soil."[106] More than anyone else, Ortiz knew that Industrial School health professionals and inmates alike needed to be reminded of these themes or exposed to them for the first time if the rehabilitative ideal he advanced in the institution was to manifest itself in the attitudes, comportment, and lives of everyone involved.

By the early 1960s, Hindu philosophy became a regular feature of Industrial School literature. *Horizontes* was succeeded by another mimeographed magazine during this period, called *Rumbos*. In this new periodical, Ortiz continued to translate pieces that he believed would intellectually stimulate and spiritually edify readers inside and outside the Industrial School. He drew the pieces from newsletters and magazines like *Yoga-Vedanta Forest Academy Weekly*, *Divine Life*, and *Wisdom Light*, publications that trafficked in midcentury Hinduism. The work of Sivananda Saraswati, a Hindu spiritual teacher and proponent of Yoga and Vedanta who had served in British Malaya as a physician before taking up monasticism, for example, prominently graced the pages of *Rumbos* for more than a year.

The articles by Saraswati published in *Rumbos* spanned a variety of religious and spiritual topics. Several of them focused on the beatitudes announced by Jesus Christ in his Sermon on the Mount (in the Bible, Matthew 5–7). In a March 1960 article, Saraswati emphasized the distinctiveness of Jesus's proclamations. True beatitude, he asserted, was a "condition in which the Spirit of God seizes man's heart, distancing him from worldly things and transforming him into a divine being."[107] Individualism ceased in such people, and they became instruments—indeed part of—God himself, doing his will by leading righteous lives and representing him on Earth.

In subsequent editions of *Rumbos*, Ortiz translated more of Saraswati's writings. These covered other themes, practices, attributes, and virtues developed in Jesus Christ's Sermon on the Mount, such as prayer and weeping, humility and meekness, divine law and justice, mercy, peacemaking, and humanitarianism.[108] His general advice about the importance of adaptation and gratitude, measures for detachment, the intersection of matter and spirit, the Spirit of Christ, and messages addressed to young people were also published.[109] Ortiz reproduced messages to the youth, in particular, because he was running an institution dedicated to building their skill sets, resocializing them, and achieving their rehabilitation. In a November 1960 article, for example, Saraswati encouraged young people to "know the source of life, what life means, the end you pursue, and the manner in which to reach that end."[110] Divinely ordained laws, duties, privileges, and routes to develop a sound body, mind, and intellect were everywhere for he who had ears to hear and eyes to see. The lesson could not be any clearer for Industrial School residents. They only needed to shed their egos and tap into available religious and spiritual options to reset their trajectories.

With this realization in hand, parallel steps included recognition of an authority greater than oneself and self-control. Ortiz connected Hindu themes to the needs of Industrial School youths and presented them through prisms magazine readers could grasp. In a February 1961 piece published in *Rumbos*, Saraswati elaborated on the concept of dharma (meaning moral order, divine law, or correct pious conduct), "the seed from which rises the powerful Artha tree or worldly prosperity, that provides the fruit of Kama or rather joy. This marvelous tree of life, that grows from the seed of virtue, in the end, proportions you with the delicious mana called freedom, of which once you have eaten, you will cease being hungry."[111] On one level, this passage would have been familiar to Industrial School inmates with Christian backgrounds (e.g., Jesus Christ's pronouncement in John 6 that he is the bread of life). On another level, the freedom referred to by Saraswati represented the culmination of noble and pure aspirations, not freedom gone awry. There was no need to dwell on mismanaged freedom. Rather, "have dominion over your mind," Saraswati stressed.[112] This could be achieved by "disciplining the senses," "cleansing your animal nature," and becoming "the owner of your destiny."[113] In other words, self-control would position Industrial School youths to exercise freedom in productive rather than self-destructive ways, *if* they could rein in their flesh. True healing transcended healing the physical body. The mind and soul also required attention and investment.

Ortiz did not pick excerpts to include in *Rumbos* at random or by chance. He calculated the impact they could potentially have on those living in the Industrial School in conjunction with the fluid health-care regimen installed there by the late 1950s and early 1960s.[114] Through Saraswati and others, Ortiz hoped to put Industrial School youths on a path that led to the creation of a new civilization. Therapeutic religion and spirituality had roles to play in this regard. The Hinduism that circulated in the Mayagüez Industrial School did not simulate cherished rituals like walking on hot coals for goddesses, summoning the spirits of the dead, or honoring Muslim martyrs, insofar as we can tell from *Horizontes* and *Rumbos*. There is little evidence of Hindu priests attending to the spiritual needs of incarcerated adherents in Puerto Rico, if there were any, as was the case in Trinidad and Tobago.[115] Instead, Hinduism was intellectualized and deployed in a way that reinforced an interdenominational Christian project of redemption and rehabilitation. It is difficult to measure the actual consumption of Hinduism in midcentury Puerto Rican carceral settings, but there is no doubt that Hindu philosophy made waves, complicating precisely where in the Caribbean it was supposed to thrive.

Conclusion

Caribbean convicts approached religion and spirituality from multiple angles and generally viewed these as healthy, practical extensions of cultures of rehabilitation. They often depended on religious and spiritual logics and practices and found meaning, belonging, stability, and healing in them. For every believer or benefactor of some kind, however, there were also skeptics. Difficult life blows hardened many incarcerated people, spawning their spiritual disequilibrium and fanning the flames of their hostility toward social order. Because the resulting corporeal symptoms and states of mind could not be exclusively contained or remedied by biomedicine and social science, prison health authorities presupposed that religiously and spiritually stirring the consciousness of incarcerated people would prove effective in their rehabilitation.

Notions of the sacred gave prisoners a way to channel or soothe their pent-up frustrations. They had transformative power and could produce civic resilience.[116] As one convict put it, in prison "dying is living," a reference to the paradox of living death and the transition from social and civic death to intellectual and spiritual awakening.[117] Juan C.R. was clearer in this regard, suggesting that the religious aspects of his prison experience had made him "a new and distinct man."[118] Religiosities and spiritualities did not simply generate guilt in convicts for what they had done in the past. Rather, they served as durable mechanisms through which inmates came to terms with their miscalculations and could look to the future. Knowledge and rites capable of yielding penitence and empowerment in inmates were available in the mid-twentieth century. Prisoners embraced cathartic narratives and practices of all kinds, including medical and social science, but they particularly embraced religious and spiritual epistemologies and ontologies to varying degrees. Their holistic views of well-being exceeded the flesh, though, and seeped into other humanities disciplines.

In Pursuit of Awakening:
Carceral Therapeutic Humanities

In November 1947, the Mayagüez district court sentenced a thirty-three-year-old white industrial day laborer from Añasco named Rufino Inglés Caraballo to a few years in prison for extortion by threat of violence. Oso Blanco's Classification and Treatment Board reviewed the man's case in June 1948 and subsequently assigned him to the penitentiary's carpentry workshop, a skill that would benefit him when he reentered society. Board members also recommended that he enroll in evening primary school, for his civic future in the context of colonial-populist political hegemony would also depend on literacy.[1] The board complemented Inglés Caraballo's vocational training and formal education by granting him access to the prison library and encouraging him to pursue sports like volleyball. Classification and Treatment officials believed that these cumulative activities would reform the convict's undesirable habits, which included gambling, drinking, and keeping suspect company. They determined he was a "good" case for rehabilitation.[2]

To make this calculation about Inglés Caraballo's future, the Classification and Treatment Board had to understand the man's history. They learned that, growing up, he worked in the sugar and coffee industries. He also bought and sold birds and animals. Penitentiary health professionals viewed these occupations as typical *jíbaro* labor more in line with the decadent Spanish past than the progressive US present. In the late 1930s and early 1940s, Inglés Caraballo had his first run-ins with the law (for theft and assault). The US Army nonetheless drafted him, and he served in the armed forces during the latter bookend of World War II (May 1944–October 1945). In the United States and Austria, he lived much like he did when he was a bachelor in Puerto Rico. He drank, sought out sex with prostitutes, and even sustained a relationship with a "Polak woman for months."[3] When Inglés Caraballo's overseas service concluded in late 1945, he returned to Puerto Rico and became a homebody.

Marriage and children changed Inglés Caraballo's behavior and outlook. He developed an interest in reading, garnering what he could from local newspapers. Inglés Caraballo extirpated festive social gatherings and leisure settings from his life almost entirely. But finding himself unemployed and dependent on a meager veteran's pension in 1947, he started retracing old footsteps and frequenting places detrimental to his general well-being. The lure of the world landed him in prison anew, and in June 1948, Inglés Caraballo told the Classification and Treatment Board that upon completion of his sentence he hoped to take advantage of veterans' benefits and education. Board members thought he was "sincere" but "untrustworthy" given his "addiction to liquor."[4] Thus, they stressed Inglés Caraballo should be monitored to ensure that his treatment stayed on course. For this to occur, his addiction to liquor and other vices had to be replaced with more productive forms of consumption.

Inglés Caraballo was a "good" case for rehabilitation because he was receptive to the rehabilitative model of the colonial-populist state. Alongside medical and social science, social work, and religion, the humanities provided carceral health professionals with other tools with which to resurrect prisoners socially and civically. To breathe new life into Inglés Caraballo, he had to be "awakened," which meant reshaping his understandings of reality and himself through holistic penitentiary science and conditioning him to adhere and thrive under the prevailing order of things. In mid-twentieth-century Puerto Rico, the humanities were a cornerstone of rehabilitative corrections. Prison authorities and convicts alike underscored the empowering and therapeutic aspects of the humanities and how these could help awaken those incarcerated from their collective civic slumber. Inglés Caraballo pursued awakening through reading. In 1949, he borrowed forty-seven books from Oso Blanco's library. He read adventure and romance novels, biographies, history, poetry, and collections of songs and catechisms.[5] If nothing else, literature offered Inglés Caraballo an escape of sorts, an opportunity for time travel and freedom of imagination and play.

To overcome living death and salvage a sense of personhood, reconnect with the outside world, and discipline himself, Inglés Caraballo looked to literature. What Inglés Caraballo read said a lot about him without his really having to put anything into words. Convicts filled their minds with certain texts not only because others wanted to shape their consciousness, however, but because they themselves sought to be patterned in specific ways. Their personal histories often reflected the themes and content they encountered in books and other humanistic practices behind bars. This concurrently tamed and awakened them. If inmates rejected the state-provided tools at their disposal to awaken and become law-abiding citizens and better human beings, then they resigned themselves to social and civic death, and further down the road, potential recidivism. For prisoners to function and succeed, they had to conform to someone else's definition of who they were, where they went wrong, and what was best for them going forward. Yet even state control was not ironclad, and convicts exploited cracks in the system to enjoy moments of agency and liberation.

This chapter uses inmate files, reading lists, and other sources to examine how inmates experienced the humanities intellectually and therapeutically. Awakening partially annulled the social and civic death effectuated by the prison. Although humanistic self-help (or "recreation") was among the last rehabilitation therapies to be fully implemented in Oso Blanco, it was one of the most impactful, at least on the surface. The late 1940s and 1950s represented a renaissance in this regard. This was a time when convicts actively pursued awakening through their own publications, the visual arts, literature, and the performing arts. The humanities were central to the correctional style that emerged in Puerto Rico under colonial-populist rule.

Legible Awakening

Justice and health professionals operating out of Oso Blanco exposed convicts to the power of a scientific and humanistic education. They deemed it a treatment, and urged inmates to tap into science and the humanities to rise from their mental graves. Literal literacy (i.e., knowing how to read and write) was an important step in this vein. Whereas in the mid-1930s justice officials found that about half of Puerto Rico's incarcerated population was illiterate, by the late 1940s this rate dropped to about a quarter, a significant reduction.[6] Still, in the penitentiary about three in four prisoners (73 percent) were "functionally illiterate," meaning they possessed no more than a sixth-grade education.[7] The inability to read and write made prisoners ineligible for other humanistic practices (e.g., music sheets, theater scripts), which in some respects were symbolic trial runs that showcased the commitment and discipline required for eventual political participation.

This is not to suggest that cultural literacy and production and its link to political participation was exclusive to the era of rehabilitation and colonial populists. In early 1920s Cuba, for example, a political prisoner named Francisco Alonso compiled an album of literary prose, poetry, biographies, confessions, theater, artistic watercolors, drawings, caricatures, and music by anarchist intellectuals serving time in a Havana prison.[8] The creative text, known as *Album "X"*, brought together offerings of "testimony and affect" conceived by Alonso and his "brothers of misfortune," whose roots could be traced to Cuba, broader Latin America, the Middle East, and East Asia.[9] Spanish dramatist and Nobel Prize winner for Literature Jacinto Benavente y Martínez visited Castillo del Príncipe prison in January 1923, bestowing the honor of a single line to *Album "X"*, commenting that "humble sin is more pleasant to God than proud virtue."[10] The warden of the prison in 1923 even contributed a dedicatory note to the album, in which he expressed fair sentences and humane treatment forged the clearest path toward the "improvement and regeneration" of incarcerated people.[11]

A watercolor by someone using the alias "SEO" captures what it was like to carry the weight of living death in early 1920s Cuba (fig. 5.1). In it, a man, presumably incarcerated at Castillo del Príncipe, is sitting down and weeps into his hands. Nearby, his hat has settled on the ground.[12] The scene is as exquisite as it is agonizing given the kin rupture associated with incarceration and the centrality of mothers, specifically, in the overall framing of *Album "X"*.[13] Similarly, a poem about the course of a day and its expiration speaks to the life process and the misery one endures throughout, the only guarantee being the nightfall (death) that awaits all human beings. Cemetery imagery accompanies the piece (fig. 5.2), as does a portion of a poem attributed to Julio Flores in which he welcomes the grave and only asks that the gravedigger bury him and never recount that he did so to anyone.[14] In these and many other contributions to *Album "X"*, anarchist prisoners made a case for their existence, the worth of their agency and families, and their collective goal to work together despite cultural and national differences. They understood their bodies were more than canvases for state violence, and therefore pursued alternative recognitions, good relations with each other (and prison personnel), and cared for one another. Co-imagining and co-forging a shared historical narrative allowed them to do this and more.[15]

As these fragments from *Album "X"* demonstrate, prisoners did not necessarily need to be inspired by state sources or forces to awaken on their own terms. In the generation between the early 1920s and midcentury, however, states embarking on rehabilitative carceral projects increasingly integrated the kinds of cultural production that made *Album "X"* unique into their visions and programs. Interdisciplinary health professionals operating in prisons, who were state surrogates, also desired to understand and work with the dispossessed and marginalized in their midst. In Puerto Rico, prison professional Susano Ortiz—who between the 1940s and 1960s served as director

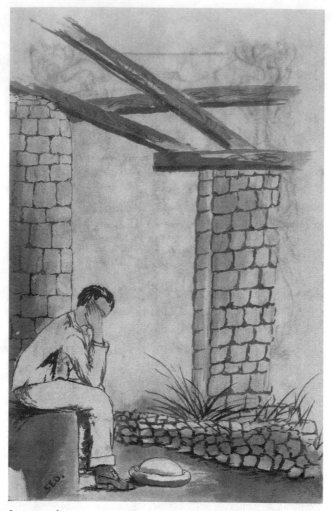

FIGURE 5.1 Incarcerated man weeping in Havana prison, by SEO. *Album "X"* (1922–23). Cuban Heritage Collection, University of Miami.

of social services in the penitentiary, and later, as director of the Industrial School for Youths in Mayagüez—helped normalize the utilization of humanistic, autoethnographic techniques in Oso Blanco.[16] During this period, he also published articles about carceral pedagogies and protocols while substantively engaging prisoners and their family members to finetune the education and care incarcerated people received. For example, Ortiz contacted Inglés Caraballo's wife shortly after the man entered prison to develop a "complete and total" understanding of his case.[17]

Most vitally, Ortiz pioneered rehabilitation curriculum in Oso Blanco. Developing this curriculum formed part of his work for the penitentiary Classification and Treatment Board. In the late 1940s, he published a series of articles in a teachers' association magazine about the historical development of welfare institutions and classification and treatment in Puerto Rico. His December 1948 article, "The Classification of Inmates," discussed holistic rehabilitation and drew from the American Prison Association's *Handbook on Classification in Correctional Institutions* (published in 1947). Ortiz understood rehabilitative logic and classificatory practice as constructive ways to achieve public safety. Incarceration was not just about confining people but also about returning them to society as the best possible versions of themselves in terms of their education, vocational capacity, and physical and mental health.[18]

Ortiz estimated that the overwhelming majority (95 percent) of convicts would return home at some point. This meant their intellectual and decision-making circuitry had to be rewired. It was the prison's responsibility to ensure that all inmates were ready for release and would refrain from going morally astray once beyond the walls. A wide-ranging strategy spanning biomedicine, psychology and psychiatry, social work, religion, and humanistic education could help achieve this goal. It was impractical and counterproductive, however, to provide all services to everyone, Ortiz claimed. Some convicts did not require or desire exposure to certain therapeutics. Further, no single scientific

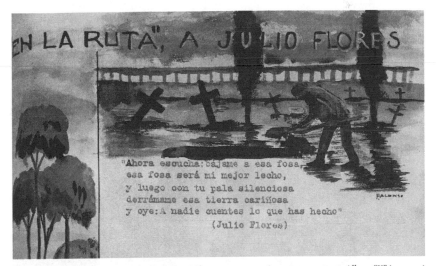

FIGURE 5.2 Cemetery imagery by Francisco Alonso accompanying a poem extract. *Album "X"* (1922–23). Cuban Heritage Collection, University of Miami.

camp enjoyed a monopoly on how to best treat convicts.[19] To treat incarcerated people effectively, authorities engaged prisoners on a case-by-case basis to unpack the complex factors shaping their individual lives, states of mind, and behaviors.

Even though disparate rehabilitative techniques reinforced one another in practice, it took time to sift through potential combinations. Administrators and health professionals had to be on the same page. Otherwise, dissonance among those charged with executing rehabilitation endangered convicts. To clarify the point, Ortiz recalled the case of a young epileptic prisoner who was assigned to work in an Oso Blanco industrial workshop when his condition illustrated that he did not belong there. To catch cases like this one preemptively, prison authorities and health professionals shifted their efforts to collaboratively developing interdisciplinary healing programs for inmates. The resulting programs reflected convict needs and were monitored for progress, revisited periodically, and altered when necessary.[20]

Oso Blanco health professionals fused the humanities to institutional treatment programs through recreation in the late 1940s through the 1950s. Humanized classification helped convicts identify their strengths. The constructive use of free time through the humanities and recreational activities set rehabilitative corrections apart from the harsher punitive regimens of the past. However, it was up to prison wardens and their professional teams to imagine and enact cutting-edge "integrated programming" that corrected deficiencies, developed talents, contributed to discipline, and lifted spirits.[21] This is precisely what occurred in midcentury Oso Blanco, at least for a time.

Developments in New York State informed Ortiz's approach. He began offering Oso Blanco convicts a course on institutional and parole problems based on Price Chenault and George Jennings's recently published text on these topics in Sing Sing penitentiary in summer 1949. In their book, Chenault and Jennings explained what prisoners needed to do to regain their freedom and thrive beyond the walls. In part, they had to conform to the prevailing conventions and character-based initiatives of the prison. These revolved around understanding one's needs, occupational training, and social interactions. The purpose of corrections education was to propose facts about the journey to reattaining societal qualification, to prepare convicts for all kinds of scenarios and contingencies.[22] Ortiz translated Chenault and Jennings's text for his course because it was "full of informative data" about life after social and civic death.[23] His translation circulated in Oso Blanco as much as Bibles and other classic literature did. Several months later, the *Revista de Servicio Social* announced that Ortiz's course had "awakened the interest and enthusiasm of the prison population."[24]

To prepare for their carceral afterlives, prisoners had to make the most of institutional life. Their primary route to doing so was via the Classification and Treatment Board. It was the board that educated inmates about therapeutic humanistic options. Ortiz reported in September 1949 that 270 prisoners had visited Oso Blanco's recreation room during the 1947–48 fiscal year. The library received 240 inmates.[25] These numbers exploded by November 1949. In a prison accommodating more than 1,600 inmates, Ortiz stated, authorities conducted 1,833 social orientation interviews, engaged 205 convicts in the educational aspect, and spoke to 795 about reading programs. Moreover, 716 borrowed books from the library, and 683 visited it. Twenty-seven prepped to take correspondence courses. Two hundred nineteen discussed music programs. Thirty-six participated in live performances. Twelve partook in radio shows transmitted from Oso Blanco. Officials interviewed 987 about religious programming, and 876 about movies. Almost 1,100 attended film screenings and cultural events, 589 joined game communities, and 6 painted.[26]

Ortiz published these findings in mainstream scholarly journals and *El Despertar*. The prisoner magazine *El Despertar* was one of the more visible initiatives authorities launched to keep the penitentiary from unraveling, at least among the institution's literate population. It shed light on carceral problems and chronicled ongoing penal reforms but ceased operation in fall 1950.[27] This coincided with the events of late October that year, when nationalists tried to start a revolution in the mountainous interior of the main island. A parallel insurgency in Oso Blanco had fatal consequences and dozens of prisoners escaped.[28] An inmate-produced periodical would not reappear until 1956 in the form of *Realidad*, another dynamic prison newspaper produced by the penitentiary chapter of Alcoholics Anonymous.

While *El Despertar* existed, the magazine was vibrant and rich in content. Its mere existence corroborates what several scholars have argued for the case of Cuba, that literary production behind bars and its circulation in society made correctional facilities "lettered prisons."[29] The prison of Havana had its own version of *El Despertar* in the 1950s, called *Superación* (*Overcoming*), which documented cultural activities and conferences carried out behind the walls.[30] Initially, Puerto Rican convicts autonomously edited *El Despertar* under the supervision of Ortiz and warden Félix Rivera.[31] By the end of 1949, inmates worked with other technical staff.[32] *El Despertar* was filled with anecdotes, analyses, and drawings about prison life. Poetry, folklore, short stories, and community histories graced its pages. It consisted of editorials, regular columns, and conveyed institutional news. Prison authorities and convicts regularly contributed articles about medicine, classification and treatment, and recreation. These reflected on people and places, religion and science, infidelity and indifference, substance abuse, charity, and the holiday season. The periodical also included puzzles and sections on humor and prison sports leagues. *El Despertar* illustrated that rehabilitation and transformation through writing and broader cultural enrichment was possible. In other words, incarcerated people defied social and civic death, decoded alternative ways to heal and empower themselves, and reclaimed their place in society through writing and interrelated humanistic practices.[33]

From the perspective of Oso Blanco, however, to awaken for the most part meant to follow a prescribed blueprint for rehabilitation. This blueprint included different forms of literacy, spectacle expression, and in the long run civic participation beyond the walls. To dig up their mental graves while incarcerated, many convicts used the humanities as a shovel. Prison authorities screened movies. Choirs and musicians visited Oso Blanco and gave performances. Artistic troupes made appearances. Convicts read classic literature and even started groups responding to their own humanistic interests, including painting and drama. While not all prisoners participated, that they had therapeutic humanistic options proved pivotal for the rehabilitation of those who did.

Visual Arts

The visual arts were among the smorgasbord of humanities circulating in Puerto Rican and other Caribbean prisons in the mid-twentieth century.[34] Film especially piqued the interest and lifted the spirits of many inmates. In February 1933, the English-language periodical *Porto Rico Progress* published an article that shed light on the role of film in convict recreation and rehabilitation. Sensorially consuming motion pictures taught inmates about the meaning of freedom and getting better. Movies also laid bare the fact that corrections had come a long way, evolving from facilities marked exclusively by inhumane conditions to new ones with "cells and other improvements," including recreational opportunities and steady access to film and the broader humanities.[35]

The accessibility of film in deteriorating prisons like La Princesa represented a bright spot in corrections because of its perceived rehabilitative function. *Porto Rico Progress* contributors observed that movies made hardened convicts vulnerable. Many inmates waxed poetic after film screenings. They followed theater, another branch of the humanities tree, and knew of certain actors (e.g., Greta Garbo, Douglas Fairbanks). Journalists viewed the 1920 Fox drama *Over the Hill to the Poorhouse* with prisoners, for instance. The movie is about a woman who has many children and never gets to enjoy life, which would have resonated with convicts coming from large rural families. *Over the Hill* incited a wave of emotion over the inmates. Prisoners despised the antagonist, who spent the money the hero of the film had sent to his mother. They wept when the hero's mother went to the poorhouse to scrub floors. Most importantly, there was a pride "by no means different from the enthusiastic pride in the free man's eyes" when "the good-bad brother met the bad-good brother over the hill."[36]

Other favorites at the prison cinema included Nick Stuart and Lois Moran in the 1929 Fox melodrama *Joy Street*, a film about an unsophisticated American girl who inherits a fortune while attending boarding school abroad and starts living wildly and recklessly. It takes a serious car accident for her to come to her senses, settle down, and marry a decent fellow. Prisoners smiled at Victor McLaglen's performance in the 1928 Fox drama *The River Pirate*, a film about a convict who is assigned to a reform school to teach sail making as part of his sentence. They were proud of Helen Twelvetrees in the 1929 Fox drama *Blue Skies*, a movie based on a short story by screenwriter Frederick Hazlitt Brennan. Promotional material for this film reads, in part: "It tells blissfully how an orphanage yard becomes the Garden of Eden for two fetching youngsters . . . A crowd of lively, unforgettable children swarm through feast, famine—recreation, rebellion—jaundice, joy. A likeable lad defies the matron and his own advantage for the sake of a charming sweetheart—and who wouldn't? *Blue Skies* will smile away your blues."[37] Each of these films taught prisoners about the consequences of actions and specific themes: living within their means in orderly fashion, vocational progress, and perseverance in good and bad times.

In addition to drama, convicts were exposed to comedy and romance. These genres, too, reminded them of aspects of their lives and carceral circumstances. Prisoners laughed watching Sammy Cohen in the 1928 Fox comedy *Why Sailors Go Wrong*, a film about a pair of seamen who are shipwrecked on an island inhabited by hungry cannibals. They enjoyed Barry Norton in the 1929 Fox comedy *The Exalted Flapper* and Will Rogers in the 1929 Fox comedy *They Had to See Paris*, which concerns a wealthy Oklahoman oil tycoon who travels to France with his family despite not really wanting to go. Charles Farrell and Mary Duncan were lovely in the 1930 Fox romance drama *City Girl*, a film based on a play (Elliot Lester's "The Mud Turtle") about a waitress who falls for a farmer and decides to lead a Midwestern country life. However, prisoners insisted Farrell and Janet Gaynor did it better in the 1929 Fox romance drama *Lucky Stars*, a movie about the impact of war on a farm girl and a returning soldier. Frank Borzage's 1929 Fox silent film *The River*, a romantic idyll between a country boy and an experienced city girl, caused a sensation among convicts.[38]

Of all the stars of the era, however, La Princesa convicts singled out Englishman Charlie Chaplin as the greatest figure in film. *Porto Rico Progress* writers announced that Chaplin "has never received a token of admiration in his life equal to that bestowed on him by the living dead at El Presidio."[39] Prisoners only regretted the long intervals between his movies. The themes of Chaplin's films piqued the curiosity of inmates while entertaining and challenging them intellectually. Between the late 1920s and 1940 alone, convicts would have seen films like *Metropolis* (1927), *City Lights* (1931), *Modern Times* (1936), and *The Great Dictator* (1940), movies that reflected a changing and increasingly urban, technological world. These kinds of films foreshadowed what the Puerto Rican experience would entail in the 1940s and 1950s, as the island economy transitioned into an industrial mode under colonial populism.[40]

By the 1940s and 1950s, film screenings were routine in Puerto Rican prisons. The attorney general Enrique Campos del Toro reported in 1946 that "movie-picture films of educational character were shown" in prisons across the main island.[41] Further evidence of screenings emerges in a convict drawing published in the July-August 1950 edition of *El Despertar*. In the image, dozens of Oso Blanco inmates are engrossed by a movie scene in which a man wearing a trench coat and sporting a hat robs a chubbier man at gunpoint. The victim's arms are raised in the air.[42] Additionally, prisoners had access to a "recreation room" where they could watch films and listen to music.[43] Inglés Caraballo, for instance, "watched movies every week" in this room.[44] At the Industrial School for Youths in Mayagüez, administrators screened films and episodes of television series on a weekly basis. These included comedy, crime, and historical dramas, adventure, biblical, fantasy, foreign, musical and war films, and comic-book shows.[45] Notably, in late 1954, Mayagüez sanitary expert Lolita Villeros telecasted a film about uncinariasis for Industrial School inmates. A discussion of the movie and questions followed.[46]

Notwithstanding the value of film behind bars, Oso Blanco health professionals also expressed reservations about what convicts might take away from films. Parole official Tomás Rosario's 1946 assessment of a twenty-four-year-old "passive sexual invert" from Jayuya named Armando Rivera Colón is a case in point. After interviewing Rivera Colón, Rosario described him as a "pale, skinny" individual with a "faint voice" and an "effeminate walk." The parole official recommended that prison psychologists delve into the convict's "emotions," especially given his affinity for "romantic movies."[47] Rosario and other legal officials drew a figurative line between Rivera Colón's demeanor and recreational preferences to explain not only his crime but also how film might serve a nontherapeutic function by affirming his idiosyncrasies and deviance.

Compared to film, it took traditional expressions of art a bit longer to gain an official foothold in Oso Blanco. Nonetheless, several convicts aspired to become artists. The work of some of these prisoners (e.g., paintings, hand-crafted toys) got exposure in the mainstream press.[48] Several cultivated their artistic talent by producing it for *El Despertar*. One striking image is on the back cover of the August 1949 edition of the magazine (fig. 5.3). It is of a man (presumably a prisoner either before incarceration or contemplating going home while incarcerated) overlooking an agriculturally developed valley bordered by foothills and mountains. Prisoners also drew pictures of different aspects of the classification and treatment process, publishing portraits every edition. Other convicts wrote articles about art. Before arriving at the penitentiary for the first time, inmate José M.N. wondered whether the facility boasted improvised or formal art studios.[49] He believed prisoners could use art to rethink their personal narratives and add value to the world. However, when José M.N. arrived at Oso Blanco, he learned that the institution lacked artistic spaces.[50]

José M.N. wondered why modern Puerto Rico, under the auspices of the United States, did not have access to a robust range of humanistic options. He explained that prison guards and administrators, including warden Rivera, respected art. Further, convicts produced art where they could, even if temporarily on prison walls. These circumstances inspired José M.N. to publicly question why convicts were bereft of formal spaces for activities that contributed to their rehabilitation. An image accompanies José M.N.'s article (fig. 5.4). In the image, a prisoner paints an unidentified woman. The portrait in progress is supported by a stand about equal in height to the inmate. Everything he needs is within arm's reach: an easel, brushes, paint, rags. Two other paintings adorn the wall in the background. The window, however, is barricaded.[51] Practices of artistic liberation like painting in a prison confirmed the elusive and illusory nature of freedom and the power and limits of awakening.

Like film, art did not exist in isolation in prisoners' minds. José M.N. cast Oso Blanco's library as a potential hub of artistic creativity and congregation. He viewed it as more than a repository of books. Artists planned to rendezvous there in mid-February 1950 but ultimately met in a nearby hallway to discuss their aspirations. José M.N. wrote that they asked prison authorities for materials but finding a space inside the prison to create art remained an obstacle. Therefore, José M.N. proposed projects wherever the Justice Department needed labor, including outside the prison. Pursuing painting beyond

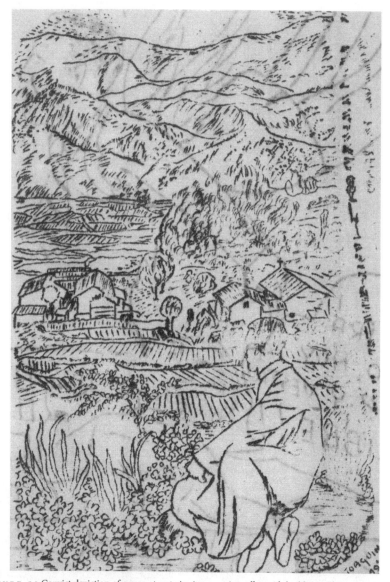

Oso Blanco's walls, he insisted, would expose convicts to vocational training, earning an honest living, and humanistic treatment.[52] These activities, many prison authorities and inmates believed, could prepare incarcerated people for life after living death and the challenge of altering public perceptions when they returned home.

FIGURE 5.3 Convict depiction of a man at rest viewing a quaint valley with buildings. *El Despertar* 1, no. 4 (August 1949). Biblioteca y Hemeroteca Puertorriqueña, Universidad de Puerto Rico–Río Piedras.

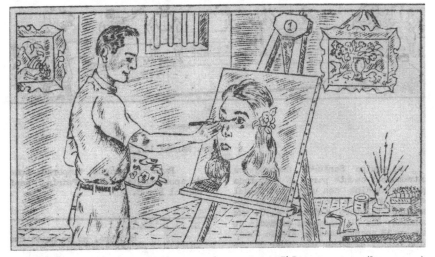

FIGURE 5.4 Convict depiction of an incarcerated man painting. *El Despertar* 1, no. 9 (January 1950). Biblioteca y Hemeroteca Puertorriqueña, Universidad de Puerto Rico–Río Piedras.

Libraries and Literature

Libraries have long been perceived as places of healing. As Megan Sweeney has observed, reading has been touted for its curative powers since ancient times. In the United States, prison authorities adopted a therapeutic model of reading in penitentiaries in the early nineteenth century. Bibliotherapy—the treatment of a patient through selective reading—gained national prominence in medical and library circles in the 1930s and in penological circles from midcentury through the 1970s. Mid-twentieth-century guidelines and manuals trumpeting the benefits of reading habits and programs identified the prison library as an instrument of education and mental health. According to Sweeney, prison personnel mostly used bibliotherapy to control without punishment. They deemed it a "normalization technique, strictly monitoring prisoners' reading and treating them as passive recipients of literary medicine."[53] Overseeing what convicts read, officials postulated, dictated who they would become in the future.

In the mid-twentieth century, United States prison libraries had three primary objectives: education, therapy, and recreation.[54] This logic extended to Puerto Rico and other corners of the Caribbean. Oso Blanco's 1933 *Reglamento*, the body of rules and regulations governing the penitentiary, decreed three articles concerning the institutional library. Article 110 stipulated that official and specific donations of books would form the library's foundation. Prison authorities purchased texts and aspired to keep them under lock and

key. Article 111 gave the warden the power to exclude certain books, magazines, and newspapers, especially those having nothing to do with the educational and moral rehabilitation of convicts. Functionaries examined all books
entering the prison. They censored certain material so that library content
mirrored state standards.[55] Sometimes this meant reducing the circulation
of the press.[56] Article 112 detailed the librarian position, which was filled by
a trusted convict who created a registry and supervised the general flow of
books.[57]

Despite the early attention that local and federal justice bureaucrats granted
to the humanities in Puerto Rican prisons, it took more than a decade for a
culture of reading to flourish.[58] In 1933, *Porto Rico Progress* writers declared
that bibliotherapy in main island prisons was stranger than fiction. Despite
having access to some classic literature, La Princesa's library, for example,
lacked enough texts overall. Among the most popular available books there,
however, were novels about the politics of incarceration and redemption.
Convicts read Victor Hugo's *Les Misérables* and Eduardo Zamacois's *Los vivos
muertos* (*The Living Dead*). Hugo's was "probably the best-known novel at El
Presidio."[59]

Zamacois's novel, "a book for strong souls," details prison life in Miguel
Primo de Rivera's Spain and the limits of convict redemption.[60] The novel
formed part of a series of works chronicling the foundations of the Spanish
Civil War. *Los vivos muertos* estimates that 30 percent of Spanish prisoners
at the time did not belong in prison.[61] To write *Los vivos muertos*, Zamacois
visited and lived in Spanish prisons for brief stints.[62] Zamacois's methodol-
ogy earned him the respect of Puerto Rican inmates. His evenhanded por-
trayal of the convict experience struck a chord with them. One Puerto Rican
prisoner asserted that "except for the unavoidable differences on account of
environment, conditions in the insular penitentiary are like those described
by Zamacois."[63]

Los vivos muertos was a popular read in Oso Blanco and other Puerto
Rican prisons in the 1930s not only because it accurately narrated prison conditions, but also because it illustrated that a desire for justice in an unjust
society and political system (in this case, Spain) could land one in prison. In
Puerto Rico, "equivalent" disenfranchisement would have been the persecution of the poor, nationalists, and other activists. *Los vivos muertos* also shows
the extent to which convicts depend on memory and hope to survive incarceration. But tragically, the protagonist of the novel, Martín Santoyo, exits
prison after serving twenty-eight years only to learn that most of his family
and friends are dead and he has no employment prospects. He returns to San
Miguel de los Reyes prison in Valencia in search of work, and there he realizes

that "the prison had killed him and he did not even know it."[64] In *Los vivos muertos*, incarcerated people struggle to overcome social and civic death.

The trope of living death traversed the Atlantic world in the 1930s. René Belbenoît's *Dry Guillotine*, for instance, also cast convicts as living dead. This memoir recounts Belbenoît's fifteen-year prison term at Cayenne (or Devil's Island) in French Guiana, a penal colony from where he tried to escape five times. *Dry Guillotine* portrays the legal unmaking of prisoners and the horrid conditions in which they lived subject to hunger, disease, wildlife, and torture. Of the eighty thousand men sentenced to the French penal colony, a majority are believed to have died there.[65] Belbenoît's and Zamacois's works increased awareness about the collective plight of inmates around the Atlantic. Their respective versions of living death contrast sharply with the experiences of convicts like Inglés Caraballo, among others, who leaned on reading and other humanities activities in prison to try to defeat social and civic death.

Bibliotherapy could potentially heal but incarcerated people in Oso Blanco and elsewhere did not have access to well stocked libraries until the late 1940s.[66] In Trinidad and Tobago, for example, libraries with plentiful, varied books were maintained at all prisons and little or no restriction was practiced in their issuing to inmates. Chaplains supervised the issuing of books and arranged for a supply of United Kingdom magazines to be on hand for general use.[67] Calls for members of the Puerto Rican public to send books to the district jail closest to them appeared in the local press around the same time.[68] The *Revista de Servicio Social* documented in July 1949 that a group of Polytechnic Institute students visited Oso Blanco and concluded that the institutional library warranted expansion.[69] In the September 1949 edition of *El Despertar*, magazine editors highlighted a list of new books the prison library had just received. Twenty-two of the books were authored by the French novelist, playwright, and poet Jules Verne.[70] Verne's adventure and science-fiction novels appealed to Oso Blanco convicts because of how they warped time. In addition to novels by Verne, eleven works by the self-help guru Orison Swett Marden became part of the penitentiary library's collection.[71] Swett Marden, who had passed away in 1924, was a US-based inspirational author who wrote about achieving success in life through commonsense principles and virtues. Many of his ideas were rooted in New Thought philosophy, which holds that sickness originates in the mind and that "right thinking" has a healing effect.[72]

Religious texts also circulated in Oso Blanco. One prisoner read a book about the life of the prophet Muhammad.[73] In general, however, such books tended to reflect the hegemonic faith in Puerto Rico—Catholicism. Inglés Caraballo, for example, read a compendium of Catholic sacred histories.[74]

Inmates mentally consumed non-Catholic Christian works as well. Penitentiary recreation director Manuel López de Victoria promoted a book by the
Seventh-Day Adventist pioneer Ellen G. White called *El deseado de todas las
gentes* (*The Desire of Ages*), which traces the life of Jesus Christ and reflects on
the precepts of his ministry. In the tradition of cigar-factory readers, an Oso
Blanco cell-block leader read portions of the book aloud every night so that
convicts could have "spiritual edification."[75]

On the other end of the content spectrum, a nineteen-year-old mulatto
shoemaker from Carolina named Salvador Alamo Rivera read a biography of
governor Luis Muñoz Marín.[76] This prisoner often carried the books he was
reading to his meetings with Classification and Treatment Board officials. In
so doing, he intended to communicate to them how serious he was about
his rehabilitation program. Board members had a mixed reaction, however.
Alamo Rivera impressed them as "cooperative," "communicative," and "academically prepared," but they also doubted his ability to interpret the heavier
literature he read, such as Miguel de Cervantes's early seventeenth-century
novel *Don Quijote* and Benito Pérez Galdós's late nineteenth-century novel
Marianela.[77] The board did not insinuate the same thing about the Muñoz
Marín biography, which was a better fit for Alamo Rivera because it went
to great lengths to inspire the next potential generation of colonial-populist
constituents.

A steady stream of secular and religious books, among other materials,
expanded Oso Blanco's library in 1949. By summer 1950 the library was thriving. Book classification and distribution improved. An eclectic mix of novels and periodicals entertained, educated, and consoled convicts.[78] Because
of regional social networks, some materials even arrived from neighboring
countries, such as the Cuban magazine *Bohemia*.[79] The inmate Joaquín R.B.V.
suggested in a summer 1950 article that such a diverse collection of books,
newspapers, and magazines, enough to meet the needs of the attending public, was indicative of a fine library. Convicts visited the library to forget about
"what brings them down" and to unfurl their "mental horizons."[80] Classification and Treatment health professionals often agreed. When prisoners expressed that they had a history of or interest in reading, board members authorized library services and administrators let them borrow books.[81] They
hoped convicts would become book "aficionados," as López de Victoria described Inglés Caraballo in February 1949.[82] As inmates made the reading
habit part of their everyday routines, acquiring books became less burden-
some. It is also not far-fetched to assume that prisoners who checked out
books informally circulated them to interested peers, spreading the gospel of
reading in the process.

Convicts understood the library as a focal point of psychological orientation and rehabilitation. In the September 1950 edition of *El Despertar*, prisoner José A.M.S. noted that incarcerated people who pursued awakening through the humanities could be compared to spiritual travelers wandering in a desert of trials and tribulations. They were victims of the inclement sun and had no choice but to accept the difficulty of finding the liquid gold that would quench their thirst. The sun burning their bodies was repentance. The missing water represented the lack of stimulus and miseducation in their lives. The desert equated their hearts' desires, which landed many of them in Oso Blanco. Penitent travelers found refuge in the prison library, a place that protected them from perverted thoughts and that redirected them toward renaissance thinking and the recovery of their innocence. The library was a fountain of wisdom. Whoever bathed in its waters with faith and love could change, for big ideas dwelled in libraries. José A.M.S. praised the ancient teachers in whose works rested the culture of past, current, and future generations.[83]

The knowledge and wisdom of antiquity and modernity could be found in prison library books. Inglés Caraballo read widely about Spain and the Spanish colonial past. His imaginary bookshelf included Santa Teresa de Jesús's *El libro de la vida* (*The Book of Life*), the reflections of a sixteenth-century Spanish nun, and a text about Santa Rosa de Lima, a seventeenth-century Puerto Rican–Peruvian colonist and charitable lay member of the Dominican Order.[84] A seventeen-year-old *trigueño* convict named Enrique Morales Carrasquillo similarly (re)discovered the Spanish colonial past through physician Manuel Zeno Gandía's *La charca* (*The Pond*), a historical novel about impoverished and infirm life in the remote and mountainous coffee regions of Puerto Rico. The novel details the injustices suffered by poor farmhands and peasants under the thumb of rich landowners. *La charca* formed part of Zeno Gandía's "chronicles of a sick world," a series of books about Puerto Rico in the late nineteenth century.[85] A young dark-skinned convict named Ramón Rosa Rodríguez, for his part, read the classic novels of the French Caribbean author Alexandre Dumas and the Colombian writer Jorge Isaacs.[86] When considered together, penitentiary library reading lists spanned a proverbial Who's Who of Caribbean, Latin American, and global cosmopolitan writers: Enrique Amorim (Uruguay), Milli Dandolo (Italy), Rubén Darío (Nicaragua), Luz Echavarría (Dominican Republic), Vicente Moreno (Ecuador), Eugène Sue (France), Ivan Turgenev (Russia), Ramón del Valle Inclán (Spain), and Hugo Wast (Argentina), among many others.[87] The book excerpts that Carmelina Freyre habitually submitted to *El Despertar* included the work of the Canadian author of inspirational books Grenville Kleiser,

Irish New Thought spiritual leader Emmet Fox, and Lebanese writer and artist Kahlil Gibran, in particular Gibran's *The Prophet*, a text of poetry fables
discussing the human condition.[88]

José A.M.S. pondered whether readers would find his notion of intellectual genealogies absurd, especially given that Oso Blanco offered more practical vocations to pursue. He argued that one could be renewed by the prison
library, a space that allowed men to confront their passions. Books were of
no value if they did not teach one how to do this. Convicts possessing will
could learn to read and write and therefore control their natures and express
themselves in a different format. The library made this possible by entrusting
classic and rare texts to prisoners.[89] While José A.M.S. found intellectual freedom in the library and hoped other inmates would as well, Freyre's column
brought pieces of the library to convicts.

Across the Mona Passage in the Dominican Republic, prisoners had less
access to library books. Despite the glaring censorship advanced by the Trujillo regime, Dominicans were as curious about literature and other reading materials as their Puerto Rican counterparts. The memoir of a scholar-
physician incarcerated in the 1930s compared the conditions in Dominican
prisons to those prevailing in Cuba and Russian author Fyodor Dostoyevsky's
late nineteenth-century novel *The House of the Dead*.[90] This novel portrays
convict life and relationships in a Siberian prison labor camp. Dostoyevsky
himself had survived such a camp following his involvement in the Petra-
shevsky Circle, a surreptitious cross-class coalition of progressive commoner-
intellectuals based in St. Petersburg who opposed tsarist autocracy. The narra-
tor of the novel, the nobleman Aleksandr Petrovich Goryanchikov, gradually
overcomes his difficult circumstances and disdain for the lower classes and
undergoes a spiritual awakening that culminates in his release from prison.
Goryanchikov, and by extension Dostoyevsky, conclude that the prison is not
only tragic but cannibalistic. It perpetuates death—physical, social, and civic.

The nationalist Heriberto Marín Torres, who in the mid-twentieth century served an extended sentence across several Puerto Rican penitentiaries
for revolutionary activity, echoed Dostoyevsky's interpretation of living death
by observing the timeless truth that incarceration is hard and not everyone
can take it: "Being locked up in a six-by-six cell is maddening. You do not
know what to do. You walk back and forth for hours. You lie down in the
bunk staring at the ceiling and the four walls that surround you and feel suffocated. . . . A week feels like a century. You cannot sleep, nor are you hungry,
nor can you smile. It is as if you are confined to a grave."[91] He also critiqued
the limits of Oso Blanco's library, especially the absence of political literature.[92] As Marín Torres attests, living death affected the mental health and

inner beings of incarcerated people in deleterious fashion. During the era of rehabilitative corrections, however, classification and treatment specialists and others viewed the prison as a place where the living dead could be raised. It is important to recognize that literature and the broader humanities also served as instruments of redemption and uplift for those incarcerated, not just as accoutrements of their entombment.

Performing Arts

Through *El Despertar* and other humanities innovations, Oso Blanco inmates exercised a modicum of control over their own hearts and minds. This agency was not low-hanging fruit, however. As we know today, the deprived space of the prison inhibits the creativity and emotional expression of incarcerated people, which in turn negatively affects their well-being. Artistic practices help convicts cope with prison life, instill a sense of confidence in them, and enable them to manage stress by making them feel productive, normal, and human.[93] But well in advance of our own times, prototype versions of contemporary arts programs therapeutically benefited prisoners in penitentiaries like Oso Blanco.[94]

The performing arts gained momentum in Oso Blanco in the mid-twentieth century. Local churches exposed prisoners to plays like "Who Gives This Feast?" as early as 1933.[95] By 1939, University of Puerto Rico–Río Piedras artists such as José Luis Torregrosa, Hernán Nigaglioni, and Rosita González Ginorio performed plays and offered musical theater at the penitentiary.[96] University artists continued to do so through the 1940s. In 1947, for instance, Ángel Florencio Rivera and José Luis Marrero of the campus drama circle coproduced a comedy titled *The Perfect Match*.[97] In a similar vein, inmate Cándido R.M. recalled that music accompanied graduation ceremonies and poetry interpretations in the penitentiary.[98] Still, convicts did not create their own drama club until the summer of 1949. Prisoner Carmelo Ch.M., an aspiring playwright and the drama club's president, insisted the group's establishment improved the spiritual outlook of inmates. Acting, music, and dance—what Carmelo Ch.M. called "high manifestations of art"—affected convicts in profound ways.[99] For three weeks in October 1949, the drama club managed to do just this by offering rehearsals of performances in Oso Blanco. López de Victoria, who helped start the group alongside several social workers, supervised its activities during this period. As Carmelo Ch.M. saw it, the drama club served a dual purpose. It made everyone involved culturally literate and provided convicts with the space to pursue therapeutic "spiritual expansion" through their craft.[100] By January 1950, the club offered two theater performances, exhibiting skills across genres from comedy to drama.[101] Staging theatrical productions empowered club members by letting them assert their humanity and capabilities, build community, attain skills, and maintain hope, as Ashley Lucas has observed for the contemporary moment.[102]

In addition to theater, the humanities ambiance of Puerto Rican prisons included music. Since 1936, the University of Puerto Rico choir began its concert season in nearby welfare institutions like Oso Blanco before touring the big island and other carceral facilities.[103] The choir visited the penitentiary and delivered a particularly rousing performance in July 1944. Twelve hundred prisoners, officials, and guests witnessed the spectacle. The choir performed religious songs in Latin, such as the sixteenth-century sacred music composer Giovanni Pierluigi da Palestrina's "Tenebrae factas sunt" (There Was Darkness) and "Adoremus te, Christe" (We Adore You, Christ). They also sang folkloric Spanish selections like "A los árboles altos," popular US songs like Stephen Foster's "Old Black Joe," danzas like Juan Morel Campos's "No me toques," and nationalistic tunes such as Rafael Hernández's "Los carreteros" and Félix Astol's "La borinqueña."[104] The choir's cosmopolitan musical range encapsulated the diverse cultural roots of the Puerto Rican people. The Santurce Baptist church choir performed for Oso Blanco inmates later in the 1940s.[105] Inmates had their own band and also welcomed individual musicians. In February 1946, university student Fico Cordero played guitar solos for an eager penitentiary audience.[106] On October 15, 1949, violinist Juan Ramón Figueroa performed several compositions on the penitentiary patio. López de Victoria had previously given Figueroa a copy of an edition of *El Despertar*, which inspired the musician to write a piece called "Mi despertar" (My Awakening). The violinist presented a version-in-progress to incarcerated people.[107]

La Princesa prison hosted a unique concert in November 1947. According to the newspaper *El Universal*, a company of artists, Mexico and Puerto Rico Sing, directed by the Mexican singer José Baladez, visited enthusiastic convicts and offered them a pleasant program. The Echevarría Sisters and San Francisco Trio opened the variety show with a Puerto Rican danza. A photograph documenting the event shows more than a hundred inmates in attendance, several of them smiling and enjoying themselves notwithstanding their incarceration. Warden Balbino González discussed the necessity of such programs and how they accelerated "the [forward] march of penal reform," bringing enchanting and purifying light to the shadows of carceral spaces.[108]

Musical dance troupes visited Oso Blanco. Puerto Rican bombshell María del Carmen Mejía's ensemble put on shows for convicts several times. Carmen Mejía graduated from San Juan High School in 1949 and was an exceptional dancer and aspiring thespian who at one point collaborated with Arturo Somohano, the founder of the San Juan Symphony Orchestra.[109] This was a significant achievement, as Somohano was an accomplished classical music composer who had made a name for himself playing the piano and directing concerts on military bases during World War II. In January 1950, *El Despertar* writers chronicled Carmen Mejía's recent holiday recital at Oso Blanco. Although she was a coveted, voluptuous apple in the eye of many convicts—a predecessor to someone like Iris Chacón—they portrayed her not as a cavorting, disheveled cabaret attraction but as a talented artist and variety performer.[110] Another woman, diva of color Conchita Turull, also occupied the minds of incarcerated people. Carmelo Ch.M., for example, exalted her quintessential Puerto Ricanness: her "golden voice," soul "rich in ambrosia," and "long braids."[111]

El Despertar contributors noted that the holiday season reminded convicts of what they had lost—freedom, family, and frivolity. Yet they were on the minds of exceptional women, including governor Luis Muñoz Marín's wife, Inés M. Mendoza, who sent them holiday booklets and pamphlets.[112] Only special people abandoned the warmth and affection of their homes during the holidays to spend time with inmates. It came as no surprise, then, that two thousand prisoners packed the penitentiary patio to see Carmen Mejía in December 1949. Convicts were stunned by the theatrical arrival of her art caravan, which announced hours of happiness. When the show commenced, they listened and bore witness religiously. *El Despertar* writers called Carmen Mejía a "crown jewel" in the flesh, one who had "fiery lips" and "eyes that explain why after 50 years of US rule we still speak Castilian [Spanish]."[113] Due to their self-described frailty, convicts could not begin to recount the exhilarating range of liberating emotions sparked by her routine. The liberation to which they referred was temporary, but therapeutic.

Carmen Mejía interpreted selections from the Spaniard Enrique Granados's piano suite *Goyescas*. She performed traditional Apache dance. Her rendition of the Russian Pyotr Ilyich Tchaikovsky's classic ballet *El lago de los cisnes* (*Swan Lake*) captivated the audience.[114] She did fun and sensual numbers like "Fantasía torera" (Bullfighter Fantasy). This latter number may have been reminiscent of the show put on by the Brazilian bombshell Rita Cadillac in the 2003 Héctor Babenco film *Carandiru*, although much less crude. In the film, the "diva of dance" performs for São Paulo convicts. She sings and dances sensually over a bottle while simulating protected intercourse with it.[115] *El Despertar* columnists concluded that Carmen Mejía's routines made both the hardest and humblest of Oso Blanco convicts unearth long buried "forgotten moments."[116] In a way, she rose them from living death. Carmen

Mejía even took the time to respond to a letter written by warden Rivera after her group's visit. She underscored the rehabilitative effects of art: "Enjoying art spectacles, [prisoners] can comprehend that there is something in the world superior to the vices and passions to which they have fallen victim and through which they have made other people victims."[117] Art provided direction that might convince them to "embark on the path of their regeneration and the salvation of their souls."[118] Carmen Mejía did not see prisoners as criminals, but as an intelligent and cultured public.

El Despertar writers assured readers they would continue following Carmen Mejía's career. She subsequently competed in the 1954 Miss America Pageant in Atlantic City, New Jersey, where she rode on a float, participated in the evening gown and swimsuit portions of the event, and danced in the talent show. Pageant officials recorded her measurements as five foot five; 118 pounds; 36, 36, 24; and with black hair, black eyes, and olive skin.[119] Gaspar Gerena Brás, who dedicated a poem to her in 1959, praised Carmen Mejía's interpretation of Oscar Wilde's play *Salomé*, which she performed as early as 1948.[120] The play is a tragedy that tells the story of Salomé, the stepdaughter of the tetrarch Herod Antipas, who requests the head of John the Baptist on a silver platter as a reward for a provocative rendition of the Dance of the Seven Veils. For incarcerated people, however, Carmen Mejía represented more than unbridled concupiscence. She helped them maintain a connection to the world beyond the walls and embodied the most appealing dimensions of the state's blended scientific and humanities rehabilitative programming. Further, on a practical level, Carmen Mejía sparked prisoners to refine their own drama club. Voice training, acting fundamentals, stage discipline, script analysis, and auditioning became points of emphasis for interested convicts. By May 1950, Oso Blanco's drama club echoed José M.N.'s earlier call for the pursuit of awakening outside the prison. They wanted to take their show to other correctional facilities and hoped that Susano Ortiz would respond to their request in the affirmative.[121]

The vision of sustained rehabilitative programming beyond Oso Blanco's walls would not be realized in the short term. Several months later, beginning with the violence of October 1950, prison insurgencies created the conditions for a moratorium on the drama club, *El Despertar*, and other manifestations of prison humanities. Oso Blanco officials straitjacketed artistic practices of liberation, which for a time had been linked to recreation, stress relief, identity reconfiguration, and community building. Convicts lost access to state-sponsored awakening, and in its place, they confronted an ambiance of paranoia and suspicion comparable to what one would have found in the prisons of neighboring Caribbean countries. It would not be until the mid-1950s that a new prisoner magazine, *Realidad*, reintroduced a forum for the articulation and dissemination of humanistic logics and practices in the Insular Penitentiary.[122]

Conclusion

In mid-twentieth-century Puerto Rico, prison officials and health professionals offered convicts a humanistic path toward healing and societal reintegration. Through the pages of *El Despertar*, books, and other humanities disciplines and artifacts, prisoners tested the limits of what they could say and do behind bars. They tapped into the humanities to negotiate structures of violence and control and to try to eke out an existence. While awakening became a reality for some convicts, their freedom was predicated on thought systems that were not entirely of their own making. Ultimately, authorship and ownership of penitentiary science rested in the hands of a colonial-populist state invested in reengineering inmates and turning them into law-abiding citizens, even as prisoners discovered ways to amend or season rehabilitative corrections as they saw fit.

Whether convicts might qualify as good citizens depended on if they conformed to the behavioral and intellectual standards of the state. An inmate like Inglés Caraballo was already predisposed to "bend the knee" considering his military background, but even he had to adapt to life behind the walls. It did not help that he had to confront issues like his wife's infidelity and the illnesses of his daughter and mother. These circumstances agitated him and disrupted his rehabilitation but did not spoil it.[123] In this case and others, Oso Blanco authorities deployed the humanities as a corrective tool. In convict hands, however, the humanities became liberating and therapeutic tools. Reading, writing, drawing, performing, and so on improved the self-esteem and communication and literacy skills of inmates, all of which they would need to thrive upon going home. Participation in humanities activities provided inmates with a social consciousness that in time redounded to their benefit, to the benefit of the penitentiary, and of the communities to which they were on the cusp of returning. Humanities opportunities and programs dovetailed with Oso Blanco's custodial purpose and regenerative mission. Constraint and agency went hand in hand.

Transitioning Oso Blanco convicts from living dead to awakened involved humanistic stimulation. Individuals deemed criminals by society proved more than capable of making society "think" and of supplementing national culture. The humanities allowed prisoners to showcase that they were more than stiff-necked, zwoddering creatures of habit defined by epicaricacy. Rather, they were imprisoned people who, like everyone else, changed throughout the course of their lives. In Oso Blanco, the transformative power of the visual and performing arts and literature were on full display. While these victories only lasted for a brief period, an important exercise played out in the work of the Classification and Treatment Board and in the pages of *El Despertar*. Oso Blanco convicts and other constituencies advocated for prison reform through the humanities. Prisoners affirmed their humanity through the humanities. Engaging the humanities represented more than their being seen or heard or exhibiting that they were doing something constructive and useful while jailed. The humanities could lead to awakening, and to pursue awakening was to sculpt one's own consciousness inside and outside the rigid parameters of the colonial-populist state.

Health Activism:
Executive Clemency on the Mona Passage

On October 26, 1951, the Mayagüez district court sentenced a twenty-eight-year-old white day laborer named Vicente Quiñones Ortiz to a maximum of four years for selling unregistered firearms to police. Three years into his sentence Quiñones Ortiz's wife, Isabel Avellanet, fell into deep despair. Between March and October 1954 she wrote multiple letters to governor Luis Muñoz Marín, pleading for her husband's exoneration or early release. She described having two young boys to provide for on her own and being debt ridden, and that Quiñones Ortiz, too, was insolvent. The only person he could count on was his elderly and infirm mother, who could do little for him in her condition. "He only has me and I only have him," Avellanet explained.[1] Imploring Muñoz Marín for a spark of hope, she asked him not to let her "die in life."[2] This could be accomplished by restoring Quiñones Ortiz's freedom. Avellanet presented her petition to "God in heaven" and Muñoz Marín "on earth," and concluded by conveying to the governor that she was also "begging Christ" to touch his heart.[3] Unfortunately for Avellanet, Quiñones Ortiz would remain behind bars a while longer.

Other documents in Quiñones Ortiz's parole file indicate that he also committed first-degree murder before entering Oso Blanco in November 1951. He was therefore slapped with a life sentence after authorities successfully prosecuted him for the illegal sale of firearms. To be eligible for parole, he would have to serve at least fifteen years of the life sentence. Quiñones Ortiz's life imprisonment and Avellanet's sufferings throw into sharp relief the extent to which living death permeated mid-twentieth-century Puerto Rico. Avellanet supplicated Muñoz Marín to help her avoid being buried alive due to the painstaking bare life she was forced to lead. For his part, Quiñones Ortiz transitioned from the cusp of release to a perpetual tomb for the living. There was a real chance he might biologically perish behind bars. Despite the challenges and odds stacked against them, Quiñones Ortiz and Avellanet persevered, although it is unclear whether they managed to secure release in the short term. The prisoner's parole file goes silent after change of custody paperwork filed in 1956.

Quiñones Ortiz's and Avellanet's well-being and life or death depended on whether they could nudge state officials into action. While medical and social scientists and social workers primarily looked to their specialized knowledge to address the health needs of incarcerated people, prisoners themselves and their extended social networks looked to more humanistic and holistic frameworks to get by and better. This is not to suggest that an impenetrable rigid line always separated the two worlds, however, for as earlier chapters have clearly established, health experts participated in religious and spiritual activities and convicts engaged and accepted scientific paradigms. Rather, regarding executive clemency, inmates and their communities tapped into a range of justifications to convince authorities of their own or their loved ones' sincere regret and to show them that matters of life and death shadowed incarcerated people both behind bars and at home.

This chapter uses the clemency letters and petitions of Caribbean prisoners, their kin, and their wider communities to trace their pursuit of well-being through health activism between the 1930s and midcentury. Materializing well-being went beyond the articulation and application of scientific and humanistic logics and practices inside prisons. Doing so transcended prison walls by necessity. Naturally, many convicts on either side of the Mona Passage maintained connections to family members and others through letters and face-to-face visits and attempted to leverage such bonds to regain freedom. In Puerto Rico, inmates even developed new bonds with health professionals stationed in the different institutions of the Río Piedras tri-institutional complex, which in some instances contributed to favorable outcomes. In the Dominican Republic, more regionalized health networks reflecting a country-wide distribution of carceral facilities were the norm. In both societies, however, the health activism of prisoners and their communities conveyed the tensions between families and total institutions while strategically merging grassroots and high politics. Household and community impetus provided a structural guarantee that total systems were contestable at the end of the day.[4] Clemency contradicted and complemented rehabilitative corrections. It was a key tool in Puerto Rican and Dominican convicts' attempts to overcome and defeat living death.

Clemency in Puerto Rico

Executive clemency has long existed in Puerto Rico. It still does and is among the powers heads of state invoke to correct judicial mistakes and show mercy to the less fortunate. Clemency in Puerto Rico was established during the Spanish colonial period. For centuries, crises-affected populations in Latin America sent petitions and requests for intervention or redress to distant monarchs in Iberia.[5] Under US rule, the tradition persisted. With common-wealth status in the mid-twentieth century, executive clemency was enshrined in Puerto Rico's US-approved constitution (Article 4). Today, it is one of the few powers of the monarch recognized by modern democratic republics.[6]

Claims making rooted in clemency should not be confused with mortuary claims making, which also circulated in Puerto Rico in the middle decades of the twentieth century. Mortuary claims making by prisoners' families often revolved around the belongings, earnings, and memories left behind by in-carcerated people when they died.[7] Regarding clemency, however, the fami-lies and extended social networks of inmates approached state officials on behalf of their incarcerated loved ones to secure parole, pardon, or the res-titution of civil rights and political privileges. Former prisoners requalified for rights and privileges at least a full year after their original sentence had been exhausted. This meant that if someone was sentenced to three years in prison and released after serving one year, for example, they usually still had to wait two more years to complete their original sentence and an additional year to apply for the restoration of rights and privileges. Releases occurred year-round but were particularly concentrated during the holiday season.[8] To advance their clemency petitions, convicts and their wider communities typi-cally contacted the governor, whether US-appointed in the 1930s and 1940s or elected by Puerto Ricans as of 1948.

Incarcerated people at Oso Blanco enjoyed access to family and friends via thousands of visits and personal letters.[9] This contact with the free world formed the basis of the health activism at the core of clemency. The po-rous boundary dividing prison and society meant that prisoners' commu-nities could be extensive. In August 1931, for instance, hundreds of Utuado townspeople—agricultural and skilled laborers, domestics, landowners, law-yers, merchants, and physicians, among others—submitted a pardon petition to governor Theodore Roosevelt Jr. in support of an elderly white tinsmith named Roque González Cruz. The man was in his seventies, in poor health (tubercular), and going blind.[10] Should González Cruz remain locked up, the townspeople averred, he would die in prison. They urged the governor to investigate his health and civic life to corroborate that he merited clemency.[11]

Although this first petition was denied, the townspeople of Utuado were not deterred. More than one hundred local students submitted their own next.[12] A pro-elder committee based in the municipality of Toa Alta followed suit in April 1932, as did González Cruz's wife, Luisa de Jesús, that October

and November, and Utuado women and men in December.[13] De Jesús implored the governor to grant clemency as a gesture of "humanity."[14] Otherwise, González Cruz's "decrepit state" in an "ergastulum" would most certainly result in biological death.[15]

De Jesús strategically used the word "ergastulum" for at least two reasons.
First, as an elderly woman who came of age in the latter decades of the nineteenth century, she would have perceived of incarceration much differently
than those exclusively bearing witness to the rise of rehabilitative corrections
in modern times. Within her life span, De Jesús beheld more archaic forms of
physical punishment alongside the ascent of the scientific penitentiary. Second, she was aware of the transition from plantation to prison or enslavement
to incarceration, but also the continuities that kept the two fused together.

An ergastulum was an ancient Roman prison, a dungeon building where
slaves were chained or punished. Usually built underground, it was large
enough for slaves to work within and contained narrow spaces in which they
slept (tombs for the living). For De Jesús to deploy the term suggests that she
continued to see incarceration through the prism of slavery. The climax of
her November 1932 letter showcased the existential continuities binding the
two forms of caging. She asseverated that prison was a "regrettable place,"
"the greatest of social abysses," and host to the "bottom of society."[16] It was a
"nefarious place where the soul is shattered and the heart is torn, where all
the hopes of man die forever until the blessed sun of freedom again kisses the
forehead that the cold slabs of captivity had muddied [and] stained with the
greatest of stigmas."[17] In addition to underscoring the misery of the prison,
De Jesús's eloquent assertions recognized that a new day was possible and left
room for the promise of redemption.

As petitions and letters in favor of González Cruz poured into Puerto
Rico's executive office, especially in 1932, the penitentiary physicians Leandro
López de la Rosa and Miguel A. Mariani reported to clemency officials that
an early release would greatly improve the convict's health and extend his
life. The attorney general Charles Winter recommended parole on December 23, 1932, and several days later, on December 27, the executive secretary
Carlos Gallardo contacted a pharmacist in Utuado who had agreed to serve
as González Cruz's adviser and help him find a job.[18] The sustained pressure
put on the state by Utuado activists produced results in this case. They faced
setbacks but built a diverse coalition that nudged state actors in the direction
they desired.

The mobilization of Utuadeños was impressive, but prisoners could also
sway the decision-making of state actors on their own or with limited backing by building support within the criminal-legal system. A young white

gardener from Santurce suffering from amblyopia named José Sotero Ortiz Cruz, for example, approached governor Blanton Winship in May 1934 about losing his vision, which he attributed to having broken human and divine laws.[19] Ortiz Cruz invited the governor to close his eyes for a moment: "you will no longer see the beauties that comprise the universe, nor the loved ones that surround you[,] and there will be sadness in your heart."[20] A few months later, Winship granted the convict a pardon on condition that he was to be confined in an asylum for the blind to receive treatment.

Ortiz Cruz's words alone did not soften Winship's heart. Months before submitting his letter, López de la Rosa told warden Sixto M. Saldaña that the prisoner's amblyopia was going to be difficult to treat in the penitentiary hospital. Therefore, he recommended that Ortiz Cruz be transferred to a facility that was better equipped to handle any intervention that may be needed.[21] Saldaña, in turn, notified legal officials, who reevaluated the case. In August 1934, the attorney general Benjamin J. Horton decided to endorse parole, in large part because trustworthy health professionals affirmed the severity of Ortiz Cruz's condition and the Health Department promised to hospitalize him in the Ponce asylum for the blind.[22]

The Ortiz Cruz saga continued in January 1935, when he again contacted governor Winship, this time requesting a full pardon as a Christmas gift. He spotlighted not having seen or heard from his mother in three years.[23] To determine whether a full pardon was appropriate, the Health Department investigated his family history and the environment where he was to reside. Beatriz Lassalle, superintendent of social services, assigned the social worker Isolina Peña Oms to carry out the research. The study revealed that Ortiz Cruz's upbringing did not raise any red flags and that his relatives in Lares were good, honest rural people who anticipated the return of their prodigal son.[24] Therefore, Lassalle recommended that he "be allowed to return to his home where family surroundings will be greatly beneficial to him."[25] The report was accompanied by blind asylum staff affirmation of Ortiz Cruz's condition; that he had totally lost vision in one eye and the other was barely stable.[26] Given these circumstances, in May 1935 then governor Horton granted Ortiz Cruz an unconditional pardon and restored his civil rights.

Whereas social workers like Lassalle and Peña Oms informally became part of Ortiz Cruz's health network, prisoners also formally cultivated relationships with government health professionals by virtue of the training they were privy to as Health Department laborers. Hundreds of prisoners put thousands of workdays into Interior Department road construction (the labor specialty of incarcerated people in Puerto Rico and elsewhere in the mid-twentieth century) and other New Deal–era and colonial-populist infrastructure projects.

They put just as many days into working for the Health Department. Their labor assignments revolved around sanitation, cleaning city streets, gardens and government offices, filling in mangrove swampland, reforestation, and combating infectious disease. On the grounds of the Río Piedras complex, labor assignments encompassed cleaning the asylum and sanatorium, burning sputum, serving as health aides, and maintaining the food and material supplies of these facilities.[27]

Incarcerated people had qualitative encounters within their health labor assignments. These enabled them to forge networks of support beyond their immediate family circles. The expansion of their activist networks indelibly marked their overall clemency experiences. For instance, in June 1937, a group of more than forty insular government Insane Asylum employees petitioned interim governor Rafael Menéndez Ramos for the restoration of the civil rights of a thirty-eight-year-old *trigueño* industrial worker from Santurce named Pablo Pacheco Cuevas, who was serving a two-year sentence for incest that was slated to be completed in the following month. According to petitioners, Pacheco Cuevas had been cleaning at the asylum for a while, showing himself to be laborious and respectful. He had earned their affection and sympathy, so they mobilized on his behalf.[28]

Pacheco Cuevas's relationship to the insane asylum transcended his work assignment, however. His Venezuelan wife, María Mateu, went crazy after he was incarcerated as she had no kin or social support in Puerto Rico. She became so nervous and depressed that she lost reason in early 1936. By June 1936, she resided in the asylum as a patient. The couple had three young children between twenty-one months and eleven years old, the two eldest having been born in New York City. The children were under the provisional care of Providencia Trinidad, a woman who rented a room in their Santurce home before their parents were incarcerated. Trinidad was also under socioeconomic duress and announced that she would transfer the children back to their father as soon as he exited prison. In her own letter to authorities, Trinidad contextualized the circumstances of Pacheco Cuevas's alleged crime—that he had another daughter with a previous partner and that daughter was at the center of the incest case. In other words, a relationship gone sour and familial bitterness, rather than an actual deed, might explain what really transpired. The eldest children, for their part, expressed that their father hoped to sell their house and with the proceeds return to New York, where their mother could receive the best treatment and he could work to provide for them.[29]

The insane asylum petitioners, a group that included the future penitentiary psychiatrist José R. Maymí Nevares, implored the acting governor to "fill part of the void that exists in [Pacheco Cuevas's] soul" by restoring his civil rights, which would allow him to access employment and other opportunities.[30] As a result, his innocent children would not have to bear the brunt of the civic living death that often characterized the experiences of ex-prisoners when they reentered society. The attorney general Benigno Fernández García carefully reviewed the case and found no legal grounds on which to make a favorable recommendation, however. Pacheco Cuevas would have to wait at least a full year after exhausting his original sentence to have a shot at restitution of his civil rights.

More than most, Pacheco Cuevas's experience illustrates how understanding confinement requires more than a consideration of spaces of enclosure. In this case, carcerality operated on at least three levels. First, Pacheco Cuevas's own family, or more specifically his previous partner, obligated him to account for his alleged violation of their daughter. She was certainly upset about him abandoning her and did everything she could to make his life miserable, for Pacheco Cuevas ended up in New York City, where he married another woman with whom he had three children. Regardless of the rationale for accusing Pacheco Cuevas of incest, the point is that the demand for punishment came from below. Interpersonal or community justice came first, and state justice rode its coattails.[31]

Second, carcerality emerged as expected, in conjunction with medicalizing institutions. Pacheco Cuevas's deviance was treated in the penitentiary. The accusations against him and the material aftermath of tearing asunder his family drove his wife María mad and orphaned their children. María landed in the insular insane asylum near Oso Blanco, and clearly Pacheco Cuevas was able to visit and communicate with her because of his labor assignment. But they could not do so whenever they desired. Even this crack in the system was not enough to annul the policing of their movement, let alone alleviate the psychosocial burdens they endured as a broken family. The tri-institutional complex was supposed to repair and heal them, but it also subjugated them in the sense that they had little real control to resolve their most pressing problems on their own.

Third, the Puerto Rican state extended and normalized dubious confinement practices by limiting Pacheco Cuevas's reacquisition of freedom. The state's role in separating this family belies the notion that midcentury state-building projects were exclusively patriarchal. If midcentury states in the Caribbean and elsewhere were merely interested in reproducing patriarchal relations, they would have done much more to preserve the integrity of the scores of nuclear families that became the collateral damage of incarceration. Moreover, even when Pacheco Cuevas was on the cusp of maxing out his sentence and being released, the state blocked the return of his civil rights, which he needed if he was going to successfully rebuild his life and secure the well-being of his family. The state failed to meet expectations then, and academic assumptions now.

The disconnect between state rhetoric and practice helps explain why incarcerated people constructed networks outside the immediate jurisdiction and purview of legal authorities. Some prisoners tapped into their health networks from every possible angle over the course of years, from one governor to the next. In August 1937, the mother of a young *trigueño* barber from San Juan named Graciano Arroyo Rivera, who was serving fifteen years for second-degree murder, set off a chain reaction of clemency letters.[32] Arroyo Rivera subsequently wrote to Governor Winship directly, accentuating that his anguished and afflicted mother and sisters were vulnerable without his assistance and protection. His most fervent desire, he professed, was to return home and sustain those who depended on him.[33] Arroyo Rivera's mother Amelia followed suit with additional letters in the early 1940s. Together, these highlighted her hardships and that there were caring people willing to aid her son so that he could, in turn, care for her.[34]

The community of care to which Amelia referred included the Health Department engineer José Culpeper, who stated that the prisoner had observed exemplary conduct while incarcerated. Therefore, he was amenable to providing him with a job as a day laborer on water drainage projects and serving as his mentor.[35] Although these early bids to free Arroyo Rivera fell on deaf ears, he was granted parole by acting governor José Gallardo in August 1941. A few months later, however, he began showing signs of mental illness, so his postrelease adviser had him admitted to the insular insane asylum for treatment.[36] The psychiatrist Carlos L. Massanet reported to clemency officials in April 1942 that the ex-convict was "in a state of psychomotor arousal, with fleeting ideas, impairment in voluntary attention, and emotional exaltation."[37] It is unclear how long Arroyo Rivera stayed at the asylum, but it appears he did so for an extended period as he was able to cultivate relationships with local health professionals. By 1947, he had expanded his clemency network. That March, a team of Río Piedras medical experts based at a children's sanatorium, an insular home for children, and in nursing circles collectively approached governor Jesús T. Piñero to ask that he "rehabilitate" Arroyo Rivera's civil rights and political privileges.[38] Piñero acquiesced and finished raising the ex-prisoner from civic death that September.

In some cases, health activism circumgyrated corporeal understandings of the body but in others it operated holistically. Religious and spiritual concerns powerfully shaped clemency processes. The health networks that mobilized on behalf of prisoners often included people of faith. In July 1940, for example, a mulatto stonemason in his thirties from Bayamón named Emilio Arroyo Rivera, who had just exhausted a five-year sentence for a crime against nature, wrote to authorities about the restoration of his civil rights, making clear that without them a person "does not amount to anything."[39] For all intents and purposes, then, an ex-convict like him remained living dead even after release precisely because he had no civic life. Arroyo Rivera had been paroled in May 1937, in large part because his partner Emilia Cantre repeatedly visited the executive mansion in Old San Juan with their three surviving children to plead for his pardon. They all appeared "undernourished" and Cantre herself suffered "from some disease."[40] The hunger and symbolic nudity of Cantre and the children throws into sharp relief that living death enveloped Arroyo Rivera's wider family.

The next month, in August 1940, Arroyo Rivera's pastor, Reverend Ramón Fontaine Morales of the Pentecostal Church of God, submitted a letter of support on his behalf. Fontaine Morales celebrated the ex-convict's exemplary conduct both inside and outside the congregation. The pastor insisted that Arroyo Rivera lived honestly with his wife and children. Using his knowledge of construction, he helped build the Pentecostal Church of God temple. For these and other reasons, the body of Christ to which he pertained was interested in the swift resolution of his case.[41] That December, Arroyo Rivera once again wrote to authorities for the return of his civil rights, which he believed would allow him to support his family more easily.[42] His petition was denied, however, because he failed to wait at least a full year after completely extinguishing his original sentence before applying for their restitution. Arroyo Rivera would have to show more patience, a central tenet of his faith, to achieve his goal.

Not only were prisoners the beneficiaries of the support of religious and spiritual partners, religious and spiritual leaders themselves engaged the clemency process *as* inmates. In January 1951, Reverend Carlos López Arellano of Caguas contacted governor Muñoz Marín about Crescencio Espinosa, an Evangelical minister who was imprisoned in the Humacao district jail for failing to support an alleged daughter.[43] This jeopardized the well-being of Espinosa's wife and six children, who like orphans were enduring material and spiritual miseries and deprivations.[44] López Arellano's letter made an impact. Muñoz Marín forwarded Espinosa's case to the Clemency (or Pardons) Board.[45] When the governor announced on January 25 that he would not be able to pardon Espinosa because of certain legal precedents, however, the pastor's allies regrouped and renewed their efforts.[46]

Given its high-profile nature, Espinosa's case regularly appeared in the mainstream newspaper *El Mundo* between 1949 and 1954. López Arellano's

letter therefore provides but a snapshot of the legal forces and moving parts
that fashioned clemency processes and the long-term commitment required
to see them through to their conclusions. Verily, Espinosa's ordeal took a
number of twists and turns. At one point, new evidence and testimonies
turned the case on its head.[47] Puerto Rico's Supreme Court intervened several
times.[48] On at least one occasion, members of Espinosa's flock protested outside Humacao court.[49] He would be released only to be incarcerated again.[50]
When he was definitively freed, the faithful crowded the vicinity of Humacao jail to escort him to their uninaugurated temple.[51] While Espinosa's legal process officially drew to a close in early 1954, a great deal of organizing
and patience characterized his network's activism for more than four years.[52]
Their collective perseverance spiritually nourished Espinosa, for he remained
active behind bars crafting hymns and sermons he later disseminated.

As this sample of cases makes evident, convict health networks in midcentury Puerto Rico often reflected the medical priorities of the Río Piedras
tri-institutional complex and the precepts of rehabilitation more broadly.
In addition to prisoners and their families, health and science professionals
of all kinds, people of faith, union leaders, politicians of different persuasions, reconstruction officials, and many others contributed to advancing
and investigating clemency petitions.[53] Nevertheless, Puerto Rico's colonial-
populist state insisted on having a certain bar met before confirming the parole, pardon, or return of rights of incarcerated people. Clemency was not
easy to come by for most prisoners. However, it was an important option for
convicts and their families as they confronted the vorticing crises of the era,
starting with the interpersonal ones that permeated their immediate lives.

Clemency in the Dominican Republic

Like Puerto Rico, executive clemency formed part of Spanish and Haitian
Santo Domingo's legal landscapes. During the era of dictator Rafael Trujillo, the prevailing Dominican constitution (Article 29) vested in presidents
the authority to pardon prisoners. Trujillo and other Dominican presidents
made a habit of pardoning mostly common but also political prisoners before, on, or up to several days after national holidays, such as February 27
(Independence Day), August 16 (Restoration Day), September 24 (Our Lady
of Mercedes Day), October 24 (Trujillo's birthday), December 25 (Christmas),
and so on. The total number of convicts pardoned and released per decree
on any given holiday between 1935 and 1942, for instance, was between nine
and thirty-nine.[54] In 1944, the government pardoned and released more than
2,000 prisoners from twenty prisons, largely on the strength of celebrating

the centennial of independence from Haiti.[55] The next year, 1945, the number of convicts pardoned and released dropped dramatically.[56] In 1946 and 1947, pardons remained low compared to 1944, but authorities pointed to sixty-seven and sixty-one cases of medical clemency, respectively.[57]

Pardonable women and men resided in prisons all over the Dominican Republic. As of 1936, the Dominican carceral archipelago consisted of a public jail in the national district (then Ciudad Trujillo, now Santo Domingo), the Nigua penitentiary on the outskirts of the capital in San Cristóbal, and at least eleven district jails or regional prisons located in Santiago, La Vega, San Francisco de Macorís, Puerto Plata, San Pedro de Macorís, Montecristi, Azua, Moca, Barahona, El Seibo, and Samaná.[58] By the late 1930s and early 1940s, the Trujillo regime ordered the reconstruction and expansion of the country's carceral infrastructure. This entailed converting the Nigua penitentiary into an insane asylum and founding institutions for women and youths.[59] An extensive network of jails, prisons, reformatories, asylums, and hospitals dotted the Dominican landscape by midcentury; nineteen of these were prisons.[60] A new scientific (or model) penitentiary with rehabilitative components, La Victoria, opened in 1952.[61]

Although Dominican prisons under Trujillo are often cast as sites of cruel and unusual punishment and political violence, in the mid-twentieth century rehabilitation began pervading many of the country's carceral spaces.[62] According to Félix Bernardino, who at one point served time in Santo Domingo's Fort Ozama (a public jail built during the Spanish era), the evolution of Dominican prisons was palpable. Using the military as the core executor of his vision, Trujillo instituted reforms that turned "dens of pain" like Ozama—once replete with torture instruments, epidemic disease, hunger, and abusive forced labor—into "correctional schools" that exposed prisoners to different vocations.[63] Convicts applied the vast knowledge they acquired through diverse labor assignments, ranging from public works projects and the construction of military airfields and bases to cleaning barracks and participating in agricultural production. Regime officials visited Ozama to monitor the progress of reforms, examine the food supply, and inquire about the treatment inmates received at the hands of guards and health personnel, for in the end, the point was to return reformed and useful people to society. The era in which prisons turned their occupants into less than human was, in theory, over.[64] By midcentury, penologist Leoncio Ramos lent his vast criminological and legal expertise to the reorganization of the Dominican penitentiary system.[65]

In this context, clemency represented yet another route to achieve the humanization and rehabilitation of incarcerated people. Hundreds of clemency letters and petitions arrived at the Dominican National Palace in the middle decades of the twentieth century. These began pouring into Trujillo's executive office as soon as he assumed power. Prisoners, their families, and their wider communities took the time to engage the clemency process for multiple reasons, the most prominent being to articulate health issues of one kind or another, bodily and otherwise. While incarcerated people and their extended networks did not always receive an affirmative response from state officials, they practiced a form of health activism that improved their chances of at least being heard.

Dominican prisoners and their communities used health as a rhetorical device in the clemency letters and petitions they submitted to authorities. Elaborating on health gave them a precise and timely vocabulary with which to generate impactful imagery that indicated why they were asking for their own or someone else's pardon. Moreover, they often fused health lexicon and imagery with notions of the sacred. In a December 1930 letter, for example, the elderly Ramona, mother of an inmate, identified herself as an "invalid" and "almost blind, stammering" woman.[66] She did so to convey how much she needed her son Domingo Nolasco around. Only he could sustain her and serve as her eyes. Ramona compared the good work Trujillo could do to the advent of Jesus Christ. While it is unclear if officials ultimately pardoned Nolasco, for many surviving clemency letters randomly appear in the archival record and fail to include decisions, Ramona's mindset is evident. She fused a description of her ailing, failing body to a spiritual epistemology believing this was the best way to convince Trujillo of the redemptive role he could play in Nolasco's story, which was also the Dominican story.

Luis Dorville Torres, serving ten years for murder in the public jail of Ciudad Trujillo, similarly cited his own poor health as justification for pardon. He wrote to Trujillo in the summer of 1940 stating that he was "an old man, continually afflicted by health problems which little by little sap me of life."[67] The overwhelming weight of the prison's walls, he added, would soon cave in on him if no one intervened in his situation. Dorville Torres placed the responsibility of Christlike salvific intervention in Trujillo's hands. Should he be pardoned and released, his primary goal was to prepare his children for the future. Citing health problems, referring to spiritual precedent, and sharing a life plan would not be enough, however. The attorney general Diógenes del Orbe rejected Dorville Torres's petition due to the nature of his crime and the fact that he had served only a short portion of his sentence to date.

Clemency petitioners highlighted the frail health of loved ones both beyond and behind prison walls and connected the resolution of their plight to the assumed divine humanity of Trujillo. Carmencita Tavarez, the sister of a young convict named Juan Humberto, contacted the president underscoring the advanced age of their parents. The relentless "precarity" in which they lived demanded his "humanitarian" consideration.[68] Juan A. Lockward approached Trujillo concerning his elderly incarcerated father, Luis, warning that prolonged reclusion could prove fatal in his case. He was "visibly weak" and in a "deplorable" state, no doubt due to his conscience eating him alive for what he had done.[69] Lockward supplicated the president to move his "generous hand" to "mitigate pain and appease suffering," as he had done countless times before.[70] In 1936, an elderly father of thirty-two children named Julio Pérez construed his imprisonment in the public jail of San Cristóbal as "difficult and irritating."[71] He hoped Trujillo would look upon his ordeal with "pious eyes" and grant clemency.[72]

Traveling vast distances was sometimes the only way to obtain clarity about the health status of imprisoned kin. In summer 1940, Monte Cristi resident Rosa Castro went to see her son Julio César Ricardo at the agricultural penal colony of Pedernales, an encampment located on the southernmost tip of the border with Haiti. She traveled more than two hundred miles to get there and found him "extremely infirm" with "chronic malaria."[73] Castro decided to stay and care for him since, in her view, he was not getting sufficient medical attention from the state. Having regained a bit of strength, a few weeks later Ricardo himself submitted a clemency letter to Trujillo in which he stressed family and military connections that merited consideration, his ill health, and the fact that he had a job waiting for him when released. He even compared his fate to those of bees and wasps should he not return to society "regenerated": "A bee stings and dies. A wasp stings and should die."[74] Ricardo anticipated not doing any harm whatsoever, thereby avoiding both scenarios.

As these cases illustrate, in midcentury Dominican Republic health issues saturated the clemency process though there was no carceral compound resembling the tri-institutional complex at Río Piedras. A cluster of institutions on the outskirts of Santo Domingo, in San Cristóbal, came the closest to approximating Puerto Rico's carceral geography in the 1930s, specifically. There, authorities planted the Nigua penitentiary, a leper colony, and eventually a youth reformatory, for example, albeit at different junctures. Nigua's transition into an insane asylum after its closure in April 1938 also restrained the making of a long-term scientific corridor in San Cristóbal.[75] Regardless, carceral spaces overlapped on Dominican soil, just as much as they were differentiated.

The overlap and gulf between the prison and the asylum emerge in the clemency letters of Dominican convicts. Víctor Puesan, for instance, who was serving a short sentence in the public jail of Ciudad Trujillo, believed a pardon would clear the prejudiced aura surrounding his case. He conveyed to Trujillo that the opprobrium he endured was attributable to his brief seclusion in the Padre Billini asylum before his current sentence.[76] An inmate named Leonte Martínez charted his carceral trajectory in reverse. His sentence began in San Pedro de Macorís prison in March 1945, but for "health reasons" he was transferred to the Padre Billini asylum in July 1948.[77] A key continuity bridged the two experiences for him: his wife and children found themselves in dire economic straits.

Whereas Puesan and Martínez blurred the boundary between prison and asylum, other petitioners distinguished between carceral spaces, attributing aggravation or healing to each accordingly. A woman from Puerto Plata named Felicita Recio, for instance, implored Trujillo to pardon her son Carlos Ruiz o Almonte because he was gravely ill. "His poor health cannot be addressed in prison," she contended.[78] Therefore, Recio urged the president not to take her word for it, but to seek out available medical certificates that corroborated Ruiz o Almonte's "incurable and contagious" condition and to facilitate his admission to a hospital.[79] In Recio's mind, a prison infirmary paled in comparison to one of the state-of-the-art hospitals being erected around the country.[80]

Many Dominican clemency letters and petitions were matters of life and death. The families of prisoners beseeched Trujillo to reunify their kin units not simply out of some aesthetic concern to preserve the integrity of the nuclear family, but because their lives depended on it. Natividad Vázquez of La Vega expressed to the president that in the nine months her son Rafael had been incarcerated, she barely nourished her old, infirm, perishing body. If Trujillo pardoned Rafael, however, that act of mercy might "prolong my sad life by a few days."[81] But these circumstances were not the preserve of the impoverished and downtrodden. A former police officer named Juan Montalvo, for example, who was serving time in San Pedro de Macorís prison for inadvertently shooting a suspect, made plain to Trujillo that his health status demanded that he be moved to a hospital for a surgery. On top of this, his children were starving to death. A pardon would begin to resolve both issues.[82]

The considerable mental anguish associated with incarceration colored the clemency experiences of Montalvo and many other similarly positioned convicts. An inmate named Adón Mona, who was serving one year in San Francisco de Macorís prison for abducting a young girl, for instance, underscored how incarceration deteriorated his psyche. The prison disrupted his peace of mind and buried him alive with "anxiety."[83] Such mental health crises could have physical symptoms. In 1951, Eulalia Medina de Javier of Yamasá implored Trujillo to free her daughter Carmen Acevedo, who was serving a one-year sentence for performing an abortion. Acevedo's "emaciated" body bore the evidence of her suffering behind bars.[84] Additionally, the uncertainty associated with incarceration impacted the mental health of the families of prisoners. Lidia Adames pleaded with Trujillo to pardon her mother, Providencia. While Providencia sat in the public jail of Ciudad Trujillo, her children struggled to survive.[85] The material, psychic, and emotional burden therefore fell on her eldest daughter, Lidia, who had to figure out where and how to secure food, clothing, shelter, and other resources.

Despite the dire realities described by Dominicans in their clemency letters and petitions, hope persisted and they connected this hope to their understanding of nation. Emilia Grullón Santana of Moca, for example, appealed to Trujillo on behalf of her son, Juan Tomás Grullón Salcedo, in August 1951. Her letter shed light not only on her circumstances but also on those affecting her immediate family. As a family unit, they shared living death—Emilia physically, her children as mechanistic laborers, and Grullón Salcedo as a convict: "I am an old and sick woman, so sick that the belief my death draws near exists in my mind. I am also poor, and my children are wretched agricultural day laborers who with their arms and sweat produced by the red hot sun provide me with sustenance and medicines."[86] To fulfill his filial obligations, Grullón Salcedo moved to the capital city to improve his wages. However, the urban underworld seduced him, he fell into gambling, and he landed in prison for a year. Emilia's letter appealed to Trujillo by invoking the upcoming Restoration War holiday, which could restore dignity to her family just as the war restored sovereignty to and resurrected the Dominican nation.

Petitioners meditated on the life-death dyad, and in several instances decided that holistic health exchanges represented the most promising course of action. A mother of ten children from Santiago de los Caballeros named Cristina Jorge, for example, proposed "a prayer to God" for Trujillo's health in exchange for the release of her husband, Erasmo Rodríguez, whose return home would improve the literal well-being of his family unit. Jorge detailed her helpless situation without the aid and support of her partner, who was serving a short sentence for the clandestine manufacture of cigars. She lacked resources entirely, having even "lost the conuco [small land plot] work" that put plantains on the table.[87] Attorney General Del Orbe took these factors into consideration and recommended that Rodríguez be released. Ramona Pontier of Ciudad Trujillo reached out to Trujillo in September 1951, assuring him that she would perform "fervent acts" for his health that would coincide with Our Lady of Mercedes Day. He would have to do his part, however, and pardon her husband, Manuel María Pontier.[88] Helpless and hindered by health problems alongside her children, Ramona believed that Trujillo would hear her plea.

Similarly, an ex-lieutenant of the military named Domingo González Gutiérrez, who was serving time at the Mariano Cesteros agricultural penal colony located in Restauración on the northern border with Haiti, declared that he would offer "fervent vows to the miraculous Virgin of Altagracia" in favor of Trujillo's health at an upcoming prison church service in exchange for his freedom.[89] However, González Gutiérrez also linked agricultural labor therapy and rehabilitation. Since arriving at the agricultural penal colony, he had developed "a well-cultivated plot of land of more than 40 hectares of minor fruits," which prepared him for future success should he be released.[90] Executive clemency and rehabilitative corrections were not always separate endeavors. They could interface with and reinforce each other.

Prisoners, their families, military officers, community members, and other social conglomerations intervened in Dominican clemency processes. In addition to health crises and issues, they cited labor and party affiliation, mutual-aid principles, science, military and property credentials, and so on, to legitimize their calls for pardon.[91] Health networks and activism in midcentury Dominican Republic were holistic in the sense that many petitioners blended material and immaterial knowledges in their attempts to compel authorities to affirmatively respond to their requests and demands. This happened in the Dominican capital and beyond, notwithstanding the deeply regionalized distribution of carceral institutions in the country. Although populist dictatorship marked the Dominican case, and colonial populism the Puerto Rican case, in both places emotional ties and everyday pressures resulted in new strategies and forms of accommodation between ordinary people, their communities, and (neo)colonial states.

Conclusion

In midcentury Puerto Rico and Dominican Republic, executive clemency was a crucial option for incarcerated people in their quests for parole, pardon, or the restitution of their civil rights and political privileges. On both sides of the Mona Passage, incarcerated people, their families, and their wider communities linked clemency to well-being, broadly defined. In engaging the state through a constitutional mechanism, prisoners and their networks developed and practiced a form of health activism. They received an education in the rule of law and government bureaucracy while pursuing justice through clemency letters and petitions. Clemency was not guaranteed. Nor was it unfathomable.

Notwithstanding the factors that integrated Puerto Rican and Domini-can approaches to clemency, there were also important differences between the two societies. The Puerto Rican experience tended to orbit "stable," cen-tralized health care, most prominently the tri-institutional complex at Río Piedras and what was fast becoming the San Juan metropolitan area. Mean-while, an ever-shifting carceral geography—one with borderland dynamics and institutional closures to consider—fashioned the Dominican experience. Although Trujillo centralized state power, health care itself was regionalized. Still, in both the Dominican Republic and Puerto Rico incarcerated people and their relations deployed clemency letters and petitions to make claims, voice health grievances, and insist on pardon. The groundswell of claims making from below demonstrated that the living dead could only be buried alive for so long.

For many petitioners, clemency was a matter of life and death. In a sense, the health vocabulary and imagery used by petitioners amounted to a sy-cophantic performance, one reflecting what governments and heads of state desired to see and hear. Knowing what was at stake—pardon, and by exten-sion a tempered freedom and all that entailed—it is to be expected that those seeking clemency would blend fact and fiction in their narratives. However, that desperate health logic necessarily and repeatedly conditioned activist ef-forts and authorities often contested or at worst rejected these efforts is sug-gestive of how genuine the claims were in the first place. Clemency laid bare the (un)seen structural violence and exposed the limits of rehabilitative cor-rections as the novel model of punitiveness was institutionalized in the mid-twentieth century.[92] But it also showed how individual contexts and choices clouded where exactly to cast blame, thereby helping make the case for fur-ther investment in and normalizing the rehabilitative paradigm. Regardless of these dialectics, repairing the health of prisoners so that they could func-tion within the prevailing social order and political economy prepared them to return to their kin and communities with fresh perspectives and refined skills. In turn, these might just allow them to circumvent the bare life and living death that awaited many of them in the "free" world.

Conclusion:
A Rehabilitative Dream
Turned Punitive Nightmare

The rise of the rehabilitative ideal in Puerto Rico's prison system coincided with the imposition of US citizenship in 1917. Its implementation commenced in La Princesa penitentiary in the years following World War I but really gained momentum at the Insular Penitentiary in the middle decades of the twentieth century. Biomedicine powerfully marked the substance of Puerto Rican corrections in the 1920s and 1930s. In the 1940s, 1950s, and part of the 1960s, social science, social work, and humanities logics and practices dominated the correctional ambiance. As the independence activist and politician Cayetano Coll Cuchí observed in 1949, this was an era of "transcendental reforms" and "results" in the penitentiary system.[1] For at least a full generation, Oso Blanco was the site of a dynamic yet flawed problem-solving-oriented culture of rehabilitative corrections.

Oso Blanco formed part of a sanitary city that included an insane asylum and a tuberculosis hospital. These welfare institutions together triply pathologized the bodies circulating on complex grounds. The penitentiary diagnosed and treated behavioral pathologies associated with crime; the asylum, the mentally infirm; and the hospital, those suffering from a debilitating infectious disease. Convicts received medical and psychiatric care within penitentiary walls, but if their cases reached a certain point of development, authorities attempted to transfer them to a corresponding institution that would best serve them. Additionally, inmates lent their labor power not only to the prison but also to the nearby asylum and hospital. Far from being enclosed, isolated spaces cut off from one another, these institutions operated in integrated fashion, forming a unique though not always fluid carceral ecology.[2]

By midcentury, the rehabilitative dream that initially defined Oso Blanco began undergoing a slow, wrenching process of transfiguration. An early manifestation of the limits of rehabilitation emerged with the short-lived nationalist rebellion of fall 1950, which spilled into the penitentiary. Prior to the insurrection, prisoners, the mainstream press, and government officials were vocal about penal reforms that did not go far enough, especially in the areas of funding, sentencing, and social and physical sustenance (e.g., visitation, overcrowding, food, water, clothing, socks, shoes, bedsheets).[3] Inmates voiced these and other concerns in El Despertar for nearly two years but lost control of the media outlet in the aftermath of the nationalist rebellion, which colonial populists branded a consequence of infectious insanity.[4] As a result, for some six years convicts lacked access to a medium that allowed them to articulate their grievances and ideas regarding rehabilitation, even as the mainstream press continued to shine a light on Oso Blanco's deficiencies.[5]

This changed in 1956, when prisoners reearned the right to publish their own magazine. Whereas El Despertar traced rehabilitation anecdotally and to a degree critiqued the structures shaping incarceration, the new periodical, Realidad, primarily took an inward view of carceral problems, emphasizing vice and personal responsibility for example. Nowhere was the shift in orientation more evident than in terms of who ran the publication: the penitentiary chapter of Alcoholics Anonymous (known as "The Last Drink"), a group that encouraged members and Oso Blanco's convict population in general to look in the mirror and evaluate self before pinning blame on others, let alone systems. Had ordinary prisoners not made this interpretive concession, which distinguished them from their nationalist and other radical counterparts, then they likely would not have been granted permission to start another publication.

Oso Blanco's educational director Juan Santana Márquez and the recreational director Manuel López de Victoria collaborated with "The Last Drink" and other Puerto Rican chapters of Alcoholics Anonymous (from San Juan, Santurce, and Cayey) to delegate the production of content for Realidad. Clearly, breaking the chains of alcoholism was a focus of the new magazine throughout its life span. Riveting articles and testimonials, poetry, short stories, local and transnational news concerning the Alcoholics Anonymous movement, and interviews with prison guards and technocrats graced its pages, providing insight into Oso Blanco's renewed rehabilitative culture. Prisoners used anthropological frameworks to understand alcohol abuse and reflected on the therapeutic utility of sports in achieving sobriety. Realidad's religious and spiritual tone and messaging indicate that convicts also persisted in drawing from belief to actualize rehabilitation.[6] Some, however, pointed to the rehabilitative ceiling of medicine and religion, as well as the collective inability of these different forms of praxis to address all cases of alcoholism.[7]

Further, relapse triggered by personality traits and external factors remained a possibility.[8] *Realidad* enabled many Puerto Rican inmates to immerse themselves in the medico-humanistic rehabilitative dream still at the core of corrections in the late 1950s and early 1960s.

Carceral afterlives characterized by transnational movement represented another possible route. Once they exited Oso Blanco and other prisons, some ex-inmates hoped for a fresh start on the United States mainland. They worked with government officials to relocate to communities in the US diaspora, such as Massachusetts, New York, Illinois, and elsewhere.[9] New York–based parolees, for instance, were supervised by Stanley Sheppard of the Salvation Army with offices at 120–130 W. Fourteenth Street.[10] In turn, Puerto Rican bureaucrats engaged their colleagues in potential host states to facilitate the movement of ex-convicts. Extensive investigations were carried out on both the Puerto Rican and US sides of the equation. Sometimes these efforts were successful; other times they failed.

While successful parole transfers shined a light on the bright side of reha-bilitation, failed parole transfers were much more dramatic and imperiled the rehabilitative ideal. It was not uncommon for ex-convicts and their commu-nities to invest copious amounts of time and energy in justifying transnational movement only to be denied by cynical mainland technocrats. In November 1953, the Connecticut State Prison parole supervisor James J. McIlduff submit-ted the results of a preparole investigation concerning Luis Rodríguez Reyes to his Puerto Rican counterpart Bibiana R. de Corneiro. McIlduff stressed that the prisoner had no definitive employment program and that the home arranged for him by his sister and brother-in-law was in a bad area of Hart-ford, where, according to Police Chief Michael J. Godfrey, many Puerto Ri-cans were causing trouble due to their unlawful conduct. There were at least five such "colonies" of Puerto Ricans in Hartford at the time, which created antagonism toward the migrant group. Therefore, the socioeconomic climate in Hartford, parole officer Robert A. Rolfe argued, may not facilitate "good parole rehabilitation" for Rodríguez Reyes.[11] Scenarios like this one, in which colonization in reverse was not tolerated, dampened popular enthusiasm and trust in rehabilitation as a viable blueprint for raising individuals from living death.

Puerto Rican authorities began reevaluating rehabilitative paradigms in the 1960s, and this despite the relative success of their rehabilitation and parole system compared to those on the US mainland.[12] This reflected, in part, con-tinued radical activism and an upswing in crime rates engendered by the con-traction of industrial manufacturing during the latter part of the decade.[13] In this context, the gradual disappearance of freedom transition mechanisms, for instance temporary passes granted to convicts so that they could visit their families beyond the walls prior to release, represented a significant rollback measure. The Popular Democratic Party governor Roberto Sánchez Vilella (1965–69) flexibilized the pass system in 1967, but according to Picó this was "the last liberal moment" for Puerto Rican corrections before authorities implemented a harsher restriction of prisoners' movements and rehabilitative prospects.[14]

A return to security-heavy approaches to incarceration in the 1970s hastened the fall of the agile rehabilitative model that appeared between the 1930s and midcentury. Within penal administration, the decision to create a corrections unit separate from the Justice Department in 1974 helped topple what was once a thriving, albeit imperfect culture of rehabilitation. Again, economic contraction—only this time in the petrochemical sector—played into rising crime rates.[15] Countering crime rates with correctional micromanagement that merely warehoused prisoners, exploited their labor power, and augmented the total penal population further distanced Puerto Rico's carceral project from the rehabilitative orientation and goals of previous generations.[16] Concurrently, multiple ongoing health crises spanning overcrowding, the lack of medical services, shortages in essential medicines, poor hygiene and ventilation, unbound infectious disease, and physical and mental abuse at the hands of guards and between convicts accelerated the deterioration of prison conditions.[17]

During this period, successive governments across Puerto Rico's party "divide" suffocated the rehabilitative ideal. The New Progressive Party governor Luis A. Ferré (1969–73) pursued policies evincing that the objective of the prison was to punish, not reform.[18] The Popular Democratic Party governor Rafael Hernández Colón (1973–77) echoed this sentiment, espousing the complete severance of prisoners from society.[19] Under the New Progressive Party governor Carlos Romero Barceló (1977–85), the carceral rehabilitative model finally collapsed notwithstanding some efforts to salvage it.[20] The bipartisan assault on rehabilitative corrections in modern Puerto Rico is a telling example of how the different political parties of our time are really a singular party that uses Kafkaesque tactics to reinforce the status quo and traditional power relations.

Like the US, where a Janus-faced uniparty also prevails to this day, the 1970s and 1980s in Puerto Rico witnessed the rise of mass incarceration. The introduction of capital-intensive, high-tech industries failed to create many new jobs in Puerto Rico, kick-starting the growth of an informal economy and triggering more crime. In response, arrests increased, and judges issued hyperbolic centuries-long sentences. Mandatory minimum sentences were affirmed. Incarcerated people increasingly served their time without any re-habilitative purpose. It was as if they existed in a parallel universe, their reality a shadow and programmed version of the world beyond prison walls.[21] In 1979, however, an inmate named Carlos Morales Feliciano and several of his peers sued the Puerto Rican government in federal court for doing nothing to address and even exasperating the adverse conditions prisoners endured. This type of case had developed through the years, since at least 1960, growing "as rivers grow—deeper, wider and with a crescendo of speed and noise as they approach the oceans."[22] Ultimately, the lawsuit obligated the state to take seriously the multifaceted well-being of incarcerated people.[23]

Through the 1980s, 1990s, and early twenty-first century, however, enclosure, security, and discipline again became the focal points of Puerto Rican (and broader global) corrections. Regardless of their political persuasion, consecutive administrations have only paid lip service to reform, rehabilitation, and harm reduction.[24] Nor has the founding of centralized, nonprofit correctional health-care services in the wake of the Morales Feliciano case improved medicine and preventive treatment for prisoners in a transformational way. Through the Morales Feliciano case, incarcerated Puerto Ricans deployed a legal strategy encompassing Puerto Rico's colonial status, the US and Puerto Rican constitutions, and the federal court system to obligate the commonwealth government to provide them with proper living conditions and health care. However, the state worked around its responsibilities in this regard, and prisoners remained entrapped by many of the same conditions against which they originally mobilized.[25] Art, film, and biographical and testimonial literature covering the post-rehabilitative era exhibits the capriciousness of modern Puerto Rican corrections in the health aspect.[26] Overcrowding and lack of medical services combined with shortages in basic equipment, the dilapidation of existing facilities, and poor nourishment to prolong carceral crises and devastate the living dead.[27] As Josué Montijo has remarked, Puerto Rican prisons became pressure cookers during this period, and then they exploded.[28]

Whereas the midcentury Puerto Rican state developed an interest in caring for prisoners, by the late twentieth century it had largely abandoned them. This structural indifference and weakness compelled prisoners to imagine and materialize their own well-being and security alternatives. Because the state could not protect them, they would have to protect themselves. Herein lie the roots of the Ñetas, an internally democratic prisoner rights association established in prisons like Oso Blanco in the late 1970s and early 1980s. The Ñetas were inspired by anti- and postcolonial intellectual currents and guided by a disciplined moral code that has since spread to other corners of the Hispanophone Atlantic world.[29] On the US mainland, however, they are often cast as a dangerous gang and persecuted for unsavory activities.

Oso Blanco finally closed in 2004, although some guards and prisoners stayed behind and served as groundskeepers for several more years. The story of these "leftovers" and the memory of the penitentiary were revived in a 2008 documentary film titled *Oso Blanco: Puerto Rico State Penitentiary*. The documentary focuses on the history of the institution since the 1970s and 1980s, when the Ñetas emerged, and follows in the footsteps of guards like César Flores and longtime prisoner Ángel L. Feliciano Hernández (known as Jíbaro). The film chronicles Jíbaro's story, the respectful relationship between Flores and Jíbaro, the latter phase of Jíbaro's rehabilitation, and his reunion with family members. In the end, it advocates for his release, which occurred in 2008.[30] The twin, not lopsided, problems of interpersonal and structural violence are prevalent throughout *Oso Blanco* and in the various forums that amplified Jíbaro's voice before his death in 2012.[31]

A few years later, in 2014, the Popular Democratic Party governor Alejandro García Padilla presented a scathing assessment of the Insular Penitentiary's history in his state of the commonwealth address. Like the 2008 documentary film, he cast Oso Blanco's history as irredeemably violent. García Padilla discussed the penitentiary's demolition, which had also started in 2014, as a socioeconomic investment: "The former prison, symbol of a time when people were afraid to leave their homes, will cease to exist, and in its place will be the City of Science. The symbols of confinement will give way to symbols of creation and creativity, of a search for life, employment—that is our debt to the future" and "the road forward."[32] As *Raising the Living Dead* has shown, however, when Oso Blanco officially opened in May 1933 it already formed part of a "City of Science," one undeniably shaped by US colonialism but more so by creole reformatory impulses. Oso Blanco was much more than a symbol of modernity and a center of raw hegemony and death. It also birthed complicated varieties of life, awakening, and consciousness.

Indeed, it is fallacious to portray Oso Blanco's history as one exclusively defined by violence. Its history was no doubt violent. That much is obvious. But it was also marked by imaginative problem solving in a society renegotiating its pluralistic identity within what many people at the time believed were more inclusive parameters. Oso Blanco was not just a site of difference-making, exploitative labor extraction, or any other number of terrible things. Complex knowledge production also unfolded in and near the prison and positioned many incarcerated people to heal, sharpen their civic swords, and empower themselves during a historical moment when colonial populists aimed to build a state that integrated large swathes of the dispossessed into a class in formation. Such insights are too easy to miss if one approaches the history of incarceration with tunnel vision. By default, one will emphasize social control, ideology from above, and the ineludibility of structures. *Raising the Living Dead* recognizes that these factors are crucial, but they are not enough for a well-rounded understanding of this history. To generate a nuanced picture of carcerality, we must also account for critical granular perspectives from the middle and below, and parallel and perpendicular to dominant discourses and practices.

The penitentiary system in Puerto Rico that took form in the Río Piedras sanitary city was not a peripheral product of the shaping of medical, psychiatric, and penal knowledge and practices, but rather an active, dynamic intersection between those circuits. The current epoch of mass incarceration and a more punitive prison system are in important ways a step back from the rehabilitative model of the 1930s to the 1960s, when the interacting and mutually malleable institutions of the sanitary city held center stage. Underscoring social control and romanticizing resistance enable us to only scratch the surface of this history. In mid-twentieth-century Puerto Rico, living death itself and the project of healing the "criminally infirm" encapsulated both control and resistance at once. Yet control and resistance themselves were polymorphous.

The constellation of redemptive logics and practices that permeated Puerto Rican prisons in the mid-twentieth century inclined but did not oblige incarcerated people to engage rehabilitative therapeutics. Colonial populism and populist dictatorship around the wider Caribbean responded unevenly to the health knowledges and claims making of prisoners and their communities. Living death could be overcome, or it could congeal. Rehabilitative corrections could restore convict bodies, minds, and spirits, but also accentuate what made them wretched and different. Incarcerated people creatively (re)defined rehabilitation on their own and in relational terms. They could raise themselves from their figurative graves or be uplifted by others, even within the architecture of a death-dealing state that was also, ironically, for a time committed to breathing new life into incarcerated people.

Acknowledgments

My interest in telling this story did not emerge after I entered graduate school or by chance. I did not discover it shooting the breeze with family and friends or theorizing with colleagues. It stems from a history hidden in plain sight, one well beyond my navel as much as it is about my navel. When I was a child, my father was arrested for several violent offenses, some of which I witnessed. In one fell swoop, he shattered my mother's and other family members' sense of security and well-being while finding himself on the receiving end of a crippling twenty-five-year sentence. And during those twenty-five years, like so many "at risk" New Jersey youths of my generation, I figured that the time would quickly come for me to either die sooner than expected or land in prison myself for an extended period.

If the numbers and those who traffic in them had their way, one of these two outcomes should have been the case. However, multiple people stepped in and contributed to piecing me back together. They helped cultivate my self-confidence and creativity, among other things, and taught me to accept that kin and community could be sources of both edification and destruction. I hope that in highlighting the experiences of incarcerated people, their complex relationships, and the variable ways in which they have attempted to work and live within and on the margins of a criminal-legal system not of their own making, the stories of people like my father and mother will be respected and understood within a narrative that affords them dignity and nuanced agency. The truth of the matter is they will continue to live and define their own stories regardless of what "experts" have to say about them.

In general, then, I and many of those in my immediate circumference have (in)directly carried this book since the triple stages of darkness, well in advance of it becoming a book published by a university press. Besides my father, Tito, my eldest siblings, Pito and Tita, have also spent considerable time behind bars, as well as other immediate family and some of my closest friends during my adolescence. None of them became political radicals, anti-structuralists, or absolutist moral relativists in the process, however. Rather, they have gone about trying to reconnect with their families and rebuild their lives as best they can. This has been the case with most people I know who have entered and exited prisons since the late 1980s and early 1990s. Why is so much energy expended on obscuring this pattern? That I pose this question at all should not be taken to suggest that incarceration is not literally or discursively violent, that prison conditions are not terrible, or that carcerality itself is not intimately linked to economic interests, exploitative structures, and the making of a hyper-surveilled world. Instead, the question should be a starting point for serious conversations about how incarceration is much more multidimensional and internally inconsistent from the ground up than we have perhaps cared to unpack up to this point.

Raising the Living Dead took initial form when I worked as a contract archivist at the General Archive of Puerto Rico in Puerta de Tierra, San Juan. There, I labored under the supervision of my dear friend Hilda M. Chicón Estrella and discovered many collections relevant to this and other projects. Oftentimes, Hilda and I worked alongside contract prisoners in the Gigante Verde (Green Giant) annex, where we had occasion to discuss some of the themes and frameworks that emerge in this book, one of which was to contemplate incarceration in as comprehensive a way as possible. After a bumpy first spell in graduate school and convinced that I would never go back, these experiences with incarcerated people, Hilda, and other beloved colleagues like the devoted María Isabel Rodríguez Matos, the indefatigable Pedro Roig Alvarado, and the steady José Charón Rivera inspired me to return to the ivory tower so that I could research incarceration further and shed light on the inconvenient truths at the core of how we understand carcerality and carceral history in our times.

I had the distinct honor of developing my early work on the history of incarceration in the Caribbean and Latin America at the University of Wisconsin–Madison. During my years there, few outside this supportive community believed in and encouraged my work. Nonetheless, my evenhanded mentors—Francisco Scarano, Steve Stern, Florencia Mallon, James Sweet, and Pablo Gómez—positioned me to persevere and achieve my degree. In the process, they revealed how caring and generous they are. Each of them continues to guide and support me in different ways, and I am grateful for their collegiality and friendship. Additionally, UW-Madison's spirited Latin American history program also shaped my work and the questions informing it from 2010 to 2017.

I would be remiss if I did not give my fellow travelers their due, particularly Carolyne Larson, Tamara Feinstein, Jessica Kirstein, Geneviève Dorais, Vikram Tamboli, Elena McGrath, Ingrid Bolívar Ramírez, Valeria Navarro Rosenblatt, Jeanne Essame, Jacob Blanc, and Bridgette Werner.

Upon graduating from UW-Madison, a series of fortunate events landed me at the University of Iowa, where Mariola Espinosa took me under her wing. Mariola and Lisa Heineman convinced the then dean Raúl Curto to put me on the tenure track, which allowed me to start carving out a space for myself in the academy. The ever-patient Mariola supervised me on the global health side of things but was also a mentor and model colleague and became my friend. Mariola was the final foundational stone—alongside Franco, Jim, and Pablo—in the formation of my "old-school" network as an early career scholar. Other colleagues have since embraced me and contributed to my academic growth in ways both large and small, including Diego Armus, Stephen T. Casper, Kristy Nabhan-Warren, Julia Rodríguez, Adam Warren, and Emilio Pantojas García. History of medicine colleagues have especially challenged my thinking and welcomed me with open arms. Meanwhile, Shennette Garrett-Scott, Ligia López López, and Sean Bloch continue to substantively engage me both academically and interpersonally when we have occasion to circle back to one another. I admire and appreciate them so much and only want to see them thrive. I will never be able to offer them enough flowers.

This book would have likely remained unwritten were it not for a Ford Foundation Postdoctoral Fellowship during the 2020–21 academic year. That pivotal year, I was a visiting researcher at the University of Puerto Rico–Río Piedras's Institute of Caribbean Studies, a dream come true for a kid born and raised in a forgotten corner of the Puerto Rican diaspora. Being a fellow gave me the time I needed to complete research and advance manuscript revisions, as well as to submit my book to the University of Chicago Press for review. The librarians Jeanmary Lugo González, Javier Almeyda Loucil, Yarelis Torres Vázquez, Ada Felicié Soto, Julio Mercado Ávila, and Mariam Feliciano García, among others, gracefully facilitated my research in the Puerto Rican Collection, the Monserrate Library, the Regional Library of the Caribbean and Latin American Studies, the *El Mundo* Project, and other collections on the UPR–Río Piedras campus. Emilio and my longtime mentor and friend Juan Giusti Cordero closely read drafts of my manuscript and gifted me precious comments and questions that have since helped me "complete" *Raising the Living Dead*. The successful parts of this book are attributable to readers like them.

In Karen Darling's expert hands, this book became a reality. I cannot say enough about her professionalism, transparency, and thoroughness. Karen's word is her bond, which there is not enough of in the academy these days.

I cannot thank Karen enough for believing in this project, and by extension Mariola, who put me into contact with Karen in the first place. The anonymous readers who sat with an earlier version of the manuscript and wrote prepublication reports for Chicago also deserve recognition. The book is much improved because of their critiques and insights. Tristan Bates, Anjali Anand, Deirdre Kennedy, Caterina MacLean, Katherine Faydash, and other Chicago colleagues shepherded me through the nuances and production phases of publication. This is no small feat. I am in awe of the behind-the-scenes work that goes into bringing a book like this to life.

Since I left Iowa and arrived at the University of Texas–Arlington, Scott Palmer and Stephanie Cole have offered me frank advice and steadfast support. The warmth of John Garrigus, Andrew Milson, Sarah Rose, and others have made my transition to Texas smooth and exciting. An American Philosophical Society Franklin Research Grant and a Library of Congress Kluge Center David B. Larson Fellowship allowed me to put the finishing touches on *Raising the Living Dead* and gave me the space and time to think through and pursue other projects. Whatever accolades I have achieved or that I may enjoy in the future are not my doing alone. They are a product and reflection of the different communities I have had the privilege of engaging since my earliest years in north Philadelphia and on Second and Elmer Streets and the Axtell housing project in Vineland, New Jersey, through the present. I can only hope—and in most cases I know for sure—that these communities and the people that constitute them accept this recognition. I am thankful for the Blue, Gibbs, Lang, and Morales families, the Pérez and Velásquez pastoral families, Trip Black and affiliated crews (who would say, "What's up with these day twos acting brand new?!"), Shakur Allah, Stephen Davis, Lisa Rosner, titi Ester, my sister Isamar and brother-in-law Byron (y ahora Marina!), the late Fernando Picó, Mauricio Tenorio Trillo, Eileen Suárez Findlay, Solsiree del Moral, Heather Erwin, my students over the years (incarcerated and traditional), and so many others who have somehow touched my life, career, and this work.

Through it all, the true and living God of the universe whose name is revealed to His children has been with me, even when, like Saul of Tarsus (Paul), I rejected and blasphemed against Him in my ignorance. The love of my life, Sherlie Ivonne, has been with me as well. Sherlie's "uncredentialed" knowledge and wisdom pervade *Raising the Living Dead*, for she has entertained many discussions about the ideas that bind the interpretive threads of this book. We have gone through countless challenges en route to publication. Yet amid the seemingly insurmountable, there have been victories and blessings, too, such as adding Ason Duke and Zeyda Lee to our clan.

I understand the deep intricacies of living death in my own life because of Sherlie. Que más puedo decirte mi amor, sino que te amo con todo mi ser. No tengo palabras suficientes, y te merece mucho más. Que privilegio es acompañarte en esta corta vida. Seguimos adelante porque en victoria estamos. De lo más vil el Señor Jesús escoge para glorificarse y deshacer la jactancia que el mundo tiene de sí mismo. Podemos testificarlo, y eso es lo clave. Me gozo en poder estar a tu lado en la senda hacia la perfección, apercibidos y reconociendo quién es el camino, la verdad, y la vida.

Notes

Preface

1. Equipo T[elemundo], "Yo era Alex Trujillo," *Telemundo Puerto Rico*, April 5, 2021, https://www.telemundopr.com/noticias/puerto-rico/equipo-t-yo-era-alex-trujillo-2/2198786/.

2. Equipo T, "Yo era Alex Trujillo."

3. Equipo T, "Yo era Alex Trujillo."

4. José Ayala Gordián, "Alex Trujillo quedó libre bajo palabra y permanecerá bajo supervisión hasta enero de 2024," *El Nuevo Día*, November 2, 2021, https://www.elnuevodia.com/noticias/tribunales/notas/alex-trujillo-quedo-libre-bajo-palabra-y-permanecera-bajo-supervision-hasta-enero-de-2024/.

5. Ernest Drucker, *A Plague of Prisons: The Epidemiology of Mass Incarceration in America* (New York: New Press, 2014).

6. Marisol LeBrón, "Puerto Rico, Colonialism, and the US Carceral State," *Modern American History* 2, no. 2 (July 2019): 170.

7. Christina Duffy Burnett and Burke Marshall, eds., *Foreign in a Domestic Sense: Puerto Rico, American Expansion, and the Constitution* (Durham, NC: Duke University Press, 2001); Sam Erman, *Almost Citizens: Puerto Rico, the US Constitution, and Empire* (New York: Cambridge University Press, 2019).

8. Gina M. Pérez, *The Near Northwest Side Story: Migration, Displacement, and Puerto Rican Families* (Berkeley: University of California Press, 2004); Carmen Teresa Whalen and Víctor Vázquez Hernández, eds., *The Puerto Rican Diaspora: Historical Perspectives* (Philadelphia: Temple University Press, 2005); Eileen J. Suárez Findlay, *We Are Left without a Father Here: Masculinity, Domesticity, and Migration in Postwar Puerto Rico* (Durham, NC: Duke University Press, 2014); Edwin Meléndez and Jennifer Hinojosa, *Estimates of Post-Hurricane Maria Exodus from Puerto Rico: Research Brief* (New York: Centro de Estudios Puertorriqueños, 2017).

9. The following works collectively touch on the most salient features of the history of race and status in Latin America and the Caribbean, and how the scholarship has evolved since the 1960s. Magnus Mörner, *Race Mixture in the History of Latin America* (Boston: Little, Brown, 1967); R. Douglas Cope, *The Limits of Racial Domination: Plebeian Society in Colonial Mexico City, 1660–1720* (Madison: University of Wisconsin Press, 1994); Matthew Restall, *The Black Middle: Africans, Mayas, and Spaniards in Colonial Yucatan* (Stanford, CA: Stanford University

Press, 2009); Joanne Rappaport, *The Disappearing Mestizo: Configuring Difference in the Colonial New Kingdom of Granada* (Durham, NC: Duke University Press, 2014).

10. Jalil Sued Badillo and Ángel López Cantos, *Puerto Rico negro* (1986; San Juan: Editorial Cultural, 2007); José Luis González, *Puerto Rico: The Four-Storeyed Country and Other Essays*, trans. Gerald Guinness (Princeton, NJ: Markus Wiener Publishers, 1993); Jay Kinsbruner, *Not of Pure Blood: The Free People of Color and Racial Prejudice in Nineteenth-Century Puerto Rico* (Durham, NC: Duke University Press, 1996); Ileana Rodríguez Silva, *Silencing Blackness: Disentangling Race, Colonial Regimes, and National Struggles in Post-Emancipation Puerto Rico, 1850–1920* (New York: Palgrave, 2012); María D. González García, *El negro y la negra libres, Puerto Rico: 1800–1873, su presencia y contribución a la identidad puertorriqueña* (San Juan: MGG Editorial, 2014); Else Zayas León, "La presencia de pardos en Toa Alta," in Gloria Tapia Ríos, ed., *Thoa Arriba, Toa Alta: Una Historia* (Toa Alta, PR: Ediciones Magna Cultura, 2021), 79–85.

11. María del Carmen Baerga, "Routes to Whiteness, or How to Scrub Out the Stain: Hegemonic Masculinity and Racialization in Nineteenth-Century Puerto Rico," *Translating the Americas* 3 (2015): 110.

12. Seymour Drescher and Stanley L. Engerman, eds., *A Historical Guide to World Slavery* (New York: Oxford University Press, 1998), 120. On how notions of place, regard for the spiritual welfare of the enslaved, different postemancipation attitudes towards African cultural retentions, and two sugar cycles (roughly one in the sixteenth century and the other in the nineteenth century) had far-reaching consequences in terms of economic diversity and in the ethnic composition of and on racial notions and relations in the Hispanic Caribbean territories, see Peter A. Roberts, *The Roots of Caribbean Identity: Language, Race and Ecology* (New York: Cambridge University Press, 2008), 264–347; Douglas Hall, "A population of free persons," in K. O. Laurence and Jorge Ibarra Cuesta, eds., *General History of the Caribbean*, vol. 4, *The Long Nineteenth Century: Nineteenth-Century Transformations* (London and Paris: Macmillan and UNESCO Publishing, 2011), 55–59; Pedro L. San Miguel, "Economic activities other than sugar: Part One The Agrarian Economies," in Laurence and Ibarra Cuesta, *General History of the Caribbean*, 4:105, 109–21.

13. My references to prison race statistics in this paragraph are drawn from *The Annual Reports of the Attorneys General to the Governors of Porto/Puerto Rico* for the years 1917–47 and 1954, and *The Annual Reports of the Secretary of Justice of Puerto Rico* for 1956–57. Most of these reports are cited in subsequent footnotes and in the bibliography, so I do not detail them here.

14. There is minimal carceral race data in justice reports for young people after 1945 because youth institutions were folded into the work of the Public Welfare Division that year. However, the "Institution for Youthful Offenders" is accounted for in the 1956 and 1957 annual Secretary of Justice reports, respectively. Awilda Palau de López and Ernesto Ruiz Ortiz, *En la calle estabas: La vida en una institución de menores* (Río Piedras, PR: Editorial Universitaria, Universidad de Puerto Rico, 1976), 21; Zenón Ortiz Colón, "La División de Bienestar Público del Departamento de Sanidad frente a la Escuela Industrial para Jóvenes en Mayagüez: Presente y perspectiva para un futuro inmediato," *Bienestar Público* 1, no. 3 (March 1946): 3, 6; Margarita Dapena de Llop, "Desarrollo histórico del programa institucional de la División de Bienestar Público," *Bienestar Público* 6, nos. 25–26 (July–December 1951): 26. Solsiree del Moral's manuscript "Street Children, Crime, and Punishment in Puerto Rico, 1940–1965," speaks to why youths of color were incarcerated at higher rates than adults of color in midcentury Puerto Rico.

15. "Población penal de Puerto Rico," *Mensuario de la División de Corrección* 2, no. 2 (March 1961): 1; Estado Libre Asociado de Puerto Rico, *Informes Estadísticos del Departamento de Justicia* for the years December 1960 to February 1966.

16. Mara Loveman and Jeronimo O. Muniz, "How Puerto Rico Became White: Boundary Dynamics and Intercensus Racial Reclassification," *American Sociological Review* 72, no. 6 (December 2007): 915–39.

17. Juan Flores, *From Bomba to Hip-Hop: Puerto Rican Culture and Latino Identity* (New York: Columbia University Press, 2000); Wakeel Allah, *In the Name of Allah*, vol. 1, *A History of Clarence 13X and the Five Percenters* (Atlanta: A-Team Publishing, 2009), 193–95. *The Problem Book* of the Five-Percent Nation of gods and earths discusses the "8-Pointed Cipher," or what Wakeel Allah refers to as the universal flag of Islam. The eight points are symbolic of eight foundational lessons. Each side has a black side and a gold side, making a total of sixteen sides. These represent the sixteen shades of black as far as skin complexion is concerned. Also consult Marisol LeBrón, *Policing Life and Death: Race, Violence, and Resistance in Puerto Rico* (Oakland: University of California Press, 2019); Ken Chitwood, "Los Musulmanes Boricuas: Puerto Rican Muslims and the Idea of Cosmopolitanism," PhD diss., University of Florida, 2019.

18. Kunlyna Tauch, "Life Inside: I Am Not Your 'Other,'" Marshall Project, July 9, 2020, https://www.themarshallproject.org/2020/07/09/i-am-not-your-other.

19. Fernando Picó, "La caducidad de la cárcel," *Revista del Colegio de Abogados de Puerto Rico* 60, no. 2 (April–June 1999): 12–15.

20. Jack Delano, *Puerto Rico mío: Cuatro décadas de cambio* (Washington, DC: Smithsonian Institution Press, 1990).

21. Nancy Scheper-Hughes, *Death without Weeping: The Violence of Everyday Life in Brazil* (Berkeley: University of California Press, 1993).

22. Angela Y. Davis, *Are Prisons Obsolete?* (New York: Seven Stories Press, 2003); Ruth Wilson Gilmore, *Golden Gulag: Prisons, Surplus, Crisis, and Opposition in Globalizing California* (Berkeley: University of California Press, 2007); Mariame Kaba, *We Do This 'Til We Free Us: Abolitionist Organizing and Transforming Justice* (Chicago: Haymarket, 2021); Victoria Law, *"Prisons Make Us Safer": And 20 Other Myths about Mass Incarceration* (Boston: Beacon, 2021); Derecka Purnell, *Becoming Abolitionists: Police, Protests, and the Pursuit of Freedom* (New York: Astra House, Penguin Random House, 2021).

23. Ben V. Olguín, *Violentologies: Violence, Identity, and Ideology in Latina/o Literature* (New York: Oxford University Press, 2021).

24. Dan Berger, Mariame Kaba, and David Stein, "What Abolitionists Do," *Jacobin*, August 24, 2017, https://jacobinmag.com/2017/08/prison-abolition-reform-mass-incarceration; Andy Douglas, *Redemption Songs: A Year in the Life of a Community Prison Choir* (San Germán, PR: Innerworld Publications, 2019).

25. William G. Martin and Joshua M. Price, eds., *After Prisons? Freedom, Decarceration, and Justice Disinvestment* (Lanham, MD: Lexington Books, 2016); Ruth Wilson Gilmore, *Abolition Geography: Essays Towards Liberation* (Brooklyn, NY: Verso, 2022).

Introduction

1. Erik Y. Rolón Suárez, "Puerto Rico's Prison Reforms Emphasize Rehabilitation," *Washington Examiner*, July 21, 2018, https://www.washingtonexaminer.com/opinion/op-eds/puerto-ricos-prison-reforms-emphasize-rehabilitation.

2. This bipartisan, federal legislation was signed into law in December 2018 by president Donald J. Trump. The act seeks to improve criminal justice outcomes, reduce the size of the federal prison population, and maintain public safety.

3. Rolón Suárez, "Puerto Rico's Prison Reforms Emphasize Rehabilitation."

4. Javier Colón Dávila, "Surgen aspirantes para vacante," *El Nuevo Día*, November 4, 2019. The board has colonial overtones. All its initial members were appointed by president Barack H. Obama. See Steven Mufson, "White House Names Seven to Puerto Rico Oversight Board," *Washington Post*, August 13, 2016, https://www.washingtonpost.com/business/economy/white -house-names-seven-to-puerto-rico-oversight-board/2016/08/31/9cee9376-6f8b-11e6-9705-2 3e51a2f424d_story.html.

5. Morales Feliciano spearheaded a class action lawsuit against the Puerto Rican government in 1979. The lawsuit claimed that the state was responsible for harmful conditions of incarceration, and that these conditions violated prisoners' constitutional rights. Feliciano v. Barcelo, 497 F. Supp. 14 (DPR 1979); Heidee Rolón Cintrón, "Aquí a los confinados nos tienen echando pipa," *El Nuevo Día*, October 11, 2019; Heidee Rolón Cintrón, "Denuncian pésimas condiciones en que viven los confinados," *El Nuevo Día*, October 12, 2019.

6. Michael Lapp, "The Rise and Fall of Puerto Rico as a Social Laboratory, 1945–1965," *Social Science History* 19, no. 2 (Summer 1995): 169–99; José Luis Méndez, *Las ciencias sociales y el proceso político puertorriqueño* (San Juan: Ediciones Puerto, 2005), 85–102, 149–202. In my article "Pathologizing the *Jíbaro*," I define "colonial populist" as a blended concept and practice of government that is inspired by policies and forms of politics that one might otherwise assume to be mutually exclusive. Many midcentury Puerto Rican populists (meaning those linked to the Partido Popular Democrático, or PPD) asserted to have a social justice–oriented vision and agenda, for example, but persecuted their competitors and political detractors in the mold of colonial-imperial powers. I use the term "populist" to underscore how the PPD appealed to and engaged ordinary people, while I also acknowledge that their political project developed within colonial constraints. This occurred against a backdrop of renewed political hostility between populists and radical nationalists, in particular. Alberto Ortiz Díaz, "Pathologizing the *Jíbaro*: Mental and Social Health in Puerto Rico's Oso Blanco (1930s to 1950s)," *The Americas* 77, no. 3 (July 2020): 415.

7. José G. Pérez, *Puerto Rico: US Colony in the Caribbean* (New York: Pathfinder Press, 1976); Pedro A. Cabán, *Constructing a Colonial People: Puerto Rico and the United States, 1898–1932* (Boulder, CO: Westview Press, 1999); César J. Ayala and Rafael Bernabe, *Puerto Rico in the American Century: A History since 1898* (Chapel Hill: University of North Carolina Press, 2007).

8. Kyle B. T. Lambelet, *¡Presente! Nonviolent Politics and the Resurrection of the Dead* (Washington, DC: Georgetown University Press, 2019).

9. An emphasis on the carceral state is especially prevalent in American Studies and US historiography. The Urban History Association's "Disciplining the City" series (2019–20) provides an excellent introduction to recent carceral history scholarship from a US perspective.

10. Nelson Miranda Sánchez, *El Jíbaro: Víctima o culpable del sistema correccional* (Naguabo, PR: Extreme Graphics, 2008), 6. In this text, the decay and stench of rehabilitation in the early 2000s and the importance of dedicated personnel to advancing rehabilitation are detailed in chapter 6.

11. Martín Ergui, "Puerto Rican Penitentiary," *Journal of Criminal Law and Criminology* 24, no. 6 (March–April 1934): 1119. A similar discourse concerning the relationship between incarceration and regeneration circulated in Brazil around the same time. See Mozart Vergetti de Menezes, "A Escola Correcional do Recife (1909–1929)," in Clarissa Nunes Maia, Flávio de Sá Neto, Marcos Costa, and Marcos Luiz Bretas, eds., *História das prisões no Brasil*, Vol. 2 (Rio de Janeiro: Editora Rocco, 2009), ch. 16.

12. The Spanish established La Princesa in 1837, but by the early twentieth century the facility had fallen into deterioration. *First Annual Report of Charles H. Allen, Governor of Porto Rico* (Washington, DC: Government Printing Office, 1901), 84, 406–7; *Second Annual Report of the Governor of Porto Rico* (Washington, DC: Government Printing Office, 1902), 66, 73–75, 316; María de los Ángeles Castro Arroyo, *Arquitectura en San Juan de Puerto Rico, siglo XIX* (San Juan: Editorial de la Universidad de Puerto Rico, 1980), 304; Edwin R. Quiles Rodríguez, *San Juan tras la fachada: Una mirada desde sus espacios ocultos, 1508–1900* (San Juan: Instituto de Cultura Puertorriqueña, 2003), 12; Pedro Malavet Vega, *El sistema de justicia criminal en Puerto Rico* (Ponce: Ediciones Lorena, 2005), 424.

13. Ricardo D. Salvatore and Carlos Aguirre, eds., *The Birth of the Penitentiary in Latin America: Essays on Criminology, Prison Reform, and Social Control, 1830–1940* (Austin: University of Texas Press, 1996).

14. Carlos Aguirre and Robert Buffington, eds., *Reconstructing Criminality in Latin America* (Wilmington, DE: Scholarly Resources Inc., 2000); Robert Buffington, *Criminal and Citizen in Modern Mexico* (Lincoln: University of Nebraska Press, 2000); Ricardo D. Salvatore, Carlos Aguirre, and Gilbert M. Joseph, eds., *Crime and Punishment in Latin America: Law and Society Since Late Colonial Times* (Durham, NC: Duke University Press, 2001); Peter Becker and Richard F. Wetzell, eds., *Criminals and Their Scientists: The History of Criminology in International Perspective* (New York: Cambridge University Press, 2006); Gerardo González Ascencio, *Los orígenes de la criminología en México: La recepción del positivismo y los gabinetes antropométricos en las cárceles de la Ciudad de México, 1867–1910* (Saarbrücken, Germany: Editorial Académica Española, 2012); Salvatore and Aguirre, *Birth of the Penitentiary in Latin America*, xvi.

15. Studies that focus on the prison-environment nexus, prison health care, and rehabilitative corrections are rare, but multiplying, albeit in a Western-centric way. Volker Janssen, "Convict Labor, Civic Welfare: Rehabilitation in California's Prisons, 1941–1971," PhD diss., University of California–San Diego, 2005; Michael Dow Burkhead, *The Treatment of Criminal Offenders: A History* (Jefferson, NC: McFarland, 2007); Margaret Lynn Charleroy, "Penitentiary Practice: Healthcare and Medicine in Minnesota State Prison, 1855–1930," PhD diss., University of Minnesota, 2013; Greg Eghigian, *The Corrigible and the Incorrigible: Science, Medicine, and the Convict in Twentieth-Century Germany* (Ann Arbor: University of Michigan Press, 2015); Raymond L. Gard, *Rehabilitation and Probation in England and Wales, 1876–1962* (London: Bloomsbury, 2016); Clair Dahm, "Community Corrections: The Rise and Fall of the Rehabilitative Ideal in Postwar St. Louis," PhD diss., Brandeis University, 2017; Clarence Jefferson Hall, Jr., *A Prison in the Woods: Environment and Incarceration in New York's North Country* (Amherst: University of Massachusetts Press, 2020); Ryan C. Edwards, *A Carceral Ecology: Ushuaia and the History of Landscape and Punishment in Argentina* (Oakland: University of California Press, 2021); Brad Stoddard, *Spiritual Entrepreneurs: Florida's Faith-Based Prisons and the American Carceral State* (Chapel Hill: University of North Carolina Press, 2021), 18–26.

16. Edward M. Peters, "Prison before the Prison: The Ancient and Medieval Worlds," in Norval Morris and David J. Rothman, eds., *The Oxford History of the Prison: The Practice of Punishment in Western Society* (New York: Oxford University Press, 1995), 3–43.

17. Benjamin David Weber, "America's Carceral Empire: Confinement, Punishment, and Work at Home and Abroad, 1865–1946," PhD diss., Harvard University, 2017; Dario Melossi and Massimo Pavarini, *The Prison and the Factory: Origins of the Penitentiary System* (Basingstoke, UK: Palgrave Macmillan, 2018).

18. Michael S. Hindus, *Prison and Plantation: Crime, Justice, and Authority in Massachusetts and South Carolina, 1767–1878* (Chapel Hill: University of North Carolina Press, 1980); Diana

Paton, *No Bond but the Law: Punishment, Race, and Gender in Jamaican State Formation, 1780–1870* (Durham, NC: Duke University Press, 2004); Reynaldo Ortiz-Minaya, "From Plantation to Prison: Visual Economies of Slave Resistance, Criminal Justice, and Penal Exile in the Spanish Caribbean (1820–1886)," PhD diss., State University of New York-Binghamton, 2014; Kelly Lytle Hernández, *City of Inmates: Conquest, Rebellion, and the Rise of Human Caging in Los Angeles, 1771–1965* (Chapel Hill: University of North Carolina Press, 2017); Dawn P. Harris, *Punishing the Black Body: Marking Social and Racial Structures in Barbados and Jamaica* (Athens, GA: University of Georgia Press, 2017).

19. Alex Lichtenstein, *Twice the Work of Free Labor: The Political Economy of Convict Labor in the New South* (New York: Verso, 1996); David M. Oshinsky, *"Worse Than Slavery": Parchman Farm and the Ordeal of Jim Crow Justice* (New York: Free Press, 1997); Douglas A. Blackmon, *Slavery by Another Name: The Re-Enslavement of Black Americans from the Civil War to World War II* (New York: Random House, 2008); Michelle Alexander, *The New Jim Crow: Mass Incarceration in the Age of Colorblindness* (New York: New Press, 2010); Cecilia A. Green, "Local Geographies of Crime and Punishment in a Plantation Colony: Gender and Incarceration in Barbados, 1878–1928," *New West Indian Guide* 86, nos. 3–4 (2012): 263–90; Dennis Childs, *Slaves of the State: Black Incarceration from the Chain Gang to the Penitentiary* (Minneapolis: University of Minnesota Press, 2015); Talitha LeFlouria, *Chained in Silence: Black Women and Convict Labor in the New South* (Chapel Hill: University of North Carolina Press, 2015); Robert T. Chase, *We Are Not Slaves: State Violence, Coerced Labor, and Prisoners' Rights in Postwar America* (Chapel Hill: University of North Carolina Press, 2020).

20. Michel Foucault, *Discipline and Punish: The Birth of the Prison*, trans. Alan Sheridan (1975; New York: Vintage, 1995).

21. Cesare Beccaria, *On Crimes and Punishments and Other Writings*, ed. Jeremy Parzen and Aaron Thomas (Toronto: University of Toronto Press, 2006); Stoddard, *Spiritual Entrepreneurs*, 19.

22. Miriam Williford, *Jeremy Bentham on Spanish America: An Account of his Letters and Proposals to the New World* (Baton Rouge: Louisiana State University Press, 1980); Anna Vemer Andrzejewski, *Building Power: Architecture and Surveillance in Victorian America* (Knoxville: University of Tennessee Press, 2008); Jeremy Bentham, *Panopticon, or, The Inspection House* (1791; Whithorn, UK: Anodos Books, 2017).

23. Michel Foucault, *Madness and Civilization: A History of Insanity in the Age of Reason*, trans. Richard Howard (1965; New York: Vintage, 1988); Michel Foucault, *The Birth of the Clinic: An Archeology of Medical Perception*, trans. A. M. Sheridan Smith (1973; New York: Vintage, 1994); Foucault, *Discipline and Punish*.

24. Alberto Ortiz, "Redeeming Bodies and Souls: Penitentiary Science and Spirituality in Twentieth-Century Puerto Rico and the Dominican Republic," PhD diss., University of Wisconsin–Madison, 2017, 86. Also see the Bennett, Parsons, and Frost case file at the Archivo de Arquitectura y Construcción de la Universidad de Puerto Rico. A similar emphasis on how carceral institutions or spaces are often enveloped in contexts of movement and openness, rather than total enclosure or isolation, is developed in Clare Anderson, ed., *A Global History of Convicts and Penal Colonies* (London: Bloomsbury, 2018), 9, 22; Edwards, *A Carceral Ecology*. On "total institutions," see Erving Goffman, "On the Characteristics of Total Institutions," in *Asylums: Essays on the Social Situation of Mental Patients and Other Inmates* (New York: Anchor, 1961), 1–124.

25. David Garland, *Punishment and Modern Society: A Study in Social Theory* (Chicago: University of Chicago Press, 1990); Philip Smith, *Punishment and Culture* (Chicago: University

of Chicago Press, 2008); Michael Welch, *Escape to Prison: Penal Tourism and the Pull of Punishment* (Oakland: University of California Press, 2015), 9–16.

26. Mary Gibson, "Global Perspectives on the Birth of the Prison," *American Historical Review* 116, no. 4 (October 2011): 1040–63; Mary Gibson, *Italian Prisons in the Age of Positivism, 1861–1914* (London: Bloomsbury, 2019); Edwards, *A Carceral Ecology*, 10.

27. Gibson, *Italian Prisons in the Age of Positivism*.

28. Or what came to be known as the Auburn and Pennsylvania systems. Stoddard, *Spiritual Entrepreneurs*, 20. The reformatory ideology put in motion by the Elmira system in New York, which centered individualization and civic regeneration through industrial work, classification, treatment, and aftercare, among other components, was just as consequential in the late nineteenth century and into the twentieth. Ricardo D. Salvatore and Carlos Aguirre, "The Birth of the Penitentiary in Latin America: Toward an Interpretive Social History of Prisons," in *The Birth of the Penitentiary in Latin America: Essays on Criminology, Prison Reform, and Social Control, 1830–1940 (Austin: University of Texas Press, 1996)*, 6–7, 10, 17, 27. For a critical interpretation of Elmira, see Alexander W. Pisciotta, *Benevolent Repression: Social Control and the American Reformatory-Prison Movement* (New York: New York University Press, 1994).

29. Salvatore and Aguirre, *Birth of the Penitentiary in Latin America*, xi, xvi–xviii.

30. Carlos Aguirre, *The Criminals of Lima and Their Worlds: The Prison Experience, 1850–1935* (Durham, NC: Duke University Press, 2005).

31. Fernando Salla, *As prisões de São Paulo, 1822–1940* (São Paulo: Annablume, 1999); Pablo Piccato, *City of Suspects: Crime in Mexico City, 1900–1931* (Durham, NC: Duke University Press 2001), ch. 8; Amy Chazkel, "Social Life and Civic Education in the Rio de Janeiro City Jail," *Journal of Social History* 42, no. 3 (Spring 2009): 697–731; Clarissa Nunes Maia, Flávio de Sá Neto, Marcos Costa, and Marcos Luiz Bretas, eds., *História das prisões no Brasil*, 2 Vols. (Rio de Janeiro: Editora Rocco, 2009); Lila M. Caimari, "Remembering Freedom: Life as Seen from the Prison Cell (Buenos Aires Province, 1930–1950)," in Salvatore, Aguirre, and Joseph, *Crime and Punishment in Latin America: Law and Society since Late Colonial Times* (Durham, NC: Duke University Press, 2001), 391–414.

32. Luz E. Huertas, Bonnie Lucero, and Gregory J. Swedburg, eds., *Voices of Crime: Constructing and Contesting Social Control in Modern Latin America* (Tucson: University of Arizona Press, 2016).

33. David Garland, *Punishment and Welfare: A History of Penal Strategies* (Aldershot, UK: Gower, 1985); Stoddard, *Spiritual Entrepreneurs*, 21–22.

34. A notable exception is Kelvin Santiago-Valles, "'Bloody Legislations,' 'Entombment,' and Race Making in the Spanish Atlantic: Differentiated Spaces of General(ized) Confinement in Spain and Puerto Rico, 1750–1840," *Radical History Review* 96 (Fall 2006): 33–57.

35. Blanca G. Silvestrini, *Violencia y criminalidad en Puerto Rico, 1898–1973: Apuntes para un estudio de historia social* (Río Piedras, PR: Editorial Universitaria, Universidad de Puerto Rico, 1980); Fernando Picó, "Esclavos y convictos: Esclavos de Cuba y Puerto Rico en el presidio de Puerto Rico en el siglo XIX," in *Al filo del poder: Subalternos y dominantes en Puerto Rico, 1739–1910* (San Juan: Editorial de la Universidad de Puerto Rico, 1996), 115–32; Kelvin Santiago-Valles, *"Subject People" and Colonial Discourses: Economic Transformation and Social Disorder in Puerto Rico, 1898–1947* (Albany: State University of New York Press, 1994); Ché Paralitici, *Sentencia impuesta: 100 años de encarcelamientos por la independencia de Puerto Rico* (San Juan: Ediciones Puerto, 2004); Nahomi Galindo-Malavé, "Cuerpos truculentos y 'desviados': Las confinadas de la Escuela Industrial para Mujeres de Vega Alta," *Identidades* 8 (November 2010): 11–34; Suset L.

Laboy Pérez, "Minor Problems: Juvenile Delinquents and the Construction of a Puerto Rican Subject, 1880–1938," PhD diss., University of Pittsburgh, 2014; José Lee Borges, *Los chinos en Puerto Rico* (San Juan: Ediciones Callejón, 2015), ch. 3; Heriberto Marín Torres, *Eran ellos* (San Juan: Editorial Patria, 2018); Josefina V. Tejada Vega, *Vagos, desertores y presos políticos en el Presidio Provincial de Puerto Rico, siglo XIX* (Las Vegas, NV: Ediciones Nóema, 2021).

36. Del Moral, "Street Children, Crime, and Punishment in Puerto Rico, 1940–1965."

37. Salvatore and Aguirre, "The Birth of the Penitentiary in Latin America," 9–15.

38. Col. J. Bascom Jones, *Livre bleu d'Haïti* (New York: Klebold Press, 1919), 45; Rogerio Zayas Bazán, *El Presidio Modelo* (Havana: n.p., 1928); José E. Embade Neyra, *El gran suicida (apuntes de una época revolucionaria): Obra escrita en el Presidio Modelo* (Havana: Imp. y Lib. "La Propagandista," 1934), 19–34; Pablo de la Torriente Brau, *Presidio Modelo* (Havana: Instituto del Libro, Editorial de Ciencias Sociales, 1969); Nancy D. Arnison, *Health Conditions in Haiti's Prisons* (Boston: Physicians for Human Rights, 1992), 6; Bernardo Vega, "Juan Bosch narra sobre su experiencia en una prisión en 1934," *Hoy*, July 16, 2007, https://hoy.com.do/juan-bosch-narra -sobre-su-experiencia-en-una-prision-en-1934/; Alejandro Paulino Ramos, "Los centros de torturas de la dictadura de Trujillo: La cárcel de Nigua," *Acento*, January 20, 2018, https://acento.com.do /politica/los-centros-torturas-la-dictadura-trujillo-la-carcel-nigua-2-8528544.html.

39. Rufus Hardy, "The Canal Zone Penitentiary," *Prison World* 8, no. 2 (March–April 1946): 4–5, 30.

40. See, e.g., T. S. Simey, *Principles of Prison Reform: Development and Welfare in the West Indies, Bulletin No. 10* (Bridgetown, Barbados: n.p., 1944); S. G. Benson (Trinidad and Tobago Prisons Department), *Administration Report of the Superintendent for the Year 1949* (Port of Spain: Government Printer, 1951); S. G. Benson (Trinidad and Tobago Prisons Department), *Administration Report of the Superintendent of Prisons for the Year 1950* (British West Indies: Government Printing Office, 1952); Sub-Committee of the Howard League of Jamaica, *The After-Care of Discharged Prisoners in Jamaica* (Kingston: Farquharson Institute of Public Affairs, 1968).

41. Lila M. Caimari, "Psychiatrists, Criminals, and Bureaucrats: The Production of Scientific Biographies in the Argentine Penitentiary System," in Mariano Plotkin, ed., *Argentina on the Couch: Psychiatry, State, and Society, 1880 to the Present* (Albuquerque: University of New Mexico Press, 2003), ch. 4; Lila M. Caimari, *Apenas un delincuente: Crimen, castigo y cultura en la Argentina, 1880–1955* (Buenos Aires: Siglo Veintiuno Editores, 2004); Julia Rodríguez, *Civilizing Argentina: Science, Medicine, and the Modern State* (Chapel Hill: University of North Carolina Press, 2006), ch. 7.

42. Lila M. Caimari, "Whose Criminals Are These? Church, State, and Patronatos and the Rehabilitation of Female Convicts (Buenos Aires, 1890–1940)," *The Americas* 54, no. 2 (October 1997): 185–208.

43. Aguirre, *Criminals of Lima and Their Worlds*, 1, 4.

44. Sidney Mintz's meditation on resistance in the history of enslavement remains evocative and captures what I am trying to say here. Limiting oneself to the study of violence, resistance, or other "natural-fit" frameworks in the history of incarceration averts our eyes from the fact that most life then, like most life now, was spent living. See Sidney Mintz, "Slave Life on Caribbean Sugar Plantations: Some Unanswered Questions," in Stephan Palmié, ed., *Slave Cultures and the Cultures of Slavery* (Knoxville: University of Tennessee Press, 1995), 13.

45. See, e.g., Jennifer L. Lambe, *Madhouse: Psychiatry and Politics in Cuban History* (Chapel Hill: University of North Carolina Press, 2017); Claire E. Edington, *Beyond the Asylum: Mental Illness in French Colonial Vietnam* (Ithaca, NY: Cornell University Press, 2019); Adria L. Imada,

An Archive of Skin, An Archive of Kin: Disability and Life-Making during Medical Incarceration (Oakland: University of California Press, 2022).

46. Mariola Espinosa, *Epidemic Invasions: Yellow Fever and the Limits of Cuban Independence, 1878–1930* (Chicago: University of Chicago Press, 2009); James Sweet, *Domingos Álvares, African Healing, and the Intellectual History of the Atlantic World* (Chapel Hill: University of North Carolina Press, 2011); Thomas Cole, Nathan Carlin, and Ronald Carson, *Medical Humanities: An Introduction* (New York: Cambridge University Press, 2015); Pablo Gómez, *The Experiential Caribbean: Creating Knowledge and Healing in the Early Modern Atlantic* (Chapel Hill: University of North Carolina Press, 2017). A more comprehensive sample of this dynamic, growing scholarship across temporalities is in Diego Armus and Pablo Gómez, eds., *The Gray Zones of Medicine: Healers and History in Latin America* (Pittsburgh, PA: University of Pittsburgh Press, 2021), 211–13nn6–9.

47. The "gray zones of medicine," meaning the interstitial, fluid spaces between official and unofficial medicine. Michel Foucault, "Panopticism" from *Discipline and Punish: The Birth of the Prison*, in *Race/Ethnicity: Multidisciplinary Global Contexts* 2, no. 1 (Autumn 2008): 8; Armus and Gómez, *Gray Zones of Medicine*, 3–10.

48. Sonja M. Kim, *Imperatives of Care: Women and Medicine in Colonial Korea* (Honolulu: University of Hawai'i Press, 2019); Anne-Emanuelle Birn and Raúl Necochea López, eds., *Peripheral Nerve: Health and Medicine in Cold War Latin America* (Durham, NC: Duke University Press, 2020); Imada, *Archive of Skin, Archive of Kin*, 8–10.

49. 1 Corinthians 15 (Reina-Valera 1960); Jan Assmann, "Resurrection in Ancient Egypt," in Ted Peters, Robert John Russell, and Michael Welker, eds., *Resurrection: Theological and Scientific Assessments* (Grand Rapids, MI: William B. Eerdmans Publishing, 2002), 124–35; Jane Gilbert, *Living Death in Medieval French and English Literature* (New York: Cambridge University Press, 2014); Sarah Juliet Lauro, *The Transatlantic Zombie: Slavery, Rebellion, and Living Death* (New Brunswick, NJ: Rutgers University Press, 2015).

50. Thomas Mathews, *Puerto Rican Politics and the New Deal* (Gainesville: University Press of Florida, 1960); Emilio Pantojas-García, "Puerto Rican Populism Revisited: The PPD during the 1940s," *Journal of Latin American Studies* 21, no. 3 (October 1989): 521–57; Manuel Rodríguez, *A New Deal for the Tropics: Puerto Rico during the Depression Era* (Princeton, NJ: Markus Wiener, 2010); Geoff G. Burrows, "The New Deal in Puerto Rico: Public Works, Public Health, and the Puerto Rico Reconstruction Administration, 1935–1955," PhD diss., Graduate Center, City University of New York, 2014.

51. Orlando Patterson, *Slavery and Social Death: A Comparative Study* (Cambridge, MA: Harvard University Press, 1982); Assman, "Resurrection in Ancient Egypt"; Gilbert, *Living Death in Medieval French and English Literature*; Lauro; *The Transatlantic Zombie*. On living death and Caribbean storytelling, see Lorenzo Araujo, *Muertos que viven: Cuentos con refranes, decires, creencias, y costumbres del alto sur de la República Dominicana* (Bloomington, IN: Palibrio, 2013).

52. Nicola Harrington, *Living with the Dead: Ancestor Worship and Mortuary Ritual in Ancient Egypt* (Oakville, CT: Oxbow Books, 2013).

53. Patrick J. Greary, *Living with the Dead in the Middle Ages* (Ithaca, NY: Cornell University Press, 1994).

54. Claude Lecouteux, *The Return of the Dead: Ghosts, Ancestors, and the Transparent Veil of the Pagan Mind* (Rochester, VT: Inner Traditions, 2009).

55. Gilbert, *Living Death in Medieval French and English Literature*.

56. James B. Twitchell, *The Living Dead: A Study of the Vampire in Romantic Literature* (1981; Durham, NC: Duke University Press, 1997).

57. Mimi Sheller, *Consuming the Caribbean: From Arawaks to Zombies* (London: Routledge, 2003), ch. 5; Lauro, *Transatlantic Zombie*.

58. Vincent Brown, *The Reaper's Garden: Death and Power in the World of Atlantic Slavery* (Cambridge, MA: Harvard University Press, 2010), 4–5.

59. Lauro, *Transatlantic Zombie*.

60. Among others, see Blair Niles, *Condemned to Devil's Island: The Biography of an Unknown Convict* (New York: Harcourt, Brace, and Co., 1928); William Clemens, dir., *Devil's Island* (Warner Brothers, 1939); Lew Landers, dir., *I Was a Prisoner on Devil's Island* (Columbia Pictures, 1941); Christian Nyby, dir., *Hell on Devil's Island* (Regal Films, 20th Century Fox, 1957); Francis Lagrange, *Flag on Devil's Island: The Autobiography of One of the Great Counterfeiters and Art Forgers of Modern Times* (Garden City, NY: Doubleday, 1961).

61. Gordon Sinclair, *Loose among Devils: A Voyage from Devil's Island to Those Jungles of West Africa Labelled "the White Man's Grave"* (Toronto: Doubleday, Doran & Gundy, 1935).

62. Multiple reproductions of Sinclair's work appear this particular year. For example, see *Puerto Rico Ilustrado*, January 26, 1935, 4–5, 67; March 16, 1935, 4, 68; and June 1, 1935, 4.

63. René Belbenoît, *Dry Guillotine: Fifteen Years among the Living Dead* (New York: Blue Ribbon Books, 1938), 56–57, 67, 84, 127, 132, 140, 148, 203.

64. Belbenoît, 171–72.

65. Conrado Asenjo, ed., *Quién es quién en Puerto Rico*, 4th ed. (San Juan: Imprenta Venezuela, 1947), 39.

66. Carlos N. Carreras, "La vida tras las rejas: Una tarde con los 'muertos vivos,'" *Puerto Rico Ilustrado* 25, no. 1264 (May 26, 1934): 7.

67. Carreras, 8.

68. Carreras, 66.

69. Carreras, 66.

70. Lisa Guenther, *Solitary Confinement: Social Death and Its Afterlives* (Minneapolis: University of Minnesota Press, 2013).

71. Joseph-Achille Mbembe, *Necropolitics* (Durham, NC: Duke University Press, 2019).

72. Caleb Smith, *The Prison and the American Imagination* (New Haven, CT: Yale University Press, 2009).

73. Susan B. Carrafiello, *"The Tombs of the Living": Prisons and Prison Reform in Liberal Italy* (New York: Peter Lang Publishing, 1998).

74. Frank Dikötter, *Crime, Punishment, and the Prison in Modern China* (New York: Columbia University Press, 2002), 173.

75. As Dostoyevsky would put it, the "glorious moment" of being resurrected from living death. See Fyodor Dostoyevsky, *The House of the Dead*, trans. Constance Garnett (Mineola, NY: Dover, 2004), 247.

76. Francisco A. Scarano, "In a Sea of Colonial Cane: Caribbean History as Autobiography," 4–5, unpublished paper delivered at "Caribbean Pasts, Presents, and Futures: An Interdisciplinary Conference in Honor of Francisco Scarano," University of Wisconsin–Madison, April 13, 2019. Also see Francisco Scarano, *Sugar and Slavery in Puerto Rico: The Plantation Economy of Ponce, 1800–1850* (Madison: University of Wisconsin Press, 1984); Fernando Picó, *Los gallos peleados* (1983; Río Piedras, PR: Ediciones Huracán, 2003); Fernando Picó, *Libertad y servidumbre en el Puerto Rico del siglo XIX: Los jornaleros utuadeños en vísperas del auge del café* (Río Piedras, PR: Ediciones Huracán, 1983); Picó, *Al filo del poder*.

77. Fernando Picó, *El día menos pensado: Historia de los presidiarios en Puerto Rico, 1793–1993* (Río Piedras, PR: Ediciones Huracán, 1994).

78. See, for instance, Gayatri Chakravorty Spivak's classic essay, "Can the Subaltern Speak?," in Cary Nelson and Lawrence Grossberg, eds., *Marxism and the Interpretation of Culture* (Urbana: University of Illinois Press, 1988), 271–313.

79. Deborah A. Thomas, "Caribbean Studies, Archive Building, and the Problem of Violence," *Small Axe* 17, no. 2 (July 2013): 27–42; Jeannette A. Bastian, John A. Aarons, and Stanley H. Griffin, "Introduction: Decolonizing the Caribbean Record," in Jeannette A. Bastian, John A. Aarons, and Stanley H. Griffin, eds., *Decolonizing the Caribbean Record: An Archives Reader* (Sacramento, CA: Litwin Books, 2018), 2.

80. Natalie Zemon Davis, *Fiction in the Archives: Pardon Tales and Their Tellers in Sixteenth-Century France* (Stanford, CA: Stanford University Press, 1987). Also see Kathryn Burns, *Into the Archive: Writing and Power in Colonial Peru* (Durham, NC: Duke University Press, 2010).

81. Michel-Rolph Trouillot, *Silencing the Past: Power and the Production of History* (Boston: Beacon, 1995).

82. Ann Laura Stoler, *Along the Archival Grain: Epistemic Anxieties and Colonial Common Sense* (2008; Princeton, NJ: Princeton University Press, 2010).

83. Marisa J. Fuentes, *Dispossessed Lives: Enslaved Women, Violence, and the Archive* (Philadelphia: University of Pennsylvania Press, 2016).

84. Jorell A. Meléndez Badillo, *The Lettered Barriada: Workers, Archival Power, and the Politics of Knowledge in Puerto Rico* (Durham, NC: Duke University Press, 2021); LeBrón, *Policing Life and Death*; Suárez Findlay, *We Are Left without a Father Here*.

85. Lila M. Caimari, "The Archive's Moment," *Histories* 1 (July 2021): 102, 104.

86. Edington, *Beyond the Asylum*, 4–9, 16–18.

87. Imada, *Archive of Skin, Archive of Kin*, 10–20. Also see Ann Laura Stoler's classic *Carnal Knowledge and Imperial Power: Race and the Intimate in Colonial Rule* (2002; Berkeley: University of California Press, 2010).

88. Jan E. Goldstein, "Toward an Empirical History of Moral Thinking: The Case of Racial Theory in Mid-Nineteenth-Century France," *American Historical Review* 120, no. 1 (February 2015): 1–27.

89. I am working on a short piece about this dynamic tentatively titled, "Mi tío abuelo y 'el caso del machete': Family and Historical Memory in Puerto Rico and its Diaspora," forthcoming.

90. Kirsten Weld, *Paper Cadavers: The Archives of Dictatorship in Guatemala* (Durham, NC: Duke University Press, 2014).

91. Fernando Picó, "Por una historia en que la gente encuentre sus apellidos," in *Una historia de servicio*, by Universidad Interamericana de Puerto Rico (San Juan: Universidad Interamericana, 1979), 55–64.

92. Carlo Ginzburg, *The Cheese and the Worms: The Cosmos of a Sixteenth-Century Miller* (Baltimore: Johns Hopkins University Press, 1980); Sweet, *Domingos Álvares*.

93. Edington, *Beyond the Asylum*, 16–18.

94. Ángel Quintero Rivera, "La ideología populista y la institucionalización universitaria de las ciencias sociales," in Silvia Álvarez Curbelo and María Elena Rodríguez Castro, eds., *Del nacionalismo al populismo: Cultura y política en Puerto Rico* (Río Piedras, PR: Ediciones Huracán, 1993), 122–45.

95. It is worth noting, however, that the colonial-populist government aimed to uncover the political sensibilities of those who might work in the prison system, particularly guards. A

midcentury report on the politics of 90 prison guard candidates reveals that the overwhelming majority identified with the PPD, and fewer with the Puerto Rican Independence Party, Republicans, Socialists, Nationalists, and other groups combined. "Análisis de la información suministrada por la brigada de seguridad interna de la Policía Insular sobre 90 candidatos que figuran en el registro para guardias penales," Folder 645, "Penal Institutions," Caja 114, Fondo Oficina del Gobernador (hereafter FOG), Archivo General de Puerto Rico (hereafter AGPR). Throughout this book, I keep all major descriptive language for archives (e.g., boxes, record series, repositories) in the original Spanish to facilitate the research of others who might want to locate relevant materials.

96. On the timeline up to this point, see Manuel Camuñas, "Executive Departments of the Government of Porto Rico and Functions of Same," in Eugenio Fernández García, ed., *El libro de Puerto Rico* (San Juan: El Libro Azul Publishing, 1923), 165; Martín Ergui, "Penal Institutions and Reform School," 279; Francisco J. García Rodríguez, "Conformación y evolución de los sistemas administrativos de la cárcel de San Juan en la transición del régimen español al régimen estadounidense en Puerto Rico (1888 a 1910)," PhD diss., Centro de Estudios Avanzados de Puerto Rico y el Caribe, 2012; Naomi Galindo, "Decolonización de los espacios de reclusión," December 13, 2016, http://umbral.uprrp.edu/archivo-de-la-palabra/conferencia/jornada /segunda-jornada-de-reflexion-sobre-educacion-universitaria-en-la-carcel/de-colonizacion-de -los-espacios-de-reclusion/.

97. José Trías Monge, *El sistema judicial de Puerto Rico* (San Juan: Editorial de la Universidad de Puerto Rico, 1988), 93–147; "Amadeo urge cambio," *La Torre*, February 23, 1944, 1, 5.

98. Enrique Campos del Toro, *Report of the Attorney General of Puerto Rico, 1946* (San Juan: Administración General de Suministros, Oficina de Servicios, División de Imprenta, 1947), 36. Campos del Toro's vision for penal reform entailed individualized and technical approaches to the causes of crime and the "social miasma" of prisoners (56–66).

99. Luis Negrón Fernández, *Report of the Attorney General of Puerto Rico, 1947* (San Juan: Real Hermanos, 1950), 30.

100. Inmates engaged by the corporation in 1946–47 numbered nearly five thousand and received from five to thirty cents for each working day depending on the kind of labor performed. Negrón Fernández, *Report of the Attorney General of Puerto Rico, 1947*, 40.

101. Operation Bootstrap was a development policy in Puerto Rico after World War II. It achieved the rapid industrialization of the economy while diminishing agricultural production, triggering dislocation and massive emigration, and increasing economic dependence on the United States. The policy attracted industrial investments from the US mainland, especially, in exchange for corporate tax breaks and low labor costs, among other benefits. James L. Dietz, *Economic History of Puerto Rico: Institutional Change and Capitalist Development* (Princeton, NJ: Princeton University Press, 1986); Alex W. Maldonado, *Teodoro Moscoso and Puerto Rico's Operation Bootstrap* (Gainesville: University Press of Florida, 1997).

102. Frank Loveland, "Report on the Penal and Correctional Program of Puerto Rico," 5–6, 8–11, 17–27, Folder 645, "Penal Institutions," Caja 114, FOG, AGPR. The research for this multipart report was primarily carried out in 1944 but supplemented and analyzed through at least 1947. The final cumulative report was processed by Puerto Rico's executive secretary in 1949.

103. Cayetano Coll Cuchí, "Reforma penal en Puerto Rico," *Norte* 9, no. 9 (October 1949): 57, 71.

104. José Trías Monge, *Informe Anual del Secretario de Justicia para el año que terminó el 30 de junio de 1956* (San Juan: Departamento de Hacienda, Servicio de Compra y Suministro, División de Imprenta, 1961), 95; Picó, "La caducidad de la cárcel," 10, 12.

105. José Trías Monge, *Report of the Attorney General of Puerto Rico, 1954* (San Juan: Department of the Treasury, Purchase and Supply Service, Printing Division, 1958), 79, 98.

106. Juan B. Fernández Badillo, *Informe Anual del Secretario de Justicia para el año que terminó el 30 de junio de 1957* (San Juan: Departamento de Hacienda, Servicio de Compra y Suministro, División de Imprenta, 1959), 89–90. The work of the Penal Reform Committee, it seems, formed part of a larger government interest to investigate the operation and effectiveness of rehabilitation on criminals in the late 1950s. Muñoz Marín approached the University of Puerto Rico to collaborate in pursuing such a study, which was published in 1959. See Rosa Celeste Marín, Awilda Paláu de López, and Gloria P. Barbosa de Chardón, *La efectividad de la rehabilitación en los delincuentes de Puerto Rico* (San Juan: Universidad de Puerto Rico, 1959), xxv.

107. Picó, "La caducidad de la cárcel," 11.

108. Feliciano v. Barcelo, 497 F. Supp. 14 (DPR 1979). Also see Morales Feliciano v. Romero-Barcelo, 672 F. Supp. 591 (DPR 1986).

Chapter One

1. Sampayo López and others counterfeited $1 silver certificates, series 1928 A, serial no. 67418148A. The fraud network in which he participated extended from Santurce to Ponce. Expediente del confinado Juan Sampayo López, October 1935, Caja 302, Serie Expedientes de Confinados (hereafter SEC), Fondo Departamento de Justicia (hereafter FDJ), AGPR.

2. Physical examinations occurred during the penitentiary central booking or intake process, as stipulated in Justice Department (Charles E. Winter), *Reglamento para el régimen y gobierno de la Penitenciaría de Puerto Rico en Río Piedras* (San Juan: Negociado de Materiales, Imprenta y Transporte, 1933), 6. Also consult Ergui, "Penal Institutions and Reform School," in Fernández García, *El libro de Puerto Rico*, 279.

3. Asenjo, *Quién es quién en Puerto Rico*, 4th ed., 97.

4. Expediente del confinado Juan Sampayo López.

5. W. Essex Wynter, "Four Cases of Tubercular Meningitis in Which Paracentesis of the Theca Vertebralis Was Performed for the Relief of Fluid Pressure," *Lancet* 137, no. 3531 (May 2, 1891): 981–82; Heinrich Quincke, *Die Technik der Lumbalpunction* (Berlin: Urban & Schwarzenberg, 1902); Susan E. Lederer, *Subjected to Science: Human Experimentation in America Before the Second World War* (Baltimore: Johns Hopkins University Press, 1997), 62, 216; Melvin G. Alper, "Three Pioneers in the Early History of Neuroradiology: The Snyder Lecture," *Documenta Ophthalmologica* 98, no. 1 (1999): 29–49; Kalyan Bhattacharyya, "Walter Edward Dandy (1886–1946): The Epitome of Adroitness and Dexterity in Neurosurgery," *Neurology India* 66, no. 2 (March 1, 2018): 304–7; Marleide da Mota Gomes, "From the Wax Cast of Brain Ventricles (1508–9) by Leonardo da Vinci to Air Cast Ventriculography (1918) by Walter E. Dandy," *Neurologique* 176, no. 5 (May 2020): 393–96.

6. Claude Quétel, *History of Syphilis* (Cambridge: Polity, 1990); John Parascandola, *Sex, Sin, and Science: A History of Syphilis in America* (Westport, CT: Praeger, 2008); Tiadmin, "The Salvarsan Wars," *Proto Magazine* (Massachusetts General Hospital), May 3, 2010, https://protomag.com/infectious-disease/paul-ehrlich-and-the-salvarsan-wars/; John Frith, "Syphilis—Its Early History and Treatment Until Penicillin, and the Debate on Its Origins," *Journal of Military and Veterans' Health* 20, no. 4 (November 2012): 49–56; Mircea Tampa, I. Sarbu, C. Matei, V. Benea, and S. R. Georgescu, "Brief History of Syphilis," *Journal of Medicine and Life* 7, no. 1 (March 15, 2014): 4–10; Peera Hemarajata, "Revisiting the Great Imitator: The Origin and History of

Syphilis," American Society for Microbiology, June 17, 2019, https://asm.org/Articles/2019/June /Revisiting-the-Great-Imitator,-Part-I-The-Origin-a.

7. Sampayo López's inmate file does not explicitly refer to salvarsan. However, other prisoner case files do. For example, see Expediente del confinado Fernando Lassalle Concepción, June 1949, Caja 171, Serie Junta Libertad Bajo Palabra (hereafter SJLBP), FDJ, AGPR. Neo-salvarsan, a more water-soluble arsenic compound, was used as well until penicillin overtook both kinds of salvarsan in the late 1940s and early 1950s. Expediente del confinado Pedro Díaz Ortiz, December 1949, Caja 481, SEC, FDJ, AGPR. On the history of salvarsan, see J. E. Ross and M. Tomkins, "The British reception of salvarsan," *Journal of the History of Medicine and Allied Sciences* 52, no. 4 (October 1997): 398–423; K. J. Williams, "The Introduction of 'Chemotherapy' Using Arsphenamine—The First Magic Bullet," *Journal of the Royal Society of Medicine* 102, no. 8 (August 2009): 343–48; Lorenzo Zaffiri, Jared Gardner, and Luis H. Toledo-Pereyra, "History of Antibiotics: From Salvarsan to Cephalosporins," *Journal of Investigative Surgery* 25, no. 2 (April 2012): 67–77; Laurence Monnais, "From Colonial Medicines to Global Pharmaceuticals? The Introduction of Sulfa Drugs in French Vietnam," *East Asian Science, Technology, and Society: An International Journal* 3, nos. 2–3 (2009): 275–76, 278, 280.

8. Lezcano Prado was scheduled for deportation upon completing his sentence. Carreras, "La vida tras las rejas," 67.

9. Joan D. Koss, "Religion and Science Divinely Related: A Case History of Spiritism in Puerto Rico," *Caribbean Studies* 16, no. 1 (April 1976): 22–43; J. G. O'Shea, "'Two Minutes with Venus, Two Years with Mercury'—Mercury as an Antisyphilitic Chemotherapeutic Agent," *Journal of the Royal Society of Medicine* 83, no. 6 (June 1990): 392–95; Judit Forrai, "History of Different Therapeutics of Venereal Disease before the Discovery of Penicillin," in Neuza Satomi Sato, ed., *Syphilis: Recognition, Description, and Diagnosis* (Rijeka, Croatia: InTech, 2011), 37–58; Goretti Virgili López, *Guía medicinal y espiritual de plantas tropicales* (Barcelona, Spain: Angels Fortune Editions, 2017), 109–31; Frith, "Syphilis"; Tampa, Sarbu, Matei, Benea, and Georgescu, "Brief History of Syphilis."

10. Expediente del confinado Juan Sampayo López.

11. Arenal was the first woman to attend university in Spain. She published widely about charity, social problems and groups, and the prison experience in Spain and beyond. Concepción Arenal, *Cartas a los delincuentes* (La Coruña, Spain: Imp. del Hospicio, 1865); Concepción Arenal, *Estudios penitenciarios*, 2nd ed. (Madrid: Impr. de T. Fortanet, 1877); Concepción Arenal, *La cárcel llamada Modelo* (Madrid: Imp. T. Fortanet, 1877). The formulation, "Hate the sin and not the sinner," can be traced to a fifth-century letter written by St. Augustine and has since appeared in altered form in Mahatma Gandhi's 1929 autobiography.

12. Cándido R.M., "Primeras impresiones de un recluso: Segunda parte," *El Despertar* 1, no. 4 (August 1949): 21.

13. Elisa Speckman Guerra, "La identificación de criminales y los sistemas ideados por Alphonse Bertillon: Discursos y prácticas (Ciudad de México 1895-1913)," *Historia y grafía* 17 (2001): 99–129; Josh Ellenbogen, *Reasoned and Unreasoned Images: The Photography of Bertillon, Galton, and Marey* (University Park: Pennsylvania State University Press, 2012); Daniel Fessler, "El delito con rostro: Los comienzos de la identificación de delincuentes en Uruguay," *Passagens: Revista Internacional de História Política e Cultura Jurídica* 7, no. 1 (January–April 2015): 15–39.

14. Benjamín Nistal Moret, *Esclavos, prófugos y cimarrones: Puerto Rico, 1770-1870* (1984; San Juan: Editorial de la Universidad de Puerto Rico, 2004); Gerardo A. Carlo Altieri, *Justicia y gobierno: La Audiencia de Puerto Rico, 1831-1861* (Seville: Consejo Superior de Investigaciones

Científicas, Academia Puertorriqueña de la Historia, 2007), chs. 7–8; Alfred W. McCoy, *Policing America's Empire: The United States, the Philippines, and the Rise of the Surveillance State* (Madison: University of Wisconsin Press, 2009), 18, 30, 33; Kelvin Santiago-Valles, "American Penal Forms and Colonial Spanish Custodial-Regulatory Practices in Fin de Siècle Puerto Rico," in Alfred W. McCoy and Francisco A. Scarano, eds., *Colonial Crucible: Empire and the Making of the Modern American State* (Madison: University of Wisconsin Press, 2009), 87–94; Gerardo A. Carlo Altieri, *El sistema legal y los litigios de esclavos en Indias: Puerto Rico, siglo XIX* (Seville: Consejo Superior de Investigaciones Científicas, 2010); Santiago-Valles, "'Bloody Legislations,' 'Entombment,' and Race Making in the Spanish Atlantic."

15. Francisco del Valle Atiles, *El campesino puertorriqueño: Sus condiciones físicas, intelectuales y morales, causas que las determinan y medios para mejorarlas* (San Juan: Tip. de José González Font, 1887); Manuel Zeno Gandía, *La charca: Crónicas de un mundo enfermo* (Ponce: Est. Tip. de M. López, 1894); Félix Mejías, *De la crisis económica del 86 al año terrible del 87* (Río Piedras, PR: Ediciones Puerto, 1972); Carlos Vélez, Raquel Colón, and Hiram Arroyo, *Desde uncinariasis hasta estilos de vida: Crónicas de la educación para la salud en Puerto Rico* (San Juan: Delta, 1994), 7. Further elaboration of Puerto Rico's economic and social conditions during this period can be found in Salvador Brau, *Ensayos: Disquisiciones sociológicas* (Río Piedras, PR: Editorial Edil, 1972).

16. Lombroso opposed eighteenth-century Italian jurist Cesare Beccaria's emphasis on free will and instead argued that criminal behavior was determined by biological, psychological, and social factors. Like disease, criminals required examination, observation, and treatment. Lombroso's text *Criminal Man* circulated widely in Europe and was translated into multiple languages between 1876 and 1895. Cesare Lombroso, *Criminal Man*, ed. Mary Gibson and Nicole Hahn Rafter (Durham, NC: Duke University Press, 2006), 2–3, 6, 29, 350–51; Salvatore, Aguirre, and Joseph, *Crime and Punishment in Latin America,* xiv–xvi; Carlos Alberto Cunha Miranda, "A fatalidade biológica: A medição dos corpos, de Lombroso aos biotipologistas," in Nunes Maia et al., *História das prisões no Brasil,* 2:281.

17. As would later be the case with eugenics, the region's intellectuals and other stakeholders adapted criminal anthropology to local circumstances. Many of their studies used inmates of different kinds as evidentiary raw material. Salvatore, Aguirre, and Joseph, *Crime and Punishment in Latin America,* 192–94, 214, 243, 346–47, 392; Salvatore and Aguirre, "The Birth of the Penitentiary in Latin America," 7, 20–21.

18. Alejandra M. Bronfman, *Measures of Equality: Social Science, Citizenship, and Race in Cuba, 1902–1940* (Chapel Hill: University of North Carolina Press, 2004), chs. 1–2.

19. Rebecca J. Scott, *Slave Emancipation in Cuba: The Transition to Free Labor, 1860–1899* (Pittsburgh, PA: University of Pittsburgh Press, 2000), 124. Also see Fernando Ortiz, *Hampa afro-cubana: Los negros brujos, apuntes para un estudio de etnología criminal* (1906; Miami: Ediciones Universal, 1973); Armando García González and Consuelo Naranjo Orovio, "Antropología, 'raza' y población en Cuba en el último cuarto del siglo XIX," *Anuario de Estudios Americanos* 55, no. 1 (1998): 267–89; Reinaldo L. Román, *Governing Spirits: Religion, Miracles, and Spectacles in Cuba and Puerto Rico, 1898–1956* (Chapel Hill: University of North Carolina Press, 2009), 7–8, 13, 18–19, 82–106; Bronfman, *Measures of Equality,* 13, 28–34, 46, 52, 59–62.

20. Kelvin Santiago-Valles, "'Forcing Them to Work and Punishing Whoever Resisted': Servile Labor and Penal Servitude under Colonialism in Nineteenth-Century Puerto Rico," in Salvatore and Aguirre, *Birth of the Penitentiary in Latin America,* 133–35.

21. Román, *Governing Spirits,* 74.

22. Román, *Governing Spirits*, 225n93.

23. Eugenic science—a scientific and social theory that advocated "race improvement" through "better breeding"—offered an interpretive framework through which to rethink and reformulate race, gender, reproduction, and public health in a time of intensified searching and longing for national identities. Nancy Leys Stepan, *"The Hour of Eugenics": Race, Gender, and Nation in Latin America* (Ithaca, NY: Cornell University Press, 1996); Laura Briggs, *Reproducing Empire: Race, Sex, Science, and US Imperialism in Puerto Rico* (Berkeley: University of California Press, 2003); Alexandra M. Stern, *Eugenic Nation: Faults and Frontiers of Better Breeding in Modern America* (Chapel Hill: University of North Carolina Press, 2005).

24. Nicole Trujillo-Pagán, *Modern Colonization by Medical Intervention: US Medicine in Puerto Rico* (Chicago: Haymarket, 2014), 2, 9-10. The term *jíbaro* does not fully account for differences within Puerto Rico's rural population. On the cultural genesis of the *jíbaro*, see Francisco A. Scarano, "The Jíbaro Masquerade and the Subaltern Politics of Creole Identity Formation in Puerto Rico, 1745-1823," *American Historical Review* 101, no. 5 (December 1996): 1398-1431. On rural differentiation in Puerto Rico, see Picó, *Los gallos peleados*; Picó, *Libertad y servidumbre*. On incarcerated jíbaros, see Ortiz Díaz, "Pathologizing the *Jíbaro*."

25. Trujillo-Pagán, *Modern Colonization by Medical Intervention*, 3, 5, 11-16. For a window into the gospel-like role of tropical medicine, specifically, consult Raúl Mayo Santana, Annette B. Ramírez de Arellano, and José G. Rigau-Pérez, eds., *A Sojourn in Tropical Medicine: Francis W. O'Connor's Diary of a Porto Rican Trip, 1927* (San Juan: Editorial de la Universidad de Puerto Rico, 2008); Raúl Mayo Santana, Silvia E. Rabionet, and Ángel A. Román Franco, *Historia de la medicina tropical en Puerto Rico en el siglo XX* (San Juan: Ediciones Laberinto, 2022).

26. Román, *Governing Spirits*, 74.

27. Mathews, *Puerto Rican Politics and the New Deal*; Rodríguez, *New Deal for the Tropics*; Burrows, "New Deal in Puerto Rico."

28. This is not to suggest that biomedicine was not important before 1933. Physician Gerónimo Carreras, for example, served as a visiting physician in La Princesa penitentiary in the early 1920s. Gerónimo Carreras, "Board of Medical Examiners," in Fernández García, *El libro de Puerto Rico*, 259. Also see the biographies of doctors Diego Biascoechea, Arturo Cadilla Cadilla, César Domínguez, and Jacinto Zaratt in Conrado Asenjo, ed., *Quién es quién en Puerto Rico*, 3rd ed. (San Juan: Cantero Fernández and Co., 1942), 40, 50-51, 81, 229.

29. On these hospitals, see César Augusto Salcedo Chirinos, *Las negociaciones del arte de curar: Los orígenes de la regulación de las prácticas sanitarias en Puerto Rico, 1816-1846* (Lajas, PR: Editorial Akelarre, 2016).

30. Justice Department (Office of the Attorney General), *Special Report of the Attorney General of Porto Rico to the Governor of Porto Rico Concerning the Suppression of Vice and Prostitution in Connection with the Mobilization of the National Army at Camp Las Casas, February 1, 1919* (San Juan: Bureau of Supplies, Printing and Transportation, 1919).

31. Eileen J. Findlay briefly discusses the campaign from the vantage point of Ponce in *Imposing Decency: The Politics of Sexuality and Race in Puerto Rico, 1870-1920* (Durham, NC: Duke University Press, 2000).

32. Howard L. Kern, *Report of the Attorney General of Porto Rico, 1919* (Washington, DC: Government Printing Office, 1919), 636-45; Harry Fielding Reid and Stephen Taber, *The Porto Rico Earthquake of 1918: Report of the Earthquake Investigation Commission* (Washington, DC: Government Printing Office, 1919).

33. Kern, *Report of the Attorney General of Porto Rico, 1919*, 647-50.

34. While the remedy for hookworm was not specified, it is likely that prison health personnel built on the treatment model of the antianemia campaigns of the early twentieth century, which involved having patients ingest chenopodium or thymol, both of which were poisonous to the worms, and then take a dose of Epsom salts to expel the chemicals and dead worms. Physicians Bailey K. Ashford and Pedro Gutiérrez Igaravídez were key players in deciphering anemia in Puerto Rico at the turn of the twentieth century. On their wider efforts, see Bailey K. Ashford, *A Soldier in Science* (1934; San Juan: Editorial de la Universidad de Puerto Rico, 1998); Bailey K. Ashford and Pedro Gutiérrez Igaravídez (Puerto Rico Anemia Commission), *Uncinariasis en Puerto Rico, un problema médico y económico* (San Juan: Bureau of Supplies, 1916).

35. Kern, *Report of the Attorney General of Porto Rico, 1919*, 649.

36. Herbert P. Coats, *Report of the Attorney General of Porto Rico, 1923* (Washington, DC: Government Printing Office, 1925), 49.

37. Coats, 50.

38. The Catholic physician and later Puerto Rico Reconstruction Administration official Pablo Morales Otero examined blood, feces, and spinal fluid obtained from La Princesa penitentiary in 1925. He identified intestinal parasites as a major problem. The hookworm infection rate in the prison reached almost 50 percent, the highest rate for any welfare institution on the big island. More than 50 percent of prisoners also had syphilis. A few years later, Morales Otero discovered that some 40 percent of inmates still tested positive for hookworm. The syphilis rate dropped but teetered between 14 percent and 19 percent depending on diagnostic method. Pablo Morales Otero, "The Work of the Biological Laboratory of the Department of Health," *Porto Rico Health Review* 1, no. 3 (August 1925): 21–25; Horace M. Towner, *Twenty-Fifth Annual Report of the Governor of Porto Rico, for the Fiscal Year Ended June 30, 1925* (Washington, DC: Government Printing Office, 1926), 333, 359; Pablo Morales Otero, "The Work of the Biological Laboratory of the Department of Health," *Porto Rico Health Review* 2, no. 9 (March 1927): 10–16. Also consult Francisco Hernández, "The Insular Biological Laboratory," in Fernández García, *El libro de Puerto Rico*, 351.

39. George C. Butte, *Report of the Attorney General of Porto Rico, 1927* (San Juan: Bureau of Supplies, Printing, and Transportation, 1927), 17–18; James R. Beverley, *Report of the Attorney General of Porto Rico, 1928* (San Juan: Bureau of Supplies, Printing, and Transportation, 1929), 13; James R. Beverley, *Report of the Attorney General of Porto Rico, 1929* (San Juan: Bureau of Supplies, Printing, and Transportation, 1929–30), 18.

40. Expediente del confinado Luciano Ayala Ramos, December 1932, Caja 223, SEC, FDJ, AGPR. Also see the chest diagram in Expediente del confinado José Álvarez Natal, July 1931, Caja 223, SEC, FDJ, AGPR.

41. James R. Beverley, *Report of the Attorney General of Porto Rico, 1931* (San Juan: Bureau of Supplies, Printing, and Transportation, 1931–32), 14, 21.

42. Charles E. Winter, *Report of the Attorney General of Puerto Rico, 1932* (San Juan: Bureau of Supplies, Printing, and Transportation, 1932–33), 19; Charles E. Winter, *Report of the Attorney General of Puerto Rico, 1933* (San Juan: Negociado de Materiales, Imprenta, y Transporte, 1934), 12, 21, 23.

43. Winter, *Report of the Attorney General of Puerto Rico, 1933*, 17–18, 23–24.

44. Ángela Negrón Muñoz, "En la penitenciaría modelo," *Puerto Rico Ilustrado* 25, 1252 (March 3, 1934): 70.

45. Conrado Asenjo, ed., *Quién es quién en Puerto Rico* (San Juan: Real Hermanos, 1933), 35; "Fue inaugurada oficialmente la nueva Penitenciaría de Puerto Rico," *El Mundo*, May 16, 1933,

2; Ernesto J. Fonfrías Rivera, "Un magno festival para la inauguración del Presidio Insular," *La Correspondencia*, May 16, 1933, 1.

46. Víctor F.F., "Departamento médico: Impresiones y comentarios de un enfermero," *El Despertar* 2, no. 2 (May 1950): 21; Winter, *Reglamento para el régimen y gobierno de la Penitenciaría de Puerto Rico*, 12–13.

47. Mutual reinforcement went beyond the realms of health and medicine, too. Economic enterprise was just as important. According to Beverley, for example, the penitentiary bakery supplied bread to Puerto Rico's broader carceral archipelago: "the San Juan district jail, the Insane Asylum, the government Orphan Asylums of Santurce, the Tubercular Hospital, and the Leper Colony. The value of the bread made during the year was $20,040.42. The cost of bread to the Government is approximately half the amount which would have to be paid in the open market." Beverley, *Report of the Attorney General of Porto Rico, 1929*, 20; Winter, *Report of the Attorney General of Puerto Rico, 1933*, 16, 18.

48. "Fue inaugurada oficialmente la nueva Penitenciaría de Puerto Rico," 2, 11; Fonfrías Rivera, "Un magno festival," 1, 3. Toledo Márquez was also involved in penitentiary economics. He initiated and organized various industrial workshops in La Princesa and Oso Blanco. Conrado Asenjo, ed., *Quién es quién en Puerto Rico*, 2nd ed. (San Juan: Real Hermanos, 1936), 161.

49. Beverley, *Report of the Attorney General of Porto Rico, 1931*, 29; Winter, *Report of the Attorney General of Puerto Rico, 1932*, 25; Winter, *Report of the Attorney General of Puerto Rico, 1933*, 23.

50. Oscar Costa Mandry and Rafael Ángel Marín, "Study of an Outbreak of Diarrhea in a Convict Camp Near San Juan," *Porto Rico Review of Public Health and Tropical Medicine* 3, no. 8 (February 1928): 311–20.

51. Such work assignments created opportunities for drinking, escape, suicide, and other activities. See, e.g., Expediente del confinado Martín Acevedo Rosa, September 1933, Caja 284, SEC, FDJ, AGPR; Benigno Fernández García, *Report of the Attorney General of Puerto Rico, 1939* (San Juan: Justice Department, 1939–40), 28; "Investigan estado de embriaguez de presos," *El Universal*, December 12, 1947, 9; "Se ahorca en Justicia," *El Imparcial*, September 19, 1949, 3.

52. Winter, *Reglamento para el régimen y gobierno de la Penitenciaría de Puerto Rico*, 12.

53. Marín Torres, *Eran ellos*, 91, 138–39.

54. For example, in 1921 prisoners participated in combatting the bubonic plague. Nearly one hundred La Princesa prisoners fought the epidemic by cleaning cities. Allegedly, none of them contracted the disease. Salvador Mestre, *Report of the Attorney General of Porto Rico, 1921* (Washington, DC: Government Printing Office, 1923), 412, 422–23. After hurricane San Felipe II in September 1928, prisoners were put to work on an emergency basis around the big island. They rendered "prompt and efficient service under the control of prison guards and of the National Guard." Several prisoners from the Arecibo district jail were permitted to work without guards, observing excellent conduct. Beverley, *Report of the Attorney General of Porto Rico, 1929*, 18. Boys detained at the Industrial School in Mayagüez helped drain and clear lowlands to control malaria. Beverley, *Report of the Attorney General of Porto Rico, 1931*, 16. Similarly, in Trinidad and Tobago incarcerated boys were also deployed to combat malaria. Benson, *Administration Report, 1949*, 51.

55. Beverley, *Report of the Attorney General of Porto Rico, 1929*, 22; Beverley, *Report of the Attorney General of Porto Rico, 1930*, 16; Beverley, *Report of the Attorney General of Porto Rico, 1931*, 16; Winter, *Report of the Attorney General of Puerto Rico, 1932*, 14; Winter, *Report of the Attorney General of Puerto Rico, 1933*, 16.

56. Ernesto Quintero, "Different Aspects of the Venereal Diseases Control Work on the Health Department," *Boletín de la Asociación Médica de Puerto Rico* 33, no. 1 (January 1941): 23. Penicillin became available in the mid-1940s as well. J. D. Porterfield, "The Present Status of the Treatment of the Venereal Diseases with Penicillin," *Boletín de la Asociación Médica de Puerto Rico* 36, no. 11 (November 1944): 473–77; Pablo Morales Otero, "La penicilina: Su descubrimiento, purificación y acción terapéutica," *Boletín de la Asociación Médica de Puerto Rico* 37, no. 2 (February 1945): 45–49.

57. Benjamin J. Horton, *Report of the Attorney General of Puerto Rico, 1934* (San Juan: Negociado de Materiales, Imprenta y Transporte, 1934), 12; Negrón Fernández, *Report of the Attorney General of Puerto Rico, 1947*, 77.

58. Expediente del confinado Justino Pacheco Cintrón, March 1943, Caja 238, SEC, FDJ, AGPR; Expediente del confinado Carlos Feliciano González, August 1946, Caja 238, SEC, FDJ, AGPR.

59. Benjamin J. Horton, *Report of the Attorney General of Puerto Rico, 1935* (San Juan: Bureau of Supplies, Printing, and Transportation, 1935), 14, 23–24; Benigno Fernández García, *Report of the Attorney General of Puerto Rico, 1936* (San Juan: Bureau of Supplies, Printing, and Transportation, 1936), 22, 24; Benigno Fernández García, *Report of the Attorney General of Puerto Rico, 1937* (San Juan: Justice Department, 1937–38), 28, 35; Benigno Fernández García, *Report of the Attorney General of Puerto Rico, 1938* (San Juan: Justice Department, 1938–39), 26, 35–36; Fernández García, *Report of the Attorney General of Puerto Rico, 1939*, 26, 28, 35–36; George A. Malcolm, *Report of the Attorney General of Puerto Rico, 1940* (San Juan: Bureau of Supplies, Printing, and Transportation, 1940), 36, 45; George A. Malcolm, *Report of the Attorney General of Puerto Rico, 1941* (San Juan: Justice Department, 1941–42), 34, 51; George A. Malcolm, *Report of the Attorney General of Puerto Rico, 1942* (San Juan: Bureau of Supplies, Printing, and Transportation, 1942), 36, 38; Oscar Costa Mandry, *Apuntes para la historia de la medicina en Puerto Rico: Reseña histórica de las ciencias de la salud* (San Juan: Departamento de Salud, 1971), 107. In the Dominican Republic in the 1940s, incarcerated people received biomedical attention in a like manner. Legal and health officials documented malaria, influenza, and sexual infections as the most common infirmities among prisoners in 1945, for example. See Víctor Garrido, *Memoria 1945 Procuraduría General de la República* (Santiago, DR: Editorial El Diario, 1945), 88, 128, 375, 377, 380, 382, 385, 387, 390, 392–93, 395–96, 398, 401, 403–4, 406–7, 409, 412, 414–17, 419–20, 422–24, 426, 429; Luis F. Thomen, *Memoria 1945 Secretaría de Estado de Sanidad y Asistencia Pública* (Ciudad Trujillo, DR: Impresora Dominicana, 1947), 2:503, 512, 525, 542–43, 556, 568, 578. This was also the case in the British Caribbean. Medical officer Ernest Brazao reported more than seventy medical conditions among incarcerated youths in Trinidad and Tobago in 1952. By June 1953, adult prisoners there were affected by eczema, bronchitis, myositis, constipation, ulcers, tooth decay, gonorrhea, and tinea. An "unusually high percentage" suffered from gonorrhea on admission but were successfully treated. See E. D. Wall (Trinidad and Tobago Prisons Department), *Administration Report of the Superintendent of Prisons for the Year 1952* (Trinidad, British West Indies: Government Printing Office, 1953), 18, 35.

60. Deaths related to Puerto Rico's death penalty are not considered here, as it was abolished in 1929. The last execution occurred in 1927. Jacobo Córdoba Chirino, *Los que murieron en la horca: Historia del crimen, juicio y ajusticiamiento de los que en Puerto Rico murieron en la horca desde las Partidas Sediciosas a Pascual Ramos* (1954; San Juan: Editorial Cordillera, 2007); María del Carmen Baerga Santini, "History and the Contours of Meaning: The Abjection of Luisa Nevárez, First Woman Condemned to the Gallows in Puerto Rico, 1905," *Hispanic American Historical Review* 89, no. 4 (November 2009): 643–73.

61. Fernández García, *Report of the Attorney General of Puerto Rico, 1936*, 67.

62. Blanton Winship, *Thirty-Sixth Annual Report of the Governor of Puerto Rico* (San Juan: Bureau of Supplies, Printing, and Transportation, 1936), 42–43; Víctor F.F., "Departamento médico," 21.

63. Víctor Gutiérrez Franqui, *Report of the Attorney General of Puerto Rico, 1951* (San Juan: Justice Department, 1951–52), 123.

64. Fernández García, *Report of the Attorney General of Puerto Rico, 1936*, 33.

65. Fernández García, *Report of the Attorney General of Puerto Rico, 1937*, 35–36.

66. Antonio Fernós Isern, *Report of the Commissioner of Health of Puerto Rico, 1942–43* (San Juan: Insular Procurement Office, Printing Division, 1944), 16, 37.

67. Such a law was approved in May 1937. See "Leyes," *Boletín de la Asociación Médica de Puerto Rico* 30, no. 5 (May 1938): 196–99; Juan A. Rosselló, *Historia de la psiquiatría en Puerto Rico, 1898–1988* (San Juan: Instituto de Relaciones Humanas, 1988), 22–23, 60–61.

68. Manuel Rodríguez Ramos, *Report of the Attorney General of Puerto Rico, 1943* (San Juan: Insular Procurement Office, Printing Division, 1943), 28, 30.

69. Enrique Campos del Toro, *Report of the Attorney General of Puerto Rico, 1945* (San Juan: Service Office of the Government of Puerto Rico, Printing Division, 1946), 22.

70. "Tres tragedias ha habido en la familia del que simuló locura," *El Universal*, November 5, 1947, 31; Asenjo, *Quién es quién en Puerto Rico*, 139–40.

71. Celeste Marín, Paláu de López, and Barbosa de Chardón, *La efectividad de la rehabilitación en los delincuentes de Puerto Rico*, ch. 1.

72. Rexford G. Tugwell, *Puerto Rican Public Papers* (San Juan: Service Office of the Government of Puerto Rico, Printing Division, 1945), 51; Frank Loveland, "Report on the Correctional Program of Puerto Rico," 1, Folder 645, "Penal Institutions," Caja 114, FOG, AGPR.

73. Loveland, "Report on the Correctional Program of Puerto Rico," 3–4.

74. Loveland, "Report on the Penal and Correctional Program of Puerto Rico," 1.

75. Loveland, "Report on the Penal and Correctional Program of Puerto Rico," 1, 3; Loveland, "Report on the Correctional Program of Puerto Rico," 8, 11.

76. Loveland, "Report on the Penal and Correctional Program of Puerto Rico," 1, 3; Loveland, "Report on the Correctional Program of Puerto Rico," 11–12.

77. Loveland, "Report on the Correctional Program of Puerto Rico," 14, 16.

78. Loveland, "Report on the Penal and Correctional Program of Puerto Rico," 1; Loveland, "Report on the Correctional Program of Puerto Rico," 14.

79. Loveland, "Report on the Penal and Correctional Program of Puerto Rico," 1–2; Loveland, "Report on the Correctional Program of Puerto Rico," 17.

80. Loveland, "Report on the Correctional Program of Puerto Rico," 17.

81. "Discurso pronunciado por el lcdo. Vicente Géigel y Polanco durante la sesión inaugural de la cuadragésima asamblea anual de la Asociación Médica de Puerto Rico," December 10, 1943, *Boletín de la Asociación Médica de Puerto Rico* 36, no. 1 (January 1944): 33.

82. Inmate file death certificates chronicle these and other causes. See, among many others, the death certificate template in Expediente del confinado Juan Soto Crespo, June 1936, Caja 184, SEC, FDJ, AGPR.

83. J. B. Kodesh is likely a reference to Jack B. Kodesh, a University of Bern graduate who appears in a Clínica Dr. Maldonado (Hato Rey) advertisement in the University of Puerto Rico *Deportes: Revista Gráfica* publication, 1, no. 2 (15 May 1946): 22–23.

84. Expediente del confinado Octavio Montilla, November 1939, Caja 221, SEC, FDJ, AGPR.

85. Loveland, "Report on the Penal and Correctional Program of Puerto Rico," 36, 42.

86. "X-Ray Traveling Unit," *Puerto Rico Health Bulletin* 8, no. 1 (January–March 1944): 22; Juan A. Pons, *Annual Report of the Commissioner of Health for the Fiscal Year 1948–49* (San Juan: Health Department, 1949), 144.

87. Campos del Toro, *Report of the Attorney General of Puerto Rico, 1946*, 44.

88. In 1946, a zoologist and a clinician conducted a filariasis study at Oso Blanco, finding that the prison's 1,300–1,500 impoverished inmates slept without screening or bed nets. The scientists learned that at least 5 percent of them were infected with the disease. Most positive cases were linked to urban areas, where it was easier for standing water to collect and mosquitoes to breed. The scientists also detected other conditions, including scabies and testicular atrophy. F. Hernández Morales and G. González Barrientos, "The Incidence of Filariasis at the Insular Penitentiary for Men," *Puerto Rico Journal of Public Health and Tropical Medicine* 22, no. 1 (September 1946): 99–101; Expediente del confinado Saturnino Rodríguez Andújar, December 1945, Caja 325, SEC, FDJ, AGPR.

89. Loveland, "Report on the Penal and Correctional Program of Puerto Rico," 29–30.

90. Luis Negrón Fernández, *Report of the Attorney General of Puerto Rico, 1948* (San Juan: Real Hermanos, 1950), 40; Ceferino A. Méndez Polo, "Departamento médico," *El Despertar* 2, no. 1 (April 1950): 19–20; Victor F.F., "Departamento médico," 21; Picó, *El día menos pensado*, 89.

91. Florencio R.S., "¿Sabía ud. que?" *El Despertar* 1, no. 4 (August 1949): 20.

92. Benjamín Santana, "La sección médica del Presidio cuenta ahora con hospital bien equipado," *El Mundo*, August 24, 1951, 18; Sergio R.R., "Una realidad," *Realidad* 2, no. 3 (September–November 1957): 19.

93. Florencio R.S., "¿Sabía ud. que?," *El Despertar* 1, no. 7 (November 1949): 20.

94. Marín Torres, *Eran ellos*, 137–38.

95. Prisoner Cándido R.M. indicates that his peers Rogelio M.C., Max P., and José E.O. founded the magazine. See Cándido R.M., "Primeras impresiones de un recluso: Tercera parte," *El Despertar* 1, no. 5 (September 1949): 14.

96. Carmelo Ch.M., "Retazo," *El Despertar* 1, no. 2 (June 1949): 12; Carmelo Ch.M., "Retazo," *El Despertar* 1, no. 4 (August 1949): 10.

97. Joaquín B., Jr., "Informe clínico," *El Despertar* 1, no. 2 (June 1949): 17.

98. Winter, *Reglamento para el régimen y gobierno de la Penitenciaría de Puerto Rico*, 13, 15; Joaquín B., Jr., "Informe clínico," 17.

99. Pneumothorax is a collection of air or gas in the space between the lungs and chest wall that uncouples the former from the latter, making it difficult to breath. Jacob Smith, "Extrapleural Pneumothorax," *Boletín de la Asociación Médica de Puerto Rico* 31, no. 3 (March 1939): 63–71; J. Rodríguez Pastor, "El neumotorax artificial como medida de salud en Puerto Rico," *Boletín de la Asociación Médica de Puerto Rico* 37, no. 12 (December 1945): 478–81.

100. Winter, *Reglamento para el régimen y gobierno de la Penitenciaría de Puerto Rico*, 15; Joaquín B., Jr., "Informe clínico," 17–18; Florencio R.S., "¿Sabía ud. que?," *El Despertar* (August 1949): 20. Marín Torres writes that nationalist convicts were deliberately deposited into certain parts of the penitentiary so as to expose them to tuberculosis. See *Eran ellos*, 185–86.

101. Winter, *Reglamento para el régimen y gobierno de la Penitenciaría de Puerto Rico*, 12–13; "Noticias médico-sociales," *Boletín de la Asociación Médica de Puerto Rico* 35, no. 11 (November 1943): 453; Oscar Costa Mandry, "Directorio médico de Puerto Rico año 1945," *Boletín de la Asociación Médica de Puerto Rico* 37, no. 8 (April 1945): 335; Méndez Polo, "Departamento médico," 19.

102. Costa Mandry, "Directorio médico de Puerto Rico año 1945," 334; Asenjo, *Quién es quién en Puerto Rico*, 4th ed., 34; Joaquín B., Jr., "Informe clínico," 18. For an example of the limits of eye care during Oso Blanco's early years and its partial outsourcing to medical professionals outside the prison, see Expediente del confinado José Sotero Ortiz Cruz, October 1937, Caja 298, SEC, FDJ, AGPR.

103. "Mi actitud hacia el programa de la institución," *El Despertar* 1, no. 5 (September 1949): 5.

104. Cachexia implies general bad health due to a specific morbid process, in this case a blend of anemia and sprue. Expediente del confinado Manuel Medina Hernández, October 1945, Caja 239, SEC, FDJ, AGPR.

105. Joaquín R.B.V., "Orientación sobre el plan de clasificación y tratamiento," *El Despertar* 2, nos. 3–4 (July–August 1950): 21–22.

106. Winter, *Reglamento para el régimen y gobierno de la Penitenciaría de Puerto Rico*, 12; Méndez Polo, "Departamento médico," 19–20.

107. Among many others, see the physical evaluation form in Expediente del confinado Justo Rivera Pabón, September 1949, Caja 477, SEC, FDJ, AGPR.

108. Florencio R.S., "¿Sabía ud. que?," *El Despertar* (August 1949): 20.

109. Méndez Polo, "Departamento médico," 19–20; Victor F.F., "Departamento médico," 21.

110. Méndez Polo, "Departamento médico," 19–20, 26.

111. Heriberto Marín Torres, *Coabey: El valle heróico* (San Juan: Editorial Patria, 2019), 108. On a similar exchange for experiment dynamic in Philadelphia, consult Allen M. Hornblum, *Acres of Skin: Human Experiments at Holmesburg Prison* (New York: Routledge, 1998).

112. Marín Torres, *Coabey*, 108–9. Marín Torres develops the experimentation line of analysis elsewhere, too, namely the drug experiments of the US military. See *Eran Ellos*, 82–83, 168–71.

113. Marín Torres, *Coabey*, 109.

114. Santana, "La sección médica del Presidio cuenta ahora con hospital bien equipado," 18.

115. Socrates Litsios, "John Black Grant: A 20th-century public health giant," *Perspectives in Biology and Medicine* 54, no. 4 (Autumn 2011): 532–49.

116. On the harm-heal dilemma as it relates to the history of medicine and psychiatry, see Richard C. Keller, *Colonial Madness: Psychiatry in French North Africa* (Chicago: University of Chicago Press, 2007).

117. Among others, see Expediente del confinado Juan Vélez Rodríguez, May 1940, Caja 238, SEC, FDJ, AGPR; Expediente del confinado Librado Roldán López, March 1943, Caja 243, SEC, FDJ, AGPR.

Chapter Two

1. In his report, Loveland proposed the penitentiary's urgent need for a classification program. See Loveland, "Report on the Correctional Program of Puerto Rico," 8–9. Also see Jesús T. Piñero, *Forty-Seventh Annual Report of the Governor of Puerto Rico for the Fiscal Year 1946–1947* (San Juan: Service Office of the Government of Puerto Rico, Printing Division, 1948), 59–60. The Classification and Treatment Board in Puerto Rico was modeled after a similar body at a federal institution in Connecticut. "Crean Junta de Clasificación de los reclusos," *El Mundo*, December 13, 1945, 1, 11; Campos del Toro, *Report of the Attorney General of Puerto Rico, 1946*, 60, 62.

2. Expediente del confinado Marcial Hernández García, January 1949, Caja 138, SJLBP, FDJ, AGPR.

3. Expediente del confinado Marcial Hernández García.

4. Expediente del confinado Marcial Hernández García. The Wechsler-Bellevue test was published in 1939, measures general intelligence and coordination in adults, and involves both verbal and performance criteria. American Psychological Association, *Directory* (Washington, DC: American Psychological Association, 1957), 351; Corwin Boake, "From the Binet-Simon to the Wechsler-Bellevue: Tracing the History of Intelligence Testing," *Journal of Clinical and Experimental Neuropsychology* 24, no. 3 (May 2002): 383–405; Patti L. Harrison and Alan S. Kaufman, "History of Intelligence Testing," in Cecil R. Reynolds and Elaine Fletcher-Janzen, eds., *Encyclopedia of Special Education*, 3rd ed. (New York: John Wiley & Sons, 2007), 1128.

5. Federal census records between 1910 and 1940 interchangeably refer to Picart as a mulatto and a person of color. His World War I draft registration card identifies him as black. "Juan B. Picart [born 1897]," Ancestry Library Edition, https://www.ancestrylibrary.com/search/?name=Juan+B._Picart&event=_puerto+rico-usa_5185&birth=1897.

6. Expediente del confinado Marcial Hernández García.

7. Celeste Marín, Paláu de López, and Barbosa de Chardón, *La efectividad de la rehabilitación en los delincuentes de Puerto Rico*, 211–24.

8. Eve Tuck and K. Wayne Yang, "R-Words: Refusing Research," in Django Paris and Maisha T. Winn, eds., *Humanizing Research: Decolonizing Qualitative Inquiry with Youth and Communities* (Thousand Oaks, CA: Sage Publications, 2014), 230.

9. Warwick Anderson, "Objectivity and Its Discontents," *Social Studies of Science* 43, no. 4 (August 2013): 557–76.

10. Anderson, 564.

11. Eugenio Astol, "Men of the Past: Celio S. Rossy," in Fernández García, *El libro de Puerto Rico*, 1051.

12. Roger Smith, *The Fontana History of the Human Sciences* (London: Fontana Press, 1997), 589–99; Lewis R. Aiken, *Tests psicológicos y evaluación*, 11th ed. (Mexico City: Pearson, 2003), 1–5; Ana María Jacó-Vilela, "Psychological Measurement in Brazil in the 1920s and 1930s," *History of Psychology* 17, no. 3 (August 2014): 237–48; John Carson, "Mental Testing in the Early Twentieth Century: Internationalizing the Mental Testing Story," *History of Psychology* 17, no. 3 (August 2014): 249–55; Frances Boulon-Díaz, "A Brief History of Psychological Testing in Puerto Rico: Highlights, Achievements, Challenges, and the Future," in Kurt F. Geisinger, ed., *Psychological Testing of Hispanics: Clinical, Cultural, and Intellectual Issues*, 2nd ed. (Washington, DC: American Psychological Association, 2015), 52.

13. Robert W. Rieber, ed., *Encyclopedia of Psychological Theories* (New York: Springer, 2012), 797–98; Boulon-Díaz, "A Brief History of Psychological Testing in Puerto Rico," 51.

14. Boulon-Díaz, "A Brief History of Psychological Testing in Puerto Rico," 51.

15. Frances Boulon-Díaz and Irma Roca de Torres, "School Psychology in Puerto Rico," in Shane R. Jimerson, Thomas Oakland, and Peter Thomas Farrell, eds., *The Handbook of International School Psychology* (Thousand Oaks, CA: Sage, 2007), 311–12.

16. Walters, a professor of education, was a specialist in the psychology of "normal" and handicapped students. Morse focused on children with disciplinary issues. Butte, *Report of the Attorney General of Porto Rico, 1927*, 17; Edith M. Irvine-Rivera, "Brief News Notes," *Porto Rico Health Review* 2, no. 12 (June 1927): 41. Compare to Silvana Vetö, "Child Delinquency and Intelligence Testing at Santiago's Juvenile Court, Chile, 1929–1942," *History of Psychology* 22, no. 3 (August 2019): 244–65.

17. Ana Isabel Álvarez, "La enseñanza de la psicología en la Universidad de Puerto Rico, Recinto de Río Piedras: 1903–1950," *Revista Puertorriqueña de Psicología* 9, no. 1 (1993): 13–29;

Guillermo Bernal, "La psicología clínica en Puerto Rico," *Revista Puertorriqueña de Psicología* 17, no. 1 (2006): 341–88; Irma Roca de Torres, "Perspectiva histórica sobre la medición psicológica en Puerto Rico," *Revista Puertorriqueña de Psicología* 19, no. 1 (2008): 11–48.

18. Ellen Herman, *The Romance of American Psychology: Political Culture in the Age of Experts* (Berkeley: University of California Press, 1995), 3–6; Roca de Torres, "Perspectiva histórica sobre la medición psicológica en Puerto Rico"; Boulon-Díaz, "A Brief History of Psychological Testing in Puerto Rico," 53–54.

19. US Department of Health, Education, and Welfare, *Bulletin No. 12: Research Relating to Children* (Washington, DC: Government Printing Office, February 1960–July 1960), 21; Irma Roca de Torres, "Algunos precursores/as de la psicología en Puerto Rico: Reseñas biográficas," *Revista Puertorriqueña de Psicología* 17, no. 1 (2006): 63–88.

20. Hussein Abdilahi Bulhan, *Frantz Fanon and the Psychology of Oppression* (New York: Plenum, 1985).

21. Allison Davis and Robert Hess, "¿Cúan justo es un examen de inteligencia?" *Bienestar Público* 6, nos. 23–24 (January–June 1951): 27–34.

22. Pablo Roca de León, *Manual escala de inteligencia Wechsler para niños* (San Juan: Departamento de Instrucción Pública, 1951); Pablo Roca de León, *Escala de inteligencia Stanford-Binet para niños* (San Juan: Departamento de Instrucción Pública, 1953); Linda H. Scott, "Measuring Intelligence with the Goodenough-Harris Drawing Test," *Psychological Bulletin* 89, no. 3 (May 1981): 483–505; Boulon-Díaz and Roca de Torres, "School Psychology in Puerto Rico"; Roca de Torres, "Algunos precursores/as"; Boulon-Díaz, "A Brief History of Psychological Testing in Puerto Rico," 54.

23. Goldstein, "Toward an Empirical History of Moral Thinking," 2.

24. Winter, *Report of the Attorney General of Puerto Rico, 1933,* 18.

25. Horton, *Report of the Attorney General of Puerto Rico, 1934,* 24.

26. Horton, *Report of the Attorney General of Puerto Rico, 1935,* 26.

27. Campos del Toro, *Report of the Attorney General of Puerto Rico, 1946,* 44.

28. Piñero, *Forty-Seventh Annual Report of the Governor of Puerto Rico,* 31, 133.

29. In the early 1900s, feeblemindedness was considered a hereditary mental disorder by prominent eugenicists like Henry Goddard (1866–1957). Goddard studied hundreds of such patients at the New Jersey Training School in Vineland and tapped Alfred Binet's mental test to analyze those in his care. In addition to being linked to low scores on intelligence tests, authorities fused feeblemindedness to promiscuity, criminality, and social dependence. Steven Noll, *Feeble-Minded in Our Midst: Institutions for the Mentally Retarded in the South, 1900–1940* (Chapel Hill: University of North Carolina Press, 1994); James W. Trent, *Inventing the Feeble Mind: A History of Mental Retardation in the United States* (Berkeley: University of California Press, 1995); Leila Zenderland, *Measuring Minds: Henry Goddard and the Intelligence Testing Movement* (New York: Cambridge University Press, 1998).

30. Ortiz Díaz, "Pathologizing the *Jíbaro,*" 429–30. As did mental health professionals in general. See, e.g., Luis M. Morales, "El problema de los tontos," *Bienestar Público* 1, no. 3 (March 1946): 31–35.

31. "Back Matter," *Yearbook of the National Council on Measurements Used in Education,* no. 11 (1953–54): xiv; Guillermo Bernal, "60 Years of Clinical Psychology in Puerto Rico," *Interamerican Journal of Psychology* 47, no. 2 (2013): 212; Bernal, "La psicología clínica en Puerto Rico," 353. Later, Picart became director of the Vocational Counseling, Training, and Adjustment Section at the Veterans Affairs Center in San Juan and published a study about the Wechsler-Bellevue test.

Juan B. Picart, "Validation of the WBIS for a Disabled Puerto Rican Veteran College Population," *Vocational Rehabilitation and Education Quarterly Information Bulletin* (January 1960): 14–15.

32. J. Antonio Alvarado, "La escuela como factor de control en el problema de la delincuencia," in *Memorias de la cuarta convención de trabajo social de Puerto Rico, marzo 1947* (Santurce: Imprenta Soltero, 1949), 57–58. Also consult Ismael Rodríguez Bou, *El analfabetismo en Puerto Rico* (San Juan: Universidad de Puerto Rico, Consejo Superior de Enseñanza, 1945).

33. Soledad Rodríguez Pastor and Maria Elisa Gómez, "La inteligencia subnormal y sus implicaciones en la delincuencia," in *Memorias de la cuarta convención de trabajo social de Puerto Rico*, 95–107. Dominican authorities propagated mental tests in juvenile reformatories in the mid-1940s. They believed these established a link between deviance, intelligence, and health. See, for instance, Víctor Garrido, *Memoria 1944 Procuraduría General de la República* (Santiago, DR: Editorial El Diario, 1944), 169; Garrido, *Memoria 1945*, 113, 118, 135.

34. Maria Elisa Gómez, "Sobre el problema de los anormales de la inteligencia en Puerto Rico," *Bienestar Público* 1, no. 2 (December 1945): 32–34. Also see Maria Elisa Gómez, "El censo de oligofrénicos," *Bienestar Público* 1, no. 3 (March 1946): 35–36; Maria Elisa Gómez de Tolosa, "El censo de oligofrénicos," *Bienestar Público* 3, no. 9 (September 1947): 6–9.

35. Expediente del confinado Santiago Ocasio Soler, January 1949, Caja 61, SJLBP, FDJ, AGPR.

36. Expediente del confinado Santiago Ocasio Soler.

37. Expediente del confinado Santiago Ocasio Soler.

38. Expediente del confinado Enrique Carmona, September 1948, Caja 73, SJLBP, FDJ, AGPR.

39. Expediente del confinado Enrique Carmona.

40. Expediente del confinado Enrique Carmona.

41. Expediente del confinado Enrique Carmona.

42. Rebecca Schilling and Stephen T. Casper, "Of Psychometric Means: Starke R. Hathaway and the Popularization of the Minnesota Multiphasic Personality Inventory," *Science in Context* 28, no. 1 (March 2015): 77–98.

43. Celeste Marín, Paláu de López, and Barbosa de Chardón, *La efectividad de la rehabilitación en los delincuentes de Puerto Rico*, 105–6.

44. A. Irving Hallowell, "The Rorschach Technique in the Study of Personality and Culture," *American Anthropologist* 47, no. 2 (1945): 195–210; Eleanor Siegel, "Arthur Sinton Otis and the American Mental Testing Movement," PhD diss., University of Miami, 1992; Damion Searls, *The Inkblots: Hermann Rorschach, His Iconic Test, and the Power of Seeing* (New York: Crown, 2017).

45. Expediente del confinado Onofre Rodríguez López, March 1950, Caja 195, SJLBP, FDJ, AGPR.

46. Expediente del confinado Onofre Rodríguez López.

47. Expediente del confinado Onofre Rodríguez López. Also see Robert E. Gibby and Michael E. Zickar, "A History of the Early Days of Personality Testing in American Industry: An Obsession with Adjustment," *History of Psychology* 11, no. 3 (September 2008): 164–84.

48. Expediente del confinado Onofre Rodríguez López.

49. Walter V. Bingham, "MacQuarrie Test for Mechanical Ability," in *Occupations: The Vocational Guidance Journal* 14, no. 3 (December 1935): 202.

50. María M. Maíz de Meléndez, "Trastornos de la personalidad," *Bienestar Público* 8, no. 33 (July-September 1953): 4–5, 20–22; James D. A. Parker, "From the Intellectual to the Non-Intellectual Traits: A Historical Framework for the Development of American Personality Research," MA

thesis, York University, Toronto, 1986; Kurt Danziger, *Constructing the Subject: Historical Origins of Psychological Research* (New York: Cambridge University Press, 1994), 158; Merve Emre, *The Personality Brokers: The Strange History of Myers-Briggs and the Birth of Personality Testing* (New York: Doubleday, 2018).

51. Expediente del confinado Antonio Hernández Alamo, April 1950, Caja 475, SJLBP, FDJ, AGPR.

52. Expediente del confinado Antonio Hernández Alamo.

53. Expediente del confinado Adolfo Ortiz Gutiérrez, July 1950, Caja 475, SJLBP, FDJ, AGPR.

54. Expediente del confinado Adolfo Ortiz Gutiérrez.

55. On trembling hands and compulsive scratching, for instance, see Expediente del confinado Cristóbal López Font, December 1948, Caja 213, SJLBP, FDJ, AGPR; Expediente del confinado Carmelo Cosme Motta, November 1950, Caja 158, SJLBP, FDJ, AGPR.

56. Expediente del confinado José Dolores Rodríguez Rolón, January 1951, Caja 400, SJLBP, FDJ, AGPR; Expediente del confinado Manuel Pagán Figueroa, May 1951, Caja 475, SJLBP, FDJ, AGPR; Expediente del confinado Antonio Batiz Santos, May 1953, Caja 484, SJLBP, FDJ, AGPR; Expediente del confinado Ceferino Santiago Maldonado, July 1953, Caja 484, SJLBP, FDJ, AGPR; Expediente del confinado José Nevarez Pérez, December 1953, Caja 484, SJLBP, FDJ, AGPR.

57. Max P., "En torno a la clasificación," *El Despertar* 1, no. 2 (June 1949): 15.

58. For example, see Susano Ortiz, "Estadísticas," *El Despertar* 1, no. 7 (November 1949): 4.

59. Here I am referring to professional and correctional psychiatry. On the circulation of earlier psychiatric knowledge in Puerto Rico, see Francisco R. de Goenaga, *Desarrollo histórico del Asilo de beneficencia y manicomio de Puerto Rico desde su creación hasta julio 31, 1929, y circulares relativas a hospitales* (San Juan: Cantero, Fernández & Co., 1929); Francisco R. de Goenaga, *Antropología médica y jurídica* (San Juan: Imprenta Venezuela, 1934). On the slow development of psychiatric facilities as of the 1950s, see Juan A. Rosselló, "Facilidades psiquiátricas en Puerto Rico," *Bienestar Público* 11, nos. 41–42 (July–December 1955): 4, 9.

60. Report of a Committee of the Southern Psychiatric Association, "Psychiatry and the National Defense," *Boletín de la Asociación Médica de Puerto Rico* 33, no. 1 (January 1941): 27–33; "Psychiatric Mobilization in the USA," *Boletín de la Asociación Médica de Puerto Rico* 33, no. 2 (February 1941): 65–67; Luis M. Morales, "Notes on the Neuroses of War in the Civilian Population" *Boletín de la Asociación Médica de Puerto Rico* 34, no. 3 (March 1942): 83–89; Lt. W. L. Holt, "Neuroses in War," *Boletín de la Asociación Médica de Puerto Rico* 35, no. 3 (March 1943): 92–104.

61. Luis M. Morales, "Mental Hygiene Problems of Students at the University of Puerto Rico," *Boletín de la Asociación Médica de Puerto Rico* 34, no. 11 (November 1942): 391–401; Louis S. London, "Psychotherapeutic Transfusions," *Boletín de la Asociación Médica de Puerto Rico* 35, no. 11 (November 1943): 414–38; Luis M. Morales, "La higiene mental del combatiente," *Boletín de la Asociación Médica de Puerto Rico* 36, no. 4 (April 1944): 186–89; Luis M. Morales, "El tratamiento de la ansiedad," *Boletín de la Asociación Médica de Puerto Rico* 37, no. 12 (December 1945): 471–77; Rosselló, *Historia de la psiquiatría en Puerto Rico, 1898–1988*, 79, 80, 88–89, 138. In the Dominican Republic, insulin and metrazol treatments and electroshock therapy were standard at the time. See Luis F. Thomen, *Memoria 1944 Secretaría de Estado de Sanidad y Asistencia Pública* (Santiago, DR: Editorial El Diario, 1944), 651–53; Thomen, *Memoria 1945*, 664–65, 668–69. By 1946 and later, Dominican mental health professionals added new drugs and treatments to their repertoire, including adrenaline, sodium amytal, penicillin, psychotherapy, and sodium pentothal, among others. Luis F. Thomen, *Memoria 1946 Secretaría de Estado de Sanidad y Asistencia Pública, Tomo I* (Ciudad Trujillo, DR: Editorial Arte y Cine, 1947), 551–54; Manuel A.

Robiou, *Memoria 1949 Secretaría de Estado de Sanidad y Asistencia Pública* (Ciudad Trujillo, DR: Editora del Caribe, 1956), 630–33; R. Espaillat de la Mota, *Memoria 1950 Secretaría de Estado de Sanidad y Asistencia Pública* (Ciudad Trujillo, DR: Editora del Caribe, 1957), 672–81.

62. Tomas G.D., "Mi historial," *Realidad* 1, no. 4 (December 1956–February 1957): 5–6; Suzanne P. Johnson, *An American Legacy in Panama* (Washington, DC: Department of Defense, 1995), 72–73; Susan I. Enscore, Suzanne P. Johnson, Julie L. Webster, and Gordon L. Cohen, *Guarding the Gates: The Story of Fort Clayton* (Champaign: US Army Corp of Engineers, 2000).

63. Rosselló, *Historia de la psiquiatría en Puerto Rico, 1898–1988*, 124–32. Luis M. Morales's studies are perhaps the best known of his generation. In the 1940s and 1950s, he was active in debunking "myths" about mental health, insanity, and psychiatry. He advocated for perceiving individual human minds as part and parcel of entire persons, not just specific to certain bodily organs, systems, and functions. Luis M. Morales, "Corrigiendo conceptos erróneos sobre las enfermedades mentales," *Revista de Servicio Social* 5, no. 4 (October 1944): 7; Luis M. Morales, *Psiquiatría, neurología e higiene mental* (San Juan: Secretaría de Instrucción Pública del Estado Libre Asociado de Puerto Rico, 1953).

64. José R. Maymí Nevares, "Sobre salud mental," *El Heraldo Médico* 2, no. 8 (August 1950): 207–8.

65. José R. Maymí Nevares, "Un hombre normal," *El Heraldo Médico* 2, no. 11 (November 1950): 275–76.

66. Maymí Nevares, "Un hombre normal," 276.

67. José R. Maymí Nevares, "El complejo de inferioridad," *El Heraldo Médico* 2, no. 12 (December 1950): 309–11.

68. Maymí Nevares, "El complejo de inferioridad," 309.

69. José R. Maymí Nevares, "La bebida social," *El Heraldo Médico* 3, no. 2 (February 1951): 33–34.

70. Penitentiary inmates were exposed to these kinds of ideas from other sources as well, including the German American medical professional Herman Bundesen and the French scholar Jean de Kerdeland. See Herman Bundesen, "¿Qué impulsa a una persona a tomar licores en exceso?" *Realidad* 2, no. 2 (June–August 1957): 6. The 80 percent figure is randomly cited on page 11 of this edition. Jean de Kerdeland, "¡El alcoholismo nos asesina!" *Realidad* 3, no. 2 (June–August 1958): 5–10, 12.

71. Mario, "Sobriedad mental," *Realidad* 2, no. 2 (June–August 1957): 7.

72. José R. Maymí Nevares, "Los síntomas nerviosos y sus causas emocionales," *El Heraldo Médico* 3, no. 4 (April 1951): 85; John Farquhar Fulton, *Frontal Lobotomy and Affective Behavior: A Neurophysiological Analysis* (New York: W. W. Norton & Co., 1951); Chauncey D. Leake, "Eloge: John Farquhar Fulton, 1899–1960," *Isis* 51, no. 4 (December 1960): 486, 560–62; David Healy, *The Creation of Psychopharmacology* (Cambridge, MA: Harvard University Press, 2002), 92; Bruno Etain and Laurence Roubaud, "Jean Delay, M.D., 1907–1987," *American Journal of Psychiatry* 159, no. 9 (September 2002): 1489; Eric R. Kandel, *In Search of Memory: The Emergence of a New Science of Mind* (New York: W. W. Norton and Co., 2007).

73. Bruce H. Friedman, "Feelings and the Body: The Jamesian Perspective on Autonomic Specificity of Emotion," *Biological Psychology* 84, no. 3 (July 2010): 383–93.

74. Walter Bradford Cannon, "Again the James-Lange and the thalamic theories of emotion," *Psychological Review* 38, no. 4 (1931): 281–95; Tim Dalgleish, "The Emotional Brain," *Nature Reviews Neuroscience* 5, no. 7 (July 2004): 582–89.

75. Maymí Nevares, "Los síntomas nerviosos y sus causas emocionales," 86.

76. Ergui, "Puerto Rican Penitentiary," 1119.

77. H. J. G., "¿Está abierta su puerta?," *El Despertar* 1, no. 5 (September 1949): 4.

78. For an example of an epileptic case, see Expediente del confinado Carlos Túa Cintrón, February 1949, Caja 204, SJLBP, FDJ, AGPR. Like Sampayo López, some people with epilepsy diagnosed themselves according to other or vernacular standards. On epilepsy as "el mal de botacoral," consult Expediente del confinado Sotero Castro Torres, October 1948, Caja 65, SJLBP, FDJ, AGPR.

79. Expediente del confinado Félix Calderón Parrilla, March 1943, Caja 392, SEC, FDJ, AGPR.

80. Expediente del confinado Félix Calderón Parrilla.

81. Expediente del confinado Arcadio Vargas Pagán, February 1945, Caja 414, SEC, FDJ, AGPR.

82. Expediente del confinado Arcadio Vargas Pagán.

83. Expediente del confinado Arcadio Vargas Pagán.

84. Expediente del confinado Armando Rivera Colón, November 1946, Caja 27, SJLBP, FDJ, AGPR.

85. Puerto Rican and Cuban intellectuals published several works about mental health and sexuality inside and outside of prisons in the middle decades of the twentieth century. Consult, for instance, Fernando Ordoñez y Fernández, *Influencia del instinto sexual sobre las facultades psíquicas, ensayo* (N.p.: n.p., 1936); José Chelala, *Reacciones mentales, psíquicas y sexuales en nuestras prisiones* (Havana: Editorial "La República," 1941); Sylvia Ledesma de Barceló, "El problema sexual en las prisiones," *Revista de Servicio Social* 9, no. 1 (January 1948): 22–26; Franco Ferracuti and G. B. Rizzo, "Signos sobresalientes de la homosexualidad en una población penitenciaria femenina, obtenidos mediante la aplicación de técnicas de proyección," *Revista de Ciencias Sociales* 2, no. 4 (December 1958): 469–79; Franco Ferracuti and Maria Christina Giannini, *L'incesto padre-figlia: Studio clinico-criminologico* (Río Piedras, PR: University of Puerto Rico, 1968). Marín Torres opines about sexuality and sexual abuse in midcentury Puerto Rican prisons in *Eran ellos*, 52–54, 92, 140–43.

86. For an example of a neurotic case, see Expediente del confinado Nicasio Otero Cruz, October 1947, Caja 93, SJLBP, FDJ, AGPR; Expediente del confinado Armando Rivera Colón.

87. Expediente del confinado Armando Rivera Colón.

88. José R. Maymí Nevares, "El delincuente como individual," in *Memorias de la cuarta convención de trabajo social de Puerto Rico*, 128, 136.

89. Maymí Nevares, 136.

90. Maymí Nevares, 136.

91. "Estudian un experimento de prisiones," *El Mundo*, August 8, 1948, 1, 10; "Group Psychotherapy in New Jersey Correctional Institutions," *Prison World* 10, no. 2 (March–April 1948): 12, 25. Sustained group psychotherapy and peer advising in the Puerto Rican prison system gained momentum in the 1960s. See Norman Fenton, *Manual sobre el uso de la consejería en grupos en las instituciones correccionales*, trans. Porfirio Díaz Santana (Río Piedras, PR: Centro de Investigaciones Sociales, Facultad de Ciencias Sociales, Universidad de Puerto Rico; Sacramento, CA: Instituto para el Estudio del Crimen y la Delincuencia, 1967).

92. Maymí Nevares, "El delincuente como individual," 129–34.

93. Expediente del confinado Modesto Matos Rodríguez, February 1949, Caja 205, SJLBP, FDJ, AGPR.

94. Franz Alexander and William Healy, *Roots of Crime: Psychoanalytic Studies* (New York: Knopf, 1935); José R. Maymí Nevares, "Contribución del médico neuropsiquiatra al tratamiento

individual del delincuente en un presidio," *Revista de Servicio Social* 7, no. 2 (April 1946): 42–43; Zalduondo Goodsaid, "El tratamiento individual del delincuente," *Bienestar Público* 2, no. 8 (June 1947): 2–14; Jon Snodgrass, "William Healy (1869–1963): Pioneer Child Psychiatrist and Criminologist," *Journal of the History of the Behavioral Sciences* 20, no. 4 (October 1984): 332–39.

95. In the Dominican Republic, the attorney general Víctor Garrido reported in 1945 that in youth facilities 15.6 percent of inmates were medically deficient, 9.1 percent psychically deficient, 26 percent morally deficient, and 21.6 percent socially deficient. Garrido, *Memoria 1945*, 118–19. The attorney general J. Tomás Mejías documented similar numbers the following year. J. Tomás Mejías, *Memoria 1946 Procuraduría General de la República* (Santiago, DR: Editorial El Diario, 1946), 198.

96. José R. Maymí Nevares, "El delincuente anormal ante la justicia," *Revista de Servicio Social* 10, no. 3 (July 1949): 19–20.

97. Víctor F.F., "Departamento Médico," 22.

98. R. de Goenaga, *Antropología médica y jurídica*, 39–74; Expediente del confinado David Luis Phillips, August 1951, Caja 172, SEC, FDJ, AGPR.

99. Rafael Troyano de los Ríos, "Neurosífilis," *Boletín de la Asociación Médica de Puerto Rico* 39, no. 5 (May 1947): 187–92; Rafael Troyano de los Ríos, "Pseudo-psicopatías de origen encefalítico," *Boletín de la Asociación Médica de Puerto Rico* 39, no. 6 (June 1947): 238–40.

100. Paciente J. A. S., "La limpieza en los pabellones del manicomio," *El Consultorio* 1, no. 9 (December 1946): 8; Paciente R. L., Jr., "Dr. Troyano de los Ríos, pido mi liber[t]ad en nombre de Dios," *El Consultorio* 1, no. 9 (December 1946): 14; Paciente I. P., "Al Dr. Troyano de los Ríos," *El Consultorio* 1, no. 9 (December 1946): 16; Paciente R. M. H. M., "El manicomio y el Dr. Troyano de los Ríos," *El Consultorio* 2, no. 14 (April 1947): 7; Paciente R. A., "Al Dr. Troyano de los Ríos," *El Consultorio* 2, no. 14 (April 1947): 9; Paciente M. V. O., "Al Doctor Troyano," *El Consultorio* 2, no. 14 (April 1947): 11.

101. Benjamín Santana, "Consideran La Palomilla tipo paranoíco deseoso de publicidad," *El Mundo*, June 2, 1951, 1, 14; Peter Khiss, "Troyano de los Ríos considera a Albizu un paranoíco," *El Mundo*, March 12, 1954, 1; Pedro I. Aponte Vázquez, *Locura por decreto* (San Juan: Publicaciones René, 1994); Carlos C. Gil Ayala, *Del tratamiento jurídico de la locura: Proyecto psiquiátrico y gobernabilidad en Puerto Rico* (San Juan: Editora Posdata, 2009). Other examples of mental health instability in prisons are in Marín Torres, *Eran Ellos*, 79–80, 136.

102. Troyano helped pioneer labor therapy in the Dominican Republic, which was introduced in that country in 1940 via the work of Hermann Simon in Gütersloh, Germany. Thomen, *Memoria 1944*, 649–51; Armando Ortiz, "Colonia psiquiátrica," in Congreso Médico Dominicano, *Memoria del Congreso Médico Dominicano del Centenario* (Santiago, DR: Editorial El Diario, 1945), 3:216–17; Thomen, *Memoria 1945*, 665–67. Labor therapy, some Puerto Rican mental health therapists thought, turned manual labor into a hobby, sparked a desire to learn and for sociability, and satiated aesthetic impulse. María Balado, "La salud mental," *Revista de Servicio Social* 11, no. 1 (January 1950): 14. Also see Juan Nicolás Martínez, "Las relaciones de trabajo y salud mental," *Bienestar Público* 8, no. 32 (April–June 1953): 31–34. Relating psychic diagnosis and social hygiene to bodily control and efficient labor was a central tenet of the discourse of regeneration and by extension rehabilitative corrections across the first half of the twentieth century. See Elizabeth Cancelli, *Carandiru: A prisão, o psiquiatria e o preso* (Brasília: Ed. UnB, 2005).

103. Paciente J. S., "El tratamiento de fisioterapia," *El Consultorio* 1, no. 9 (December 1946): 2–3; Paciente J. A. S., "El tratamiento de los pacientes en el manicomio," *El Consultorio* 1, no. 9 (December 1946): 11; Rosselló, *Historia de la psiquiatría en Puerto Rico, 1898–1988*, 15, 89.

104. Expediente del confinado Carlos Avilés González, August 1951, Caja 172, SEC, FDJ, AGPR.

105. Ortiz Díaz, "Pathologizing the *Jíbaro*," 435n90.

106. Joaquín R.B.V., "Orientación sobre el plan de clasificación y tratamiento," 23.

107. Maymí Nevares, "El delincuente como individual," 127, 134.

108. Expediente del confinado Domingo Rosario Santiago, January 1951, Caja 300, SJLBP, FDJ, AGPR; Expediente del confinado Antonio Enrique Lafontaine, January 1951, Caja 208, SJLBP, FDJ, AGPR; Expediente del confinado Julio Vázquez Burgos, January 1951, Caja 140, SJLBP, FDJ, AGPR; Expediente del confinado José Luis Rodríguez Galarza, January 1951, Caja 50, SJLBP, FDJ, AGPR; Expediente del confinado Rafael Llanos Resto, February 1951, Caja 111, SJLBP, FDJ, AGPR; Expediente del confinado Julio Enrique Muriel, February 1951, Caja 133, SJLBP, FDJ, AGPR; Expediente del confinado Juan López Monge, March 1951, Caja 175, SJLBP, FDJ, AGPR; Expediente del confinado Julio Ramírez Cruz, June 1951, Caja 201, SJLBP, FDJ, AGPR.

109. For example, see Expediente del confinado José Ramón Aguilar Salas, January 1951, Caja 140, SJLBP, FDJ, AGPR; Expediente del confinado Basilio Rodríguez Colón, January 1951, Caja 138, SJLBP, FDJ, AGPR; Expediente del confinado Ángel Luis Díaz, January 1951, Caja 136, SJLBP, FDJ, AGPR; Expediente del confinado Francisco Benítez Beauchamp, February 1951, Caja 132, SJLBP, FDJ, AGPR; Expediente del confinado Gilberto Quiñones Quintero, February 1951, Caja 133, SJLBP, FDJ, AGPR.

110. Expediente del confinado José Sánchez Rodríguez, May 1951, Caja 202, SJLBP, FDJ, AGPR; Expediente del confinado Ángel Miranda Ayala, August 1951, Caja 300, SJLBP, FDJ, AGPR; Expediente del confinado Lady Rosado Mercado, September 1951, Caja 210, SJLBP, FDJ, AGPR; Expediente del confinado Miguel Silva Fuentes, September 1951, Caja 270, SJLBP, FDJ, AGPR.

111. Expediente del confinado José Luis Rodríguez Galarza.

112. "Coordinación de servicios siquiátricos y penitenciarios," *Mensuario de la División de Corrección* 2, no. 10 (October 1961): 3–4; Rosselló, *Historia de la psiquiatría en Puerto Rico, 1898–1988*, 483. But surging numbers of mentally ill convicts needing care strained facilities, putting the different experts at loggerheads. Rosselló, 292–94.

113. H. J. G., "Está abierta su puerta?," 4.

114. División de Corrección (Porfirio Díaz Santana), *Boletín Informativo* 1 (December 1956): 7–8, Caja 1229, FOG, AGPR.

115. Eight different possible tests are mentioned in Expediente del confinado Alejandro Rosario Báez, September 1950, Caja 172, SEC, FDJ, AGPR. Also see Carlos D. Vázquez, "Ensayo sobre exámenes mentales de aplicación clínica," *Bienestar Público* 14, no. 53 (July–September 1958): 11–18, 39; Celeste Marín, Paláu de López, and Barbosa de Chardón, *La efectividad de la rehabilitación en los delincuentes de Puerto Rico*, 211–12.

116. Stephen Garton, "Crime, Prisons, and Psychiatry: Reconsidering Problem Populations in Australia, 1890–1930," in *Criminals and Their Scientists: The History of Criminology in International Perspective*, ed. Peter Becker and Richard F. Wetzell (New York: Cambridge University Press, 2006), 231–51.

117. Lillian Guerra, *Popular Expression and National Identity in Puerto Rico: The Struggle for Self, Community, and Nation* (Gainesville: University Press of Florida, 1998); Trujillo-Pagán, *Modern Colonization by Medical Intervention*.

Chapter Three

1. Expediente del confinado Jorge Díaz Ruiz, November 1949, Caja 450, SJLBP, FDJ, AGPR.

2. Expediente del confinado Jorge Díaz Ruiz.

3. Expediente del confinado Jorge Díaz Ruiz.

4. Loveland, "Report on the Penal and Correctional Program of Puerto Rico," 12–16; Loveland, "Report on the Correctional Program of Puerto Rico," 5–8; División de Corrección, *Boletín Informativo*, 18; Celeste Marín, Paláu de López, and Barbosa de Chardón, *La efectividad de la rehabilitación en los delincuentes de Puerto Rico*, 109–10.

5. Sol Rubin, *Planning for Correctional Progress in Puerto Rico* (New York: National Probation and Parole Association, 1951), 6–7, Folder 646, "Pardons and Parole," Caja 114, FOG, AGPR. Penologist Howard B. Gill subsequently completed a report on Puerto Rican prisons, in 1952. He stressed "the future development of corrections in Puerto Rico" would have to take into account prisons and parole but also policing and the problem of "crime control." His assertion was symptomatic of the punitive (re)turn in corrections that began to materialize in the 1960s and 1970s. Howard B. Gill, "Preliminary Report on the State of the Prisons of Puerto Rico," October 1952, 4, Folder 11, Box 42, Howard B. Gill Papers, MS 1995.018, John J. Burns Library, Boston College.

6. Loveland, "Report on the Correctional Program of Puerto Rico," 2.

7. Julienne Weegels, "Beyond the Cemetery of the Living: An Exploration of Disposal and the Politics of Visibility in the Nicaraguan Prison System," in Sacha Darke, Chris Garces, Luis Duno-Gottberg, and Andrés Antillano, eds., *Carceral Communities in Latin America: Troubling Prison Worlds in the 21st Century* (Cham, Switzerland: Palgrave Macmillan, 2021), 295–320; Caimari, "Remembering Freedom," 391–414.

8. Lydia Peña Beltrán, *30 años en las cárceles de Puerto Rico* (Río Piedras, PR: Borikén, 1995), 117.

9. Notably, there is evidence of some social workers bucking these trends and falling victims to the criminal-legal system. The nationalist-communist social worker of color Deusdedid Marrero Nazario, for example, served prison time in Arecibo and subsequently in mental hospitals in New York and Río Piedras. David Joel Viera Lozada, "Deusdedid Marrero: La criminalización del ideario comunista en Puerto Rico, 1947–1957," MA thesis, Centro de Estudios Avanzados de Puerto Rico y el Caribe, 2018; Marín Torres, *Eran ellos*, 218–19. On communism in Puerto Rico from the perspective of a black medical professional, see José A. Lanauze Rolón, *Por los caminos de la violencia: La idea comunista* (Ponce, PR: Casa Editorial América, 1932).

10. Emma Amador, "The Politics of Care: Puerto Ricans, Citizenship, and Migration after 1917" (unpublished ms.).

11. Beatriz Lassalle, "El gobierno de Puerto Rico y el trabajo social," *Revista de Servicio Social* 1, no. 1 (February 1939): 5, 7.

12. Lassalle, 8.

13. Carmen Rivera de Alvarado, "Quién es quién en trabajo social en Puerto Rico," *Revista de Servicio Social* 1, no. 1 (February 1939): 12–13; Porfirio Díaz Santana, "Nuestras actualidades en trabajo social," *Revista de Servicio Social* 1, no. 1 (February 1939): 14; Celia Núñez de Bunker, "El trabajador social y su clientela," *Revista de Servicio Social* 1, no. 2 (April–May 1939): 11.

14. Adriana Ramú de Guzmán, "Historia de la Escuela de Trabajo Social de la Universidad de Puerto Rico," *Revista de Servicio Social* 10, no. 4 (October 1949): 2–3; Julia Denoyers, "Efemérides del trabajo social en Puerto Rico," *Revista de Servicio Social* 11, no. 3 (July 1950): 21–22.

15. Núñez de Bunker, "El trabajador social y su clientela," 11–12.

16. Celia Núñez de Bunker, "El campo del trabajo social en Puerto Rico," *Revista de Servicio Social* 1, no. 1 (February 1939): 16–18; Adriana Ramú de Guzmán, "La labor de la maestra visitante en un programa de higiene mental," *Revista de Servicio Social* 1, no. 2 (April-May 1939): 8–9; Manuel Cabranes, "El trabajo social en las segundas unidades rurales," *Revista de Servicio Social*

1, no. 4 (August-September 1939): 8–9; Rafaela Espino, "Trabajo social dentro de un programa de Reconstrucción," *Revista de Servicio Social* 1, no. 5 (November–December 1939): 23–26; Nilsa M. Burgos Ortiz, *Pioneras de la profesión de trabajo social en Puerto Rico* (San Juan: Publicaciones Puertorriqueñas, 2013), 13–39, 63–86; Lassalle, "El gobierno de Puerto Rico y el trabajo social," 5–6; Rivera de Alvarado, "Quién es quién en trabajo social en Puerto Rico," 13–14; Núñez de Bunker, "El trabajador social y su clientela," 11.

17. Ergui, "Puerto Rican Penitentiary," 1119.

18. "Datos oficiales sobre la Junta Examinadora de Trabajadores Sociales de P.R.," *Revista de Servicio Social* 1, no. 4 (August–September 1939): 13–14; Felicia Boria, "¡Trabajador social: Organízate!" *Revista de Servicio Social* 1, no. 5 (November–December 1939): 5.

19. Julia Denoyers, "Nuestras actualidades en trabajo social," *Revista de Servicio Social* 1, no. 2 (April–May 1939): 14; Carmen Rivera de Alvarado, "El Departamento de Trabajo Social dentro de la reforma universitaria," *Revista de Servicio Social* 3, nos. 8–12 (October 1942): 4; René Muñoz Padín, "Es necesaria una reforma en el sistema penitenciario de Puerto Rico," *La Torre* 7, no. 195 (November 21, 1945), 2, 8; "Editorial," *Revista de Servicio Social* 9, no. 2 (April 1948): 1, 17; "Visitando las agencias," *Revista de Servicio Social* 10, no. 4 (October 1949): 23; Lassalle, "El gobierno de Puerto Rico y el trabajo social," 7; Ramú de Guzmán, "Historia de la Escuela de Trabajo Social de la Universidad de Puerto Rico," 4–5; Burgos Ortiz, *Pioneras de la profesión de trabajo social en Puerto*, 42–44.

20. Luis Adam Nazario, "Ideas del director: La cárcel de mujeres de Arecibo," *Revista de Servicio Social* 1, no. 6 (February–March 1940): 3; Burgos Ortiz, *Pioneras de la profesión de trabajo social en Puerto Rico*, 40–41.

21. Félix Rodríguez Higgins, "La delincuencia juvenil en Puerto Rico," *Revista de Servicio Social* 6, nos. 2–3 (April–July 1945): 18–24; Julia Carmen Marchand, "Los trabajos de la cuarta convención de trabajo social," *Revista de Servicio Social* 8, no. 2 (April 1947): 20–26; "Visitando las agencias," *Revista de Servicio Social* 10, no. 2 (April 1949): 25–26.

22. Loveland, "Report on the Correctional Program of Puerto Rico," 1.

23. Loveland, 2.

24. Loveland, 2.

25. Delegación Cubana, "Información general sobre problemas de delincuencia en Cuba," in *Memorias de la cuarta convención de trabajo social de Puerto Rico*, 210–16. Also see Jesús A. Portocarrero, *Proyecciones de la ciencia penitenciaria en Cuba* (Havana: Editorial Lex, 1945).

26. Carmen Adolfina Henríquez Almanzar, "La delincuencia, sus causas y posibles soluciones," in *Memorias de la cuarta convención de trabajo social de Puerto Rico*, 219–23. The Trujillo regime started deploying supervisory commissions staffed mainly by women to prisons in the mid-1930s. These commissions were a pillar of early social work in the country. See Rafael Trujillo, "Decreto Número 1747: Nombramiento de comisiones supervisoras de instituciones benéficas y afines," December 3, 1936, *Gaceta Oficial*, 4–11, in Ginetta E. B. Candelario, Elizabeth S. Manley, and April J. Mayes, eds., *Cien años de feminismos dominicanos, Tomo II* (Santo Domingo: Archivo General de la Nación, 2016), 472–78.

27. Maria Pintado Rahn, "Nuestro trabajo social en Venezuela," *Revista de Servicio Social* 1, no. 2 (April–May 1939): 6; Generosa F. de Net, "La Escuela de Servicio Social en Buenos Aires," *Revista de Servicio Social* 1, no. 3 (June–July 1939): 23; "Congreso Panamericano de servicio social," *Revista de Servicio Social* 6, nos. 2–3 (April–July 1945): 25–26; Lassalle, "El gobierno de Puerto Rico y el trabajo social," 6; Burgos Ortiz, *Pioneras de la profesión de trabajo social en Puerto Rico*, 45–46.

28. Burgos Ortiz, *Pioneras de la profesión de trabajo social en Puerto Rico*, 49.

29. Natalie Lira, *Laboratory of Deficiency: Sterilization and Confinement in California, 1900–1950s* (Oakland: University of California Press, 2021).

30. Peña Beltrán, *30 años en las cárceles de Puerto Rico*, 115.

31. Picó, "La caducidad de la cárcel," 12.

32. María Pintado Rahn, "Lillian Wald: Neighbor and Crusader," *Revista de Servicio Social* 1, no. 5 (November–December 1939): 17; Francisco J. Menchaca, "Labor salvadora sin gestos heróicos," *Revista de Servicio* 9, no. 3 (July 1948): 2–4, 16; "El hermano Pedro," *Revista de Servicio Social* 12, no. 3 (July–September 1951): 14, 31; Núñez de Bunker, "El trabajador social y su clientela," 12.

33. See, e.g., social worker Carmen Silvia García's use of biblical diction and imagery in her piece, "Surcos," *El Despertar* 2, no. 1 (April 1950): 11.

34. Absolute idealism, meaning the metaphysical view that all aspects of reality, including those we experience as disconnected or contradictory, are ultimately unified in the thought of a single all-encompassing consciousness.

35. "Consejo del Prof. Josiah Royce a los trabajadores sociales," *Revista de Servicio Social* 1, no. 5 (November–December 1939): 27.

36. Adriana Ramú de Guzmán, "El trabajo social y su relación con las ciencias sociales," *Revista de Servicio Social* 9, no. 4 (October 1948): 2–5, 20.

37. Esther Pou González, "Estudio en Presidio revela relación entre delincuencia y normas de vida," *La Torre*, March 7, 1945, 2.

38. Pou González, 2.

39. American Correctional Association, *State and National Correctional Institutions of the United States of America, Canada, England and Scotland* (New York: The Association, 1956), 39–40.

40. José Rodríguez Castro, *La embriaguez y la locura, o, Consecuencias del alcoholismo* (San Juan: Imp. del Boletín Mercantil, 1889). Also see Jesús María Amadeo y Antomarchi, *Una plaga social y la plegaria de una virgen* (San Juan: Tip. al vap. de "La Correspondencia," 1894).

41. Jesús E. Palmer, "Alcoholismo," *El Universitario*, March 12, 1947, 2.

42. Palmer, 2, 4.

43. Domingo E., ¿"Podemos librarnos del vicio del alcohol?," *El Despertar* 1, no. 4 (August 1949): 13, 34.

44. "Entrevistas," *Realidad* 1, no. 3 (September-November 1956): 9–10; Hiram R. Cancio, *Informe Anual del Secretario de Justicia al Gobernador del Estado Libre Asociado de Puerto Rico, 1963–64* (San Juan: Departamento de Hacienda, Servicio de Compra y Suministro, División de Imprenta, 1966), 42.

45. Sonia Bauza Guerra, "Labor de las trabajadoras sociales ayuda a clasificación de reclusos," *El Mundo*, August 23, 1952, 10.

46. María L. Molina, "Un programa de actividades en la Penitenciaría Insular," *El Mundo*, September 16, 1945, 15; Ledesma de Barceló, "El problema sexual en las prisiones," 22–26.

47. One of the primary critiques against the Industrial School in the mid-1940s, for example, was its poor infrastructure for effective treatment in general but particularly in the social aspect. See Ortiz Colón, "La División de Bienestar Público del Departamento de Sanidad frente a la Escuela Industrial para Jóvenes en Mayagüez," 4–5. The populist health official Antonio Fernós Isern argued that familial disintegration facilitated by parental irresponsibility, child and home abandonment, marriage problems, and substance abuse played roles in corrupting and

antisocializing Puerto Rico's youth. Antonio Fernós Isern, "Editorial," *Bienestar Público* 1, no. 2 (December 1945): 1. Also see Trías Monge, *Informe Anual del Secretario de Justicia, 1956,* 32–33.

48. Ramón Pérez de Jesús, "Clasificación de reclusos," *Revista de Servicio Social* 9, no. 2 (April 1948): 18. Marín Torres claims the classification process for nationalist and other political prisoners, in contrast, was "ridiculous." See *Eran Ellos,* 138.

49. "En hora buena," *El Despertar* 1, no. 4 (August 1949): 10; "Visitando las agencias," *Revista de Servicio Social* (October 1949): 23.

50. Susano Ortiz, "Clasificación de reclusos II," *Revista de la Asociación de Maestros de Puerto Rico* 8, no. 4 (May 1949): 124, 127; Pérez de Jesús, "Clasificación de reclusos," 19; Coll Cuchí, "Reforma penal," 57.

51. Negrón Fernández, *Report of the Attorney General of Puerto Rico, 1947,* 30.

52. Luis M.C., "Una escuela," *El Despertar* 1, no. 4 (August 1949): 19.

53. "Carta," *El Despertar* 1, no. 4 (August 1949): 5.

54. Ortiz, "Clasificación de reclusos II," 127, back cover.

55. Max P., "En torno a la clasificación," 16.

56. Frank M.Q., "El que no tenga pecado," *El Despertar* 1, no. 7 (November 1949): 10, 16.

57. Cándido R.M., "Primeras impresiones de un recluso: Tercera parte," 10.

58. Max P., "En torno a la clasificación," *El Despertar* 1, no. 4 (August 1949): 9.

59. Susano Ortiz, "El trabajo en prisiones," *El Despertar* 2, nos. 3–4 (July-August 1950): 33.

60. Max P., "En torno a la clasificación," 9.

61. Max P., 9.

62. "Estadística," *El Despertar* 1, no. 6 (October 1949): 8; Joaquín B.V., Jr., "Problemas de actualidad: Segunda parte," *El Despertar* 1, no. 7 (November 1949): 17; Rogelio M.C., "Editorial," *El Despertar* 1, no. 10 (February 1950): 3–4, 6.

63. Max P., "En torno a la clasificación," 9.

64. Benigno D.R., "Habla la voz de la experiencia," *El Despertar* 1, no. 4 (August 1949): 13.

65. Sergio V.A., "Reflexión," *El Despertar* 1, no. 10 (February 1950): 13.

66. Juan C.R., "No todos pensamos así," *El Despertar* 1, no. 5 (September 1949): 16.

67. Luis M.G., "Clasificación," *El Despertar* 1, no. 7 (November 1949): 13.

68. Luis M.G., 13.

69. "¿Cuál es su propósito? (De clasificación y tratamiento)," *El Despertar* 2, no. 1 (April 1950): 34.

70. Joaquín R.B.V., "Orientación sobre el plan de clasificación y tratamiento," 21.

71. Joaquín R.B.V., Jr., "Sobre la reforma penal," *El Despertar* 1, no. 4 (August 1949): 25.

72. Luis M.C., "Una escuela," 19.

73. Juan C.R., "La reforma penal," *El Despertar* 1, no. 7 (November 1949): 25; H. J. G., "Solamente seguridad temporal," *El Despertar* 1, no. 7 (November 1949): 12–13; "Colaboración que agradecemos mucho (de la Señora Carmelina G. Freyre)," *El Despertar* 1, no. 8 (December 1949): 15, 17–18, 20.

74. "Reforma plausible," *El Despertar* 1, no. 11 (March 1950): 28.

75. "Reforma plausible," 28.

76. Many inmate files contain department store receipts from places like La Gran Tienda in Río Piedras. The receipts log the attire prisoners received prior to being released from the penitentiary, which is suggestive of the importance and power of clothing in procuring health and citizenship making. Merchandise included suits, shoes, hats, socks, belts, neckties, and shirts. See Expediente del confinado Eulogio Cintrón Calderón, Caja 477, SEC, FDJ, AGPR; Expediente

del confinado Domingo Torres Meléndez, Caja 477, SEC, FDJ, AGPR; Expediente del confinado Juan Sampayo López. On "La Gran Tienda," consult Florencio Sáez, *Río Piedras: Estampas de mi pueblo, 1898-1945* (1988; San Juan: Editorial Palma Real, 1996), 101.

77. Joaquín R.B.V., "Comentarios en torno al Editorial publicado por 'Puerto Rico Ilustrado' en su edición del 16 de septiembre de 1950," *El Despertar* 2, no. 5 (September 1950): 9-10.

78. Susano Ortiz, "Clasificación de reclusos III," *Revista de la Asociación de Maestros de Puerto Rico* 8, no. 5 (September 1949): 147, 153.

79. Ortiz, "Estadísticas," 4.

80. Coll Cuchí, "Reforma penal," 71.

81. Social scientists like José Colombán Rosario, who pondered whether Puerto Rico had a "justice" or "injustice" system, and Jaime Toro Calder strove to hear the voices of prisoners through their research during this period as well. Toro Calder's research is particularly fascinating because of how it had an impact on colonial-populist knowledge production about incarceration from the vantage point of the US Midwest, not the headquarters of US empire in Washington, DC. Jaime Toro Calder, "Personal Crime in Puerto Rico: A Study of the Cultural Elements in Personal Crime," MA thesis, University of Wisconsin-Madison, 1950; José Colombán Rosario, *Problema de la criminalidad en Puerto Rico* (Río Piedras, PR: Universidad de Puerto Rico, Colegio de Pedagogía, 1952). Also see Roberto Pérez-Pérez, "A Survey of the Insular Industrial School for Boys at Mayagüez, Puerto Rico," MA thesis, Ohio State University, 1951. The first attorney general under governor Luis Muñoz Marín, Vicente Géigel Polanco, sent corrections official Félix Rodríguez Higgins to the 79th Congress of the American Prison Association in Milwaukee, who in turn submitted a report that was later used in carceral policymaking. Félix Rodríguez Higgins, "Informe de viaje oficial a los Estados Unidos," October 17, 1949, Folder 645, "Penal Institutions," Caja 114, FOG, AGPR. A few years earlier the Association praised Governor Piñero for beginning to modernize Puerto Rican corrections. *Proceedings of the Seventy-Sixth Annual Congress of the American Prison Association* (New York: The Association, 1946), 277.

82. Ortiz, "Clasificación de reclusos III," 147.

83. Joaquín R.B.V., "A través de los ojos de otros," *El Despertar* 1, no. 8 (December 1949): 19.

84. Ortiz Díaz, "Pathologizing the *Jíbaro*," 430-31.

85. Expediente del confinado Julio Nieves Guzmán, February 1948, Caja 33, SJLBP, FDJ, AGPR; Expediente del confinado Ramón Castro García, September 1948, Caja 168, SJLBP, FDJ, AGPR; Expediente del confinado Felipe Martínez Rodríguez, July 1949, Caja 480, SEC, FDJ, AGPR; Expediente del confinado Victor Celso Ortiz Morales, September 1954, Caja 533, SJLBP, FDJ, AGPR.

86. Expediente del confinado Pantaleon Álvarez Vélez, October 1951, Caja 210, SJLBP, FDJ, AGPR.

87. José A. Roméu, "El problema de los arrabales," *Alma Latina* no. 599 (May 24, 1947): 5. Also consult José Barbosa Aquino, "Estampas de San Juan: Los arrabales de la capital," *El Universal*, November 5, 1947, 24; Celestina Zalduondo, "El arrabal: Factor determinante en el crimen," *Bienestar Público* 9, no. 35 (January-March 1954): 19-21.

88. Expediente del confinado Pedro Díaz Ortiz.

89. Peña Beltrán, *30 años en las cárceles de Puerto Rico*, 116-17.

90. Expediente del confinado Carlos Orizal Félix, February 1951, Caja 450, SJLBP, FDJ, AGPR.

91. Expediente del confinado Carlos Orizal Félix.

92. Expediente del confinado Carlos Orizal Félix.

93. Expediente del confinado Félix Enrique Soto Vélez, October 1951, Caja 270, SJLBP, FDJ, AGPR.

94. Expediente del confinado Félix Enrique Soto Vélez.

95. Expediente del confinado Sandalio Mateo Vázquez, October 1953, Caja 484, SJLBP, FDJ, AGPR.

96. Expediente del confinado Carlos Osorio Acevedo, May 1951, Caja 400, SJLBP, FDJ, AGPR.

97. Expediente del confinado Carlos Osorio Acevedo.

98. Expediente del confinado Enrique Astacio Cruz, January 1954, Caja 493, SJLBP, FDJ, AGPR.

99. Expediente del confinado Enrique Astacio Cruz.

100. Expediente del confinado Iván Graciano Núñez, September 1947, Caja 205, SJLBP, FDJ, AGPR.

101. Emphasis in original. Expediente del confinado Iván Graciano Núñez.

102. Picó, *El día menos pensado*, 174–77.

103. Loveland, "Report on the Correctional Program of Puerto Rico," 2. Also see Edwin Cortés García, "La Libertad Bajo Palabra como período de reajuste necesario en el tratamiento del delincuente puertorriqueño," in *Memorias de la cuarta convención de trabajo social de Puerto Rico*, 78–94.

104. José S. Alegría, "La libertad condicional en Puerto Rico," 1, Folder 646, "Pardons and Parole," Caja 114, FOG, AGPR.

105. E. D. Wall (Trinidad and Tobago Prisons Department), *Administration Report of the Superintendent of Prisons for the Year 1951* (Trinidad, British West Indies: Government Printing Office, 1953), 12, 15–17; Wall, *Administration Report, 1952*, 12, 21–24.

106. Ramón Pérez de Jesús, "La libertad a prueba," *Revista de Servicio Social* 8, no. 1 (January 1947): 8; Victor F.F., "En torno a la reincidencia," *El Despertar* 2, no. 1 (April 1950): 32, 44, 46.

107. Pérez de Jesús, "La libertad a prueba," 10.

108. "Visitando las agencias," *Revista de Servicio Social* 9, no. 4 (October 1948): 17.

109. Expediente del confinado Pedro Ortiz Figueroa, February 1950, Caja 307, SJLBP, FDJ, AGPR.

110. Expediente del confinado Pedro Ortiz Figueroa.

111. Expediente del confinado Pedro Ortiz Figueroa.

112. Expediente del confinado Ismael Barnés Figueroa, March-April 1952, Caja 361, SJLBP, FDJ, AGPR.

113. Expediente del confinado Ismael Barnés Figueroa.

114. Expediente del confinado Ismael Barnés Figueroa.

115. Expediente del confinado Ismael Barnés Figueroa.

116. Expediente de la confinada Nieves Torres Santiago, October 1953, Caja 400, SJLBP, FDJ, AGPR.

117. Expediente de la confinada Nieves Torres Santiago.

118. "Mi actitud hacia el programa de la institución," 8. Society's attitude toward parolees was a key factor in their social readjustment or non-adjustment. Joaquín R.B.V., "Editorial: Actitud de la sociedad hacia el ex-confinado," *El Despertar* 2, no. 5 (September 1950): 3–4.

119. Expediente del confinado Esteban Méndez Jiménez, August 1955, Caja 520, SJLBP, FDJ, AGPR.

120. Expediente del confinado Esteban Méndez Jiménez.

121. Alegría, "La libertad condicional en Puerto Rico," 10.

122. Joaquín B.V., "El punto psicológico," *El Despertar* 1, no. 11 (March 1950): 9–10.

123. Florencio R.S., "Dos días de pase en Ponce," *El Despertar* 1, no. 11 (March 1950): 13–14.

124. Burgos Ortiz, *Pioneras de la profesión de trabajo social en Puerto Rico*, 52.

125. Vicente R.S., "Orientando al recluso sobre las condiciones bajo las cuales se concede la libertad bajo palabra," *El Despertar* 1, no. 4 (August 1949): 4; Joaquín B.V., "Los confinados bajo 'parole' o libertad bajo palabra necesitan educación," *El Despertar* 1, no. 5 (September 1949): 15, 17, 20, 22; H. J. G., "Es un buen negocio," *El Despertar* 1, no. 6 (October 1949): 6–7; Joaquín B.V., "Bosquejo sobre la propuesta escuela para los reclusos a ser puestos en libertad bajo palabra," *El Despertar* 1, no. 6 (October 1949): 13, 24; Joaquín R.B.V., "Sobre la libertad bajo palabra," *El Despertar* 2, no. 2 (May 1950): 9–10; H. J. G., "Solamente seguridad temporal," 12–13.

126. Cándido R.M., "Escuelas antes que cárceles y presidio . . . ¿porqué no?," *El Despertar* 1, no. 6 (October 1949): 9.

127. Emilio R.B., "Comentando ideas," *El Despertar* 1, no. 6 (October 1949): 14, 27.

128. Frank M.Q., "Editorial," *El Despertar* 1, no. 11 (March 1950): 3–4.

Chapter Four

1. The construction of Puerto Rico's Women's Industrial School started in 1952. It officially opened in 1954. Galindo-Malavé, "Cuerpos truculentos y 'desviados,'" 11–34. However, debates about its construction began at least a decade or so earlier, when colonial officials sought Works Progress Administration funding to complete a women's penitentiary project in Manatí. Much of the debate revolved around the presumed competition that would ensue between convict and free workers in contracting a labor force for the construction of the new prison. See George A. Malcolm to Guy J. Swope, May 12, 1941, Correspondencia General, Caja 390, FOG, AGPR.

2. The letter's handwriting is difficult to decode in places. Ribot's cursive bs and fs are easy to confuse but different enough to identify the letter recipient as most likely Rabi.

3. Although Ribot referred to Rabi as a man, it is also possible Rabi was the nickname of a fellow female inmate, for another document in Ribot's file reveals her involvement in homosexual affairs in the women's prison before she was sent to the Industrial School for Girls in Ponce. Expediente de la confinada Nereida Ribot, September 1957, Caja 7, Subfondo Escuela Industrial para Mujeres (hereafter SEIM), FDJ, AGPR.

4. Expediente de la confinada Nereida Ribot.

5. Compare to Kent R. Kerley, ed., *Finding Freedom in Confinement: The Role of Religion in Prison Life* (Santa Barbara, CA: Praeger, 2018).

6. Expediente de la confinada Nereida Ribot.

7. Mario A. Núñez Molina, "Toward an Experiential Approach for Researching Religious Experiences," *Revista Puertorriqueña de Psicología* 10, no. 1 (1995): 248; Sally Promey, ed., *Sensational Religion: Sensory Cultures in Material Practice* (New Haven, CT: Yale University Press, 2017); Gómez, *Experiential Caribbean*.

8. Luis M. Morales, "La religión y la salud mental," *Bienestar Público* 7, nos. 27–28 (January–June 1952): 29, 40. As prisoner Sergio R.N. noted, this was because penal reform functioned as a sort of religion. It tried to strengthen convicts' mental condition so they would not fall victim to "telepathic phenomena" (i.e., cryptic forms of belief that failed to improve their chances of exiting prison sooner). Sergio R.N., "Mirando El Despertar," *El Despertar* 1, no. 7 (November 1949): 22. Also consult Harold G. Koenig, Dana E. King, and Verna Benner Carson, eds., *Handbook of Religion and Health*, Second edition (New York: Oxford University Press, 2012).

9. In midcentury Cuban prisons, female inmates practiced a variety of Afro-Catholic and Spiritist religions as well. See, e.g., Ofelia Domínguez Navarro, *De 6 a 6: La vida en las prisiones cubanas* (Mexico City: n.p., 1937), 21–25, accessed at the Cuban Heritage Collection, University of Miami (hereafter CHC, UM).

10. José Manuel García Leduc, *Intolerancia y heterodoxias en Puerto Rico (siglo XIX): Protestantes, masones y espiritistas-kardecianos reclaman su espacio social, c. 1869–1898* (San Juan: Isla Negra Editores, 2009).

11. "Instrucción religiosa en la cárcel," *El Piloto*, November 14, 1942, 6; "Santa misión en la penitenciaría de distrito," *El Piloto*, January 15, 1944, 5; "Clases de doctrina en 'La Princesa,'" *El Piloto*, November 25, 1944, 6; "Una fiesta tradicional en La Princesa," *El Piloto*, January 13, 1945, 6; Campos del Toro, *Report of the Attorney General of Puerto Rico, 1946*, 43; Marín Torres, *Eran ellos*, 43, 72, 137.

12. Cronista, "Espléndida labor de misioneros Redentoristas en Instituciones Insulares," *El Piloto*, November 19, 1938, 4.

13. Winter, *Report of the Attorney General of Puerto Rico, 1933*, 58; Fernández García, *Report of the Attorney General of Puerto Rico, 1936*, 71; Fernández García, *Report of the Attorney General of Puerto Rico, 1939*, 74; Malcolm, *Report of the Attorney General of Puerto Rico, 1942*, 81; Campos del Toro, *Report of the Attorney General of Puerto Rico, 1945*, 52; Negrón Fernández, *Report of the Attorney General of Puerto Rico, 1947*, 73.

14. Expediente del confinado Santiago Casiano Ortiz, May 1948, Caja 133, SJLBP, FDJ, AGPR. Sometimes the observance of holidays happened in collective venues. The December 1949 edition of *El Despertar*, for example, commemorated the Christmas holiday.

15. Expediente del confinado Antonio Palmer Crespo, July 1949, Caja 205, SJLBP, FDJ, AGPR.

16. Expediente del confinado Justino Curbelo Mercado, May 1948, Caja 90, SJLBP, FDJ, AGPR; Expediente del confinado Fernando López Vargas, June 1948, Caja 168, SJLBP, FDJ, AGPR; Expediente del confinado Hipólito Rodríguez Oquendo, April 1950, Caja 200, SJLBP, FDJ, AGPR.

17. Expediente del confinado Miguel Ángel Estrada Sánchez, May 1950, Caja 200, SJLBP, FDJ, AGPR; Expediente del confinado Carlos Pagán Hernández, September 1950, Caja 154, SJLBP, FDJ, AGPR; Expediente del confinado Juan del Valle Serrano, November 1950, Caja 134, SJLBP, FDJ, AGPR; Expediente del confinado Eustaquio Pérez González, December 1950, Caja 161, SJLBP, FDJ, AGPR; Expediente del confinado Juan López Monge.

18. Expediente del confinado Amador Mangual Toro, January 1950, Caja 130, SJLBP, FDJ, AGPR.

19. "Colaboración de la Sra. Carmelina G. Freyre," *El Despertar* 2, no. 1 (April 1950): 30.

20. "Colaboración de la Sra. Carmelina G. Freyre," 30.

21. "Misa en la penitenciaría," *El Imparcial*, August 1, 1946, 20.

22. Cassandra Sheppard, "The Neuroscience of Singing," *Uplift: Science*, December 11, 2016, https://upliftconnect.com/neuroscience-of-singing/; Douglas, *Redemption Songs*.

23. "Una misa en el Presidio Insular," *El Mundo*, August 13, 1946, 7.

24. "En el patio del Presidio Insular asisten a misa 1,300 reclusos-Comulgan 405," *El Piloto*, May 1, 1948, 2; "Carta de reclusos del Presidio Insular," *El Piloto*, May 29, 1948, 2.

25. Padres Redentoristas, "Misión Católica en la Penitenciaría Insular," *El Despertar* 1, no. 5 (September 1949): 31.

26. In the ritual, believers travel between "stations," recite prayers, and contemplate the sacred images or scenes. The images are arranged around a church nave or along a path. The

faithful travel from image to image, in order, stopping at each station to recite select prayers. This can be done individually or in groups. Occasionally, the faithful might perform the ritual without any images. It is unclear whether images were used in the Oso Blanco Via Crucis procession of September 1949. On the history of Via Crucis, see Herbert Thurston, *The Stations of the Cross: An Account of their History and Devotional Purpose* (Charleston, SC: Nabu Press, 2010).

27. "Misión Católica en la Penitenciaría," *El Despertar* 1, no. 6 (October 1949): 15.

28. "Misión Católica en la Penitenciaría," 15.

29. "Misión Católica en la Penitenciaría," 24.

30. In the July-August 1950 edition of *El Despertar*, convicts depicted a similar scene. The only differences are that prisoners receive the sacrament individually and a piano player sets the mood through music. Joaquín R.B.V., "Orientación sobre el plan de clasificación y tratamiento," 22.

31. Marín Torres, *Coabey*, 90.

32. "Misión Católica en la Penitenciaría," 24.

33. J. Estades Rigau, "Siembran esperanza y consuelo tras las rejas: Un sacerdote católico y un ministro protestante hacen obra de ajuste moral y espiritual en nuestras prisiones," *Puerto Rico Ilustrado*, October 11, 1952, 30–33, 35, 38.

34. Luis C.S., "En comunión con Dios," *El Despertar* 2, no. 1 (April 1950): 28; Estades Rigau, "Siembran esperanza y consuelo tras las rejas," 30–33, 35, 38.

35. Margarite Fernández Olmos and Lizabeth Paravisini, eds., *Healing Cultures: Art and Religion as Curative Practices in the Caribbean and Its Diaspora* (New York: Palgrave, 2001).

36. Expediente de la confinada Lucía Ortiz, January 1958, Caja 7, SEIM, FDJ, AGPR.

37. Fernández Badillo, *Informe Anual del Secretario de Justicia, 1957*, 102.

38. Cancio, *Informe Anual del Secretario de Justicia, 1963–64*, 42.

39. "Carta del Can. Pérez Sánchez a Virgilio Trujillo Molina, secretario de Interior, Policía, Guerra y Marina, sobre visitas de evangélicos a las cárceles de San Cristóbal," September 1, 1932, in José Luis Sáez, ed., *La sumisión bien pagada: La iglesia dominicana bajo la era de Trujillo, 1930–1961, Tomo 1* (Santo Domingo: Archivo General de la Nación, 2008), 127.

40. "Discurso pronunciado por Fr. Cipriano de Utrera en la Penitenciaría de Boca-Nigua en las fiestas religiosas celebradas el 19 de agosto 1923," *Listín Diario*, August 31, 1923, 1, 5; "Acto religioso en la Penitenciaría de Nigua," *La Opinión*, May 11, 1928, 1; Photo press release, *La Opinión*, May 14, 1928, 7.

41. Juan Isidro Jimenes Grullón, *Una gestapo en América: Vida, tortura, agonía y muerte de presos políticos bajo la tiranía de Trujillo* (1948; Santo Domingo: Editora Montalvo, 1962), 171, 195.

42. Jimenes Grullón, 181–82.

43. "Sugerencia de que se efectúe la colocación del crucifijo en las cárceles," January 28–30, 1946, Caja IT: 2903478, Secretaría de Estado de Justicia e Instrucción Pública, Sección Palacio Nacional, Fondo Presidencia, Archivo General de la Nación (hereafter SEJIP, SPN, FP, AGN). Note that *IT* stands for *asignatura topográfica*, an indication of where material is in the stacks of Dominican archives.

44. Samuel Lightbourne, "Informe de la labor realizada durante el año 1944, en la cárcel de Puerto Plata," December 31, 1944, Caja IT: 8/006064, legajo 12, año 1940, Fondo Ejército Nacional (hereafter FEN), AGN.

45. "The Medical Missionary at Work: Medical Work in the West Indies," *Life and Health* 21, no. 9 (September 1906): 252–54; P. E. Brodersen, "Medical Missionary Work in South America,"

Advent Review and Sabbath Herald 104, no. 12 (March 24, 1927): 2, 14; A. R. Sherman, "Medical Work Opens Doors in Venezuela" and Dr. Raymundo Garza, "Medical Ministry Wins in Mexico," *Missions Quarterly* 34, no. 1 (First Quarter 1945): 2–3, 8–9; B. M. Heald, "Medical and Evangelistic Advances in Jamaica," *Advent Review and Sabbath Herald* 124, no. 52 (December 25, 1947): 25; S. L. Folkenberg, "Medical Work in Puerto Rico," *Advent Review and Sabbath Herald* 126, no. 31 (August 4, 1949), 18; Ellen Walsh, "'Advancing the Kingdom': Missionaries and Americanization in Puerto Rico, 1898–1930s," PhD diss., University of Pittsburgh, 2008, chs. 3, 5; Winifred C. Connerton, "Working towards health, Christianity and democracy: American colonial and missionary nurses in Puerto Rico, 1900–30," in Helen Sweet and Sue Hawkins, eds., *Colonial Caring: A History of Colonial and Post-colonial Nursing* (Manchester, UK: Manchester University Press, 2015), 126–44.

46. Glenn Calkins, "Good News from Santo Domingo," *Advent Review and Sabbath Herald* 124, no. 52 (December 25, 1947): 23; J. DeWitt Fox, "Doctor of Medicine and Doctor of Ministry" and Grant E. Ward, "Christianity and Modern Medicine," *The Ministry* 21, no. 10 (October 1948): 27–28, 30–32.

47. F. W. Steeves, "A Cry from a Prison Cell," *Inter-American Division Messenger* 8, no. 12 (December 1931): 6–7; Wesley Amundsen, "Carrying the Gospel to Those in Jail," *Inter-American Division Messenger* 25, no. 7 (September 1948): 6.

48. See *The Annual Reports of the Attorneys General to the Governors of Porto/Puerto Rico* for the years 1930–47.

49. Expediente del confinado Miguel Muñoz Guzmán, August 1948, Caja 172, SJLBP, FDJ, AGPR; Expediente del confinado Félix Medina Martínez, December 1948, Caja 168, SJLBP, FDJ, AGPR; Expediente del confinado Tomás Ramírez Santiago, February 1950, Caja 125, SJLBP, FDJ, AGPR; Expediente del confinado Domingo Rosario Santiago.

50. Expediente del confinado José Medina Berríos, November 1947, Caja 146, SJLBP, FDJ, AGPR.

51. Expediente del confinado José Luis Marrero, March 1951, Caja 283, SJLBP, FDJ, AGPR; Expediente del confinado Gilberto Quiñones Quintero.

52. Benjamín Santana, "Revelan Pedro Benejam estudia teología por correspondencia," *El Mundo*, October 1, 1952, 14; Benjamín Santana, "Un líder del motín del Presidio revela cómo se hizo religioso," *El Mundo*, October 4, 1952, 14; Benjamín Santana, "El Alcaide Jones y los reclusos interceden por una evangelista," *El Mundo*, October 8, 1952, 12; Helen V. Tooker, "Boricua indultado," *El Mundo*, October 16, 1953, 14. Norwegian American, Swedish American, and German American missionary women were active in Oso Blanco's 2 Corinthians 5:17 congregation in the late 1950s. "Giny Carlson: Completa el maravilloso trio," *Realidad* 2, no. 4 (December 1957): 11; *Experiencias cortas escogidas del ministerio de Sally Olsen: "El ángel de los prisioneros"* (San Juan: Rose of Sharon Foundation, 1976).

53. Marín Torres, *Eran ellos*, 132–33. On his Catholic faith in action while incarcerated, see Heriberto Marín Torres, "Crónica: Penitenciaría Estatal," *La Milagrosa* 36, no. 6 (March 25, 1958): 116–17.

54. Samuel Silva Gotay, *Protestantismo y política en Puerto Rico, 1898–1930: Hacia una historia del protestantismo evangélico en Puerto Rico* (San Juan: Editorial de la Universidad de Puerto Rico, 1997), 124–27.

55. Laura Fish, "Christmas in the Río Piedras Penitentiary," *Missions* 24, no. 10 (December 1933): 600.

56. *Actas de la trigésimo quinta asamblea anual de la convención de Iglesias Bautistas de Puerto Rico, celebrada en Caguas* (March 10–13, 1938), 20–21, accessed at the Seminario Evangélico de Puerto Rico (hereafter SEPR).

57. Juan Sánchez Padilla, "El pastor evangélico en las instituciones del gobierno," *Puerto Rico Evangélico* 36, no. 1000 (1947): 10; Juan Sánchez Padilla, "El pastorado evangélico en las instituciones insulares," *Puerto Rico Evangélico* 37, no. 1032 (1949): 45. In a 1957 conference report, Sánchez Padilla also shed light on clashes with the Catholic mission at a youth prison in Miramar over the use of sacred iconography. He claimed that the images made the environment "feel alien." *Actas de la quincuagésima quinta asamblea de la asociación de Iglesias Bautistas de Puerto Rico, celebrada en Ponce* (February 7–10, 1957), 67–70, 89, SEPR.

58. H. B. Lundquist, "Jottings from the Antillean Union," *Advent Review and Sabbath Herald* 122, no. 51 (December 20, 1945): 14; H. B. Lundquist, "Echoes from the Antilles," *Inter-American Division Messenger* 24, no. 5 (July–August 1947): 2.

59. Wesley Amundsen, "Look upon the Fields," *Advent Review and Sabbath Herald* 122, no. 52 (December 27, 1945): 13; Glenn Calkins, "A Survey of Our Work in Inter-America," *Inter-American Division Messenger* 23, no. 3 (March 1946): 4.

60. H. E. Rogers, "Foreign Periodicals," in *Yearbook of the Seventh-Day Adventist Denomination* (Washington, DC: Review and Herald Publishing, 1933), 273; "Our Foreign Missions," *Church Officers' Gazette* 27, no. 4 (April 1940): 32; D. D. Fitch, "A Dutch Oven Produces a Soul Winner," *Advent Review and Sabbath Herald* 120, no. 16 (April 22, 1943): 18–19; Robert M. Whitsett, "Outpouring of the Spirit in Puerto Rico," *Advent Review and Sabbath Herald* 122, no. 13 (March 29, 1945): 1.

61. By the early 1940s, Prince was traveling to US welfare institutions and charged with reviving the Adventist presence in Mayagüez. He also led Spanish-language church work in Harlem, New York. D. A. McAdams, "Spanish Work in New York City," *Advent Review and Sabbath Herald* 123, no. 58 (December 19, 1946): 18; Fitch, "Dutch Oven Produces a Soul Winner," 18–19.

62. On the longer history of station WKAQ and radio in Puerto Rico, consult José Luis Torregrosa, *Historia de la radio en Puerto Rico* (San Juan: Publicaciones Gaviota, 1991).

63. English-language *The Voice of Prophecy* radio broadcasts commenced on foreign soil in Panama City in October 1942. The first Spanish-language broadcast in Latin America was on LU4 Comodoro Rivadavia (Patagonia, Argentina). Portuguese-language broadcasts started simultaneously over five Brazilian radio stations, including one in Rio de Janeiro. M. L. Rice, "Puerto Rico Penitentiary," *Atlantic Union Gleaner* 44, no. 19 (May 11, 1945): 1–2, 7; "From behind Prison Walls," *Church Officers' Gazette* 33, no. 2 (February 1946): 20; Paul Wickman, "*The Voice of Prophecy*," *Advent Review and Sabbath Herald* 123, no. 27 (June 11, 1946): 100; Whitsett, "Outpouring of the Spirit in Puerto Rico," 1; Amundsen, "Look upon the Fields," 13.

64. Glenn Calkins, "The Inter-American Division," *Advent Review and Sabbath Herald* 123, no. 27 (June 11, 1946): 109.

65. W. E. Murray, "Radio in Puerto Rico," *Advent Review and Sabbath Herald* 121, no. 31 (August 3, 1944): 17; Whitsett, "Outpouring of the Spirit in Puerto Rico," 1.

66. S. L. Folkenberg, "A *Voice of Prophecy* Experience from Puerto Rico," *Advent Review and Sabbath Herald* 121, no. 37 (September 14, 1944): 16; M. V. Campbell, "Puerto Rico Visited," *Northern Union Outlook* 9, no. 41 (March 19, 1946): 1–2; Paul Wickman, "Radio Knows No Bounds," *Australasian Record* 56, no. 20 (May 19, 1952): 2–3; Rice, "Puerto Rico Penitentiary," 7; Whitsett, "Outpouring of the Spirit in Puerto Rico," 2.

67. Glenn Calkins, "Puerto Rico Penitentiary Interest Continues," *Advent Review and Sabbath Herald* 122, no. 51 (December 20, 1945): 17–18.

68. Calkins, "Puerto Rico Penitentiary Interest Continues," 17–18.

69. S. L. Folkenberg, "Two Days of Liberty," *Advent Review and Sabbath Herald* 123, no. 16 (April 18, 1946): 14.

70. Folkenberg, "Two Days of Liberty," 14.

71. Tommy Lee Osborn, *Puerto Rico: Revival Harvest, with Miracles of Healing* (Tulsa, OK: Voice of Faith Ministries, 1951); "To the Regions Beyond: Authentic . . . Historic . . . Epics, Unprecedented Victory of Osborn's Return to Ponce," *Voice of Healing* (June 1951): 8–9; "Documented Healings Stop Opposition in Osborn Campaigns," *Voice of Healing* (July 1951): 3, 10.

72. "To the Regions Beyond," 8.

73. "Documented Healings," 3, 10.

74. Tommy Lee Osborn, *Personal Diary Notes: The Ponce, Puerto Rico Crusade and its Significance* (Tulsa, OK: Osborn Publishers, 2007), 11.

75. In the prisoner magazine *Realidad*, Jesus's spiritual medicine is credited with healing moral and physical infirmity. See "Sally Olsen," *Realidad* 3, no. 2 (June–August 1958): 15. Also see Américo M.R., "Mi testimonio," *El Despertar* 2, nos. 3–4 (July-August 1950): 17–19.

76. Fernández Badillo, *Informe Anual del Secretario de Justicia, 1957*, 102–3.

77. Cancio, *Informe Anual del Secretario de Justicia, 1963–64*, 42.

78. Estades Rigau, "Siembran esperanza y consuelo tras las rejas," 35.

79. Alvin J. Stewart, "Sunday School in Prison," *Inter-American Division Messenger* 22, no. 12 (December 1945): 3–4; Advent Youth in Action, "A Sunday School in Prison," *Youth's Instructor* 94, no. 9 (February 26, 1946): 9.

80. Joan Koss-Chioino, *Women as Healers, Women as Patients: Mental Health Care and Traditional Healing in Puerto Rico* (Boulder, CO: Westview Press, 1992), xiii, xviii, 12; Marta Moreno Vega, "Kongo Presence in the Espiritismo of Puerto Rico," in María Elba Torres Muñoz, Mónica Cortés, and Marta Moreno Vega, eds., *Actualidad de las tradiciones espirituales y culturas africanas en el Caribe y Latinoamérica* (San Juan: Centro de Estudios Avanzados de Puerto Rico y el Caribe, 2010), 169–87; Núñez Molina, "Toward an Experiential Approach for Researching Religious Experiences," 248–49.

81. García Leduc, *Intolerancia y heterodoxias en Puerto Rico*; Román, *Governing Spirits*, 5.

82. Román, *Governing Spirits*, 72.

83. M. Camuñas, Director de Prisiones, Circular No. 1, "Sobre meetings espiritistas," August 2, 1905, Circulares, División de Prisiones, Departamento de Trabajo, Beneficencia y Correcciones, Oficina del Procurador General, AGPR.

84. "Visita a la Penitenciaría del Distrito de Ponce," *Cosmos* 9, no. 101 (October 1949): 8.

85. León Bravo directed the Havana group "Luz que Alumbra" with her husband, Lucas Pino, as well as the prestigious magazine *Urania*. Grupo Espírita Apoyo Fraterno sin Fronteras, "Personalidades relevantes a través de la história espírita en Cuba," *La Siembra: Revista Espírita* (June 2010): 9.

86. "Visita a la Penitenciaría del Distrito de Ponce," 8.

87. "Obra social espiritista," *Cosmos* 14, no. 152 (January 1954): 4.

88. "En la reclusión de mujeres en Arecibo," *Cosmos* 12, no. 128 (January 1952): 21.

89. See *The Annual Reports of the Attorneys General to the Governors of Porto/Puerto Rico* for the years 1930–47.

90. Expediente del confinado Esteban Rodríguez Marrero, December 1947, Caja 59, SJLBP, FDJ, AGPR; Expediente del confinado Mario A. Rivera del Palacio, July 1950, Caja 275, SJLBP, FDJ, AGPR.

91. Expediente del confinado Jesús Méndez Caraballo, February 1951, Caja 175, SJLBP, FDJ, AGPR.

92. Expediente del confinado Miguel Ángel Martínez García, September 1947, Caja 205, SJLBP, FDJ, AGPR; Expediente del confinado Ramón Carrasquillo González, September 1950, Caja 200, SJLBP, FDJ, AGPR.

93. Expediente del confinado Agapito Cruz Ramos, November 1948, Caja 168, SJLBP, FDJ, AGPR.

94. Expediente del confinado Ramón Molina Avilés, October 1948, Caja 173, SJLBP, FDJ, AGPR.

95. Expediente del confinado Ramón Molina Avilés.

96. "Nuestro Director entrevista a Don Eduardo Rivera, Presidente de la Casa de las Almas," *El Despertar* 1, no. 2 (June 1949): 5–7.

97. Juan B. Fernández Badillo, *Informe Anual del Secretario de Justicia para el año económico 1957–58* (San Juan: Departamento de Hacienda, Servicio de Compra y Suministro, División de Imprenta, 1964), 42.

98. A. Margenat, "'Bautizan' a 32; reclusos campamento Guavate fundan centro espiritualista," *El Mundo*, May 22, 1962, 15.

99. See *The Annual Reports of the Attorneys General to the Governors of Porto/Puerto Rico* for the years 1930–47. On religious "sects" in the penitentiary, see José B.M., "Sobre religión," *El Despertar* 2, nos. 3–4 (July-August 1950): 20.

100. Carlos D.A., "Resucitó Lazaro," *El Despertar* 2, no. 5 (September 1950): 14.

101. Winter, *Report of the Attorney General of Puerto Rico, 1933*, 58; Horton, *Report of the Attorney General of Puerto Rico, 1934*, 58; Sergio R.N., "Religión," *El Despertar* 1, no. 5 (September 1949): 18, 23.

102. A convict library reading list from 1949 indicates that a prisoner read a book about the prophet Muhammad (Washington Irving's *Vida de Mahoma*). Expediente del confinado Ramón Rosa Rodríguez, November 1949, Caja 480, SEC, FDJ, AGPR. Also consult Swami Sivananda, "Sabiduría budista," *Rumbos* 2, no. 10 (August 1961): 10.

103. Alexander Rocklin, *The Regulation of Religion and the Making of Hinduism in Colonial Trinidad* (Chapel Hill: University of North Carolina Press, 2019).

104. Amaresh Datta, *The Encyclopedia of Indian Literature, Volume Two: Devraj to Jyoti* (1988; New Delhi: Sahitya Akademi, 1996).

105. "De la oficina del director," *Horizontes* 5, no. 2 (September 1956): 10.

106. "De la oficina del director," *Horizontes* 5, no. 3 (October 1956): 5.

107. Swami Sivananda, "Las bienaventuranzas," *Rumbos* 1, no. 6 (March 1960): 10.

108. "Las bienaventuranzas," *Rumbos* 1, no. 8 (May 1960): 10; "Las bienaventuranzas," *Rumbos* 1, no. 9 (June 1960): 10; "Las bienaventuranzas," *Rumbos* 1, no. 10 (July 1960): 8; "Las bienaventuranzas," *Rumbos* 1, no. 11 (August 1960): 8; "Hijos de Dios," *Rumbos* 1, no. 12 (September 1960): 10; "Los benefactores de la humanidad," *Rumbos* 2, no. 1 (October 1960): 10.

109. "Consejos útiles," *Rumbos* 2, no. 3 (December 1960): 8; "Necesidad de una medida para el desprendimiento," *Rumbos* 2, no. 4 (January 1961): 10; "Materia y espíritu," *Rumbos* 2, no. 6 (March 1961): 10; "Espíritu de Cristo," *Rumbos* 2, nos. 8–9 (June-July 1961): 10.

110. "Perspectiva espiritual para la juventud," *Rumbos* 2, no. 2 (November 1960): 10.

111. In Hinduism, Artha is the pursuit of wealth or material advantage. It is one of four traditional aims in life. In the mythology of India, Kama is the god of love and pleasure. During Vedic times, he personified cosmic desire, or the creative impulse, and was called the firstborn of the primeval Chaos that makes all creation possible. "Perspectiva espiritual para la juventud," *Rumbos* 2, no. 5 (February 1961): 10.

112. "Perspectiva espiritual para la juventud," 10.

113. "Perspectiva espiritual para la juventud," 10.

114. The regimen highlighted social, residential, and medical services, as well as varieties of education. Susano Ortiz, "Cómo contribuye la Escuela Industrial para niños a afrontar el problema de la delincuencia juvenil," *Bienestar Público* 14, no. 55 (January–March 1959): 14–15, 18, 21.

115. Wall, *Administration Report, 1951*, 10, 24; Wall, *Administration Report, 1952*, 10, 28.

116. Rogelio M.C., "Algo sobre religión: Como afecta nuestras vidas en la penitenciaría," *El Despertar* 1, no. 9 (January 1950): 23–24.

117. José P.B.M., "Morir es vivir," *El Despertar* 2, no. 5 (September 1950): 16.

118. Juan C.R., "El presidio y mi experiencia," *El Despertar* 2, no. 1 (April 1950): 8.

Chapter Five

1. The colonial-populist government advanced multiple modernization-oriented reform projects in the 1940s and 1950s, including campaigns against illiteracy. See Eloy A. Ruiz Rivera, "La 'gran agenda del porvenir': Ruta de la reforma educativa, 1949–1960," *Revista Magisterio* 5, no. 1 (December 2015): 18–19.

2. Expediente del confinado Rufino Inglés Caraballo, December 1949, Caja 481, SEC, FDJ, AGPR.

3. Expediente del confinado Rufino Inglés Caraballo.

4. Expediente del confinado Rufino Inglés Caraballo.

5. Inglés Caraballo devoured books about Spanish romantic painter and printmaker Francisco de Goya and Venezuelan military and political leader Simón Bolívar. He engaged the work of the Spanish Catholic scholar Domingo Lázaro, including *Doctrina y vida cristiana* (*Christian Doctrine and Life*), a text that establishes the basic precepts of Marian spirituality. He borrowed Western classics like Mark Twain's *Adventures of Tom Sawyer*, William Shakespeare's *A Midsummer Night's Dream*, and Walter Scott's *Ivanhoe*. He also read travel literature, like the Spanish writer Justo González Garrido's *Bajo el cielo del oriente* (*Under the Eastern Sky*), a text about Mediterranean cities. Expediente del confinado Rufino Inglés Caraballo.

6. Horton, *Report of the Attorney General of Puerto Rico, 1935*, 62; Campos del Toro, *Report of the Attorney General of Puerto Rico, 1946*, 42; Negrón Fernández, *Report of the Attorney General of Puerto Rico, 1947*, 73.

7. Officials correlated lack of education with certain crimes, including murder, theft, and breaking and entering. "73 por ciento de reclusos en Presidio Insular son analfabetos funcionales," *El Universal*, November 3, 1947, 61. Also see Alvarado, "La escuela como factor de control en el problema de la delincuencia."

8. Among the contributors was a young Carlos Montenegro, a Spanish-Cuban writer who would later enjoy great fame in Cuban literary circles and the country in general. See Carlos Montenegro, "Penumbras" and "Simbolismo," in Francisco Alonso, *Album "X": Rari nantis in gurgite vasto* (1922–23), 31–33 and 191 according to pagination in text, CHC, UM.

9. Alonso, *Album "X"*, digital image 6 and pages 2 and 6 according to pagination in text.

10. Jacinto Benavente, "Recuerdo de mi visita al Presidio de Cuba," in Alonso, *Album "X"*, 3 according to pagination in text.

11. Alonso, *Album "X"*, digital image 17.

12. Alonso, digital image 16.

13. Alonso, digital image 6. On reverence for mothers in Puerto Rican prisons, see, e.g., Juan R.H., "Maternal amor," *El Despertar* 1, no. 7 (November 1949): 18; Rogelio M.C., "Elegía de

Nochebuena," *El Despertar* 1, no. 8 (December 1949): 11; Victor M.R., "A mi madre," *El Despertar* 1, no. 9 (January 1950); 17; Picó, *El día menos pensado*, 141–43.

14. Jesús Montalvo, "En la ruta," in Alonso, *Album "X"*, 211–12 according to pagination in text.

15. I will elaborate more on the intricacies and history of *Album "X"* in several forthcoming individual and collaborative projects. One of these is tentatively titled "Archival Mysteries: Incarceration and Anarchist Knowledge Production in Cuba in the Early 1920s."

16. US Children's Bureau, *Public Training Schools for Delinquent Children: Directory* (Washington, DC: Government Printing Office, 1955), 38; US Children's Bureau, *Directory of Public Training Schools Serving Delinquent Children* (Washington, DC: US Department of Health, Education, and Welfare Administration, 1958), 69; Puerto Rico Health Department, *Annual Report* (San Juan: Health Department, 1959), viii, 109.

17. Expediente del confinado Rufino Inglés Caraballo.

18. American Prison Association, *Handbook on Classification in Correctional Institutions* (New York: American Prison Association, 1947); Susano Ortiz, "La clasificación de reclusos," *Revista de la Asociación de Maestros de Puerto Rico* 7, no. 7 (December 1948): 220.

19. Ortiz, "La clasificación de reclusos," 220.

20. Ortiz, 220–21.

21. Ortiz, 221, 243.

22. Price Chenault and George Jennings, *Institutional and Parole Problems of Inmates* (New York: State Department of Corrections, Sing Sing School of Printing, 1945).

23. "Una nueva actividad del Sr. Ortiz," *El Despertar* 1, no. 2 (June 1949): inside front cover.

24. "Visitando las agencias," *Revista de Servicio Social* (October 1949): 23.

25. Ortiz, "Clasificación de reclusos III," 153.

26. Ortiz, "Estadísticas," 4, 14.

27. Benjamín Santana, "Plantean problemas: Reclusos publican revista en penitenciaría," *El Mundo*, September 22, 1949, 7. Also see "Felicita a los editores," *El Despertar* 1, no. 5 (September 1949): 6.

28. Gutiérrez Franqui, *Report of the Attorney General of Puerto Rico, 1951*, 59.

29. Rafael Saumell, *La cárcel letrada* (Madrid: Editorial Betania, 2012); Jorge Marturano, *Narrativas de encierro en la República cubana* (Madrid: Editorial Verbum, 2017), 17, 51, 55; Edwards, *A Carceral Ecology*, ch. 5. This phrasing is, of course, a spin on Ángel Rama's classic *The Lettered City*, trans. John Charles Chasteen (Durham, NC: Duke University Press, 1996).

30. Ángel Aparicio Laurencio, *La reforma penitenciaria en Cuba: Conferencia pronunciada en La Casa Cultural de Católicas, el día 5 de junio de 1956* (Havana: Ruiz-Castañeda, 1956), 24, CHC, UM. Mimeographed carceral magazines were common in many countries during this period. Aside from Cuba, in the US state of Texas, for example, prisoners produced a magazine called *The Echo*. See A. B. J. Hammett, *Miracle within the Walls: The Texas Prison Story* (Corpus Christi, TX: South Texas Pub. Co., 1963), ch. 11. The JSTOR Reveal Digital project "American Prison Newspapers, 1800–2020: Voices from the Inside" is bringing many more historical prison periodicals into public view.

31. *El Despertar* 1, no. 5 (September 1949): Table of Contents.

32. *El Despertar* 1, no. 8 (December 1949): Table of Contents. For more on the consequences of operating under the watchful eye of a "censorship board," see "Editorial," *El Despertar* 2, no. 2 (May 1950): 3–4.

33. Contemporary initiatives cut from similar cloth persist in Puerto Rico, and have been taken to a new level. See Edna Benítez Laborde, ed., *Desde adentro: Entre la universidad y la*

cárcel, 2nd ed. (San Juan: Desde Adentro Editores, 2015); Mara Daisy Cruz, ed., *De adentro hacia afuera: Antología de cuentos y cartas desde las prisiones* (San Juan: Divinas Letras, Instituto de Formación Literaria, 2015); Mara Daisy Cruz, ed., *Cicatrices de mi encierro: Antología de cuentos y otros escritos desde las prisiones* (San Juan: Editorial Otros, Instituto de Formación Literaria, 2018); Márel Malaret, dir., *Todos íbamos a ser reyes* (San Juan: Producciones Damiana, 2020).

34. On film screenings in Trinidad and Tobago prisons, see Benson, *Administration Report, 1949*, 9, 23; Benson, *Administration Report, 1950*, 12, 27.

35. "The Presidio," *Porto Rico Progress* 31, no. 5 (February 2, 1933): 8–9.

36. "The Presidio," 8–9.

37. "Blue Skies" (1929), The Silent Film Still Archive, https://www.silentfilmstillarchive.com /blue_skies.htm.

38. "The Presidio," 8–9.

39. "The Presidio," 8–9.

40. Francisco A. Scarano, *Puerto Rico: Cinco siglos de historia*, Cuarta edición (San Juan: McGraw-Hill, 2015), chs. 24–25.

41. Campos del Toro, *Report of the Attorney General of Puerto Rico, 1946*, 44.

42. Joaquín R.B.V., "Orientación sobre el plan de clasificación y tratamiento," 23.

43. Expediente del confinado Damaso Román Zamot, October 1947, Caja 33, SJLBP, FDJ, AGPR.

44. Expediente del confinado Rufino Inglés Caraballo.

45. "Películas a exhibirse durante los meses de mayo y junio de 1953," *Horizontes* 1, no. 2 (May 19, 1953): 10; "Comenzando el día 3 de octubre hasta el 30 de diciembre de 1953, serán exhibidas en el salón de Actos de nuestra Institución las siguientes películas," *Horizontes* 1, no. 5 (September 30, 1953): 6; "Películas a exhibirse durante los meses de febrero y marzo de 1954," *Horizontes* 2, no. 2 (February 28, 1954): 16; "Películas a exhibirse durante los días de abril 3/54 a junio 30/54," *Horizontes* 2, no. 4 (April 30, 1954): 15; "Lista adicional de películas para el mes de junio," *Horizontes* 2, no. 5 (May 1954), 17.

46. "Películas instructivas," *Horizontes* 2, no. 9 (November–December 1954): 3.

47. Expediente del confinado Armando Rivera Colón.

48. José Arnaldo Meyners, "Los artífices reales del penal," *Puerto Rico Ilustrado*, January 5, 1946, 7; Estades Rigau, "Siembran esperanza y consuelo tras las rejas," 35.

49. Later in the twentieth century and in the early twenty-first, cell walls, stairwells, and community rooms became canvases for Oso Blanco prisoners. Eduardo Lalo, *El deseo del lápiz: Castigo, urbanismo, escritura* (San Juan: Editorial Tal Cual, 2010). Poets like Francisco Matos Paoli carved their verses into cell walls, according to Marín Torres. See *Eran Ellos*, 45.

50. José M.N., "La penitenciaría y el arte de la pintura," *El Despertar* 1, no. 9 (January 1950): 27.

51. José M.N., "La penitenciaría y el arte de la pintura," 27.

52. José M.N., "El Arte," *El Despertar* 1, no. 10 (February 1950): 24.

53. Megan Sweeney, *Reading Is My Window: Books and the Art of Reading in Women's Prisons* (Chapel Hill: University of North Carolina Press, 2010), 27–29, 33–35. Also see Joanne Trautmann Banks, *Healing Arts in Dialogue: Medicine and Literature* (Carbondale, IL: Southern Illinois University Press, 1981); Mildred L. Methven, "Prisons Need Libraries," *Prison World* 2, no. 5 (September–October 1940): 7–10.

54. Anna Lila Howard, "Kentucky Prison Libraries," *Prison World* 9, no. 5 (September–October 1947): 15.

55. Winter, *Reglamento para el régimen y gobierno de la Penitenciaría de Puerto Rico*, 22.

56. Florencio R.S., "¿Sabía ud. que?," *El Despertar* 1, no. 7 (November 1949): 22.

57. Winter, *Reglamento para el régimen y gobierno de la Penitenciaría de Puerto Rico*, 22.

58. Loveland, "Report on the Penal and Correctional Program of Puerto Rico," 35, 58.

59. "The Presidio," 8–9.

60. José Rico de Estasen, "Los vivos muertos," *Puerto Rico Ilustrado* 22, no. 1087 (January 3, 1931): 5.

61. Eduardo Zamacois, *Los vivos muertos* (Madrid: Compañía Ibero-Americana de Publicaciones, 1929); José Ignacio Cordero Gómez, "La obra literaria de Eduardo Zamacois," PhD diss., Universidad Complutense de Madrid, 2007, 35, 66, 121, 436.

62. Rico de Estasen, "Los vivos muertos," 5.

63. "The Presidio," 8–9.

64. Cordero Gómez, "La obra literaria," 436–39.

65. Miranda F. Spieler, *Empire and Underworld: Captivity in French Guiana* (Cambridge, MA: Harvard University Press, 2012); Belbenoît, *Dry Guillotine*.

66. Howard, "Kentucky Prison Libraries," 15, 17.

67. Benson, *Administration Report, 1949*, 9, 23; Benson, *Administration Report, 1950*, 12, 27.

68. Carlos Rechaní Agrait, "Del palacio al capitolio," *El Universal*, November 12, 1947, 4.

69. "Visitando las agencias," *Revista de Servicio Social* 10, no. 3 (July 1949): 27.

70. "Adquisiciones de biblioteca," *El Despertar* 1, no. 5 (September 1949): 24. Spanish translations included: *Cinco Semanas en Globo, De la Tierra a la Luna, Dos Años de Vacaciones, En el País de las Pieles, Héctor Servadac, La Vuelta al Mundo en 80 Días, Los Hijos del Capitán Grant, Miguel Strogoff, El Soberbio Orinoco, Escuela de los Robinsones, El Naufragio de Cynthia, El Chancellor, Claudio Bombarnac, La Esfinge de los Hielos, La Caza del Meteoro, Los Hermanos Kip, La Casa de Vapor, La Jangada, Matías Sandorf, Ante la Bandera, Clovis Dardentor*, and *Aventuras del Capitán Hatteras*.

71. "Adquisiciones de biblioteca," 24. Works included: *Actitud Victoriosa, Energía Mental, Paz, Poder y Abundancia, Perfeccionamiento Individual, La Alegría del Vivir, Abrirse Paso, Los Caminos del Amor, Atractivos Personales, La Vida Optimista, Defiende Tus Energías*, and *La Mujer y el Hogar*.

72. Margaret Connolly, *The Life Story of Orison Swett Marden: A Man Who Benefitted Men* (New York: Thomas Crowell Co., 1925).

73. Expediente del confinado Ramón Rosa Rodríguez.

74. Expediente del confinado Rufino Inglés Caraballo.

75. "Nota del Director Recreativo," *El Despertar* 1, no. 6 (October 1949): 27; Araceli Tinajero, *El Lector: A History of the Cigar Factory Reader*, trans. Judith E. Grasberg (Austin: University of Texas Press, 2010).

76. Although not explicitly mentioned in Alamo Rivera's inmate file, the biography was likely Ángel M. Torregrosa's *Luis Muñoz Marín: Su vida y su patriótica obra* (San Juan: Editorial Esther, 1944).

77. Expediente del confinado Salvador Alamo Rivera, June 1947, Caja 468, SEC, FDJ, AGPR. Luis M.C. also read *Don Quijote*. He described the text as a useful tool for "straightening out" wayward citizens. Luis M.C., "Una escuela," 19.

78. Expediente del confinado Félix Nieves Ortiz, September 1949, Caja 84, SJLBP, FDJ, AGPR.

79. Marín Torres, *Coabey*, 90; Marín Torres, *Eran ellos*, 148.

80. Joaquín R.B.V., "Orientación sobre el plan de clasificación y tratamiento," 21–24. Similarly, inmates at the Industrial School for Youths in Mayagüez had access to a strong collection of

books, newspapers, and magazines. "Por el taller de Industrias Nativas y Biblioteca," *Horizontes* 1, no. 3 (June 3, 1953): 10.

81. Expediente del confinado Serafín Feliciano González, November 1947, Caja 33, SJLBP, FDJ, AGPR; Expediente del confinado José María Rivera Rosario, November 1947, Caja 45, SJLBP, FDJ, AGPR.

82. Expediente del confinado Rufino Inglés Caraballo.

83. José A.M.S., "En torno a la biblioteca," *El Despertar* 2, no. 5 (September 1950): 11–12.

84. Expediente del confinado Rufino Inglés Caraballo. Also see Antulio Parrilla, "Santa Rosa de Lima: Primera mística de América," *El Piloto*, September 11, 1948, 1–2, 7–8; Paniagua Serracante, "Espiritualidad de Sta. Rosa de Lima, primera santa de América" *La Milagrosa* 37, no. 16 (August 25, 1959): 444–46, 459–60.

85. Expediente del confinado Enrique Morales Carrasquillo, October 1949, Caja 478, SEC, FDJ, AGPR. Also see Ernesto Álvarez, *Manuel Zeno Gandía: Estética y sociedad* (San Juan: Editorial de la Universidad de Puerto Rico, 1987); Vivian Auffant Vázquez, *El concepto de crónicas en Crónicas de un Mundo Enfermo de Manuel Zeno Gandía* (San Juan: Publicaciones Puertorriqueñas, 1998).

86. Expediente del confinado Ramón Rosa Rodríguez.

87. Expediente del confinado Ernesto Delgado Sárraga, July 1949, Caja 475, SEC, FDJ, AGPR; Expediente del confinado Andrés Pabón Cabrera, October 1949, Caja 479, SEC, FDJ, AGPR; Expediente del confinado Félix Nieves Ortiz, December 1949, Caja 480, SEC, FDJ, AGPR; Expediente del confinado Rufino Inglés Caraballo; Expediente del confinado Enrique Morales Carrasquillo. Also see José Rial, "Elogia de la risa ingenua" and Yoryi Lockward, "Pum, poi la boca," in Lockward's *Acúcheme uté: Cuentos típicos dominicanos* (Puerto Plata: Imp. El Porvenir, A. Rodríguez D., 1941), reproduced in *El Despertar* 1, no. 4 (August 1949): inside front cover and 12; Rubén Darío, "Lo fatal (del libro *Cantos de vida y esperanza*)," *El Despertar* 1, no. 10 (February 1950): 28.

88. "Colaboración," *El Despertar* 1, no. 10 (February 1950): 15–16; "Colaboración," *El Despertar* 1, no. 11 (March 1950): 12, 22; "Colaboración," *El Despertar* 2, no. 2 (May 1950): 20.

89. José A.M.S., "En torno a la biblioteca," 11–12.

90. Jimenes Grullón, *Una gestapo en América*, 9, 17–18.

91. Marín Torres, *Coabey*, 102.

92. Marín Torres, *Eran ellos*, 137.

93. Anthony P. Travisono, *Arts in Corrections* (Washington, DC: American Correctional Association, 1978).

94. Victoria Bates, Alan Bleakley, and Sam Goodman, eds., *Medicine, Health, and the Arts: Approaches to the Medical Humanities* (London: Routledge, 2015); Fernández Olmos and Paravisini, *Healing Cultures*.

95. Fish, "Christmas in the Río Piedras Penitentiary," 600.

96. José Luis Torregrosa, "Cinco años de farándula," *La Torre*, December 13, 1939, 3.

97. "Señoritas del Pensionado ayudan resolver problemas en residencia," *La Torre*, May 14, 1947, 2.

98. Cándido R.M., "Primeras impresiones de un recluso: Segunda parte," 21–22.

99. Carmelo Ch.M., "Retazo," *El Despertar* (August 1949): 10.

100. Carmelo Ch.M., "Retazo," *El Despertar* 1, no. 6 (October 1949): 25.

101. Carmelo Ch.M., "Retazo," *El Despertar* 1, no. 9 (January 1950): 6.

102. Ashley E. Lucas, *Prison Theatre and the Global Crisis of Incarceration* (London: Bloomsbury, 2020).

103. "Diez años de labor seria," *La Torre*, April 24, 1946, 4.

104. "Coro dá cantata de despedida frente a La Torre el viernes," *La Torre*, May 3, 1944, 7; "El Coro Universitario visita la Penitenciaría Insular," *Revista de Servicio Social* 5, no. 3 (July 1944): 22–23.

105. "Visita a la Penitenciaría," *El Despertar* 1, no. 6 (October 1949): 25.

106. Lirio A. D'Acunti, "Sociales del campus," *La Torre*, February 27, 1946, 6.

107. Carmelo Ch.M., "Retazo," *El Despertar* (October 1949): 25.

108. "Programa de variedades ofrecido a los reclusos de 'La Princesa,'" *El Universal*, November 8, 1947, 28.

109. Josefina Guevara de Castañeira, "Joven artista de excepción," *El Mundo*, January 20, 1946, 10.

110. Edgardo Rodríguez Juliá, *Una noche con Iris Chacón* (Carolina, PR: Editorial Antillana, 1986), 109.

111. Carmelo Ch.M., "Retazo," *El Despertar* 1, no. 8 (December 1950): 18.

112. "Acusamos recibo," *El Despertar* 1, no. 7 (November 1949): 5.

113. "Página de arte," *El Despertar* 1, no. 9 (January 1950): 11.

114. Tchaikovsky is also known for "Sleeping Beauty" (1889) and "The Nutcracker" (1892).

115. Héctor Babenco, dir., *Carandiru* (Sony Pictures Classics/Globo Filmes, 2003).

116. "Página de arte," 11, 14.

117. "Carta a nuestro Jefe," *El Despertar* 1, no. 9 (January 1950): 5.

118. "Carta a nuestro Jefe," 5.

119. *The Miss America Pageant Centennial Year Souvenir Program*, September 1954, 12, 23–25, 41.

120. "Tendrá papel principal en la obra Salomé," *El Mundo*, April 21, 1948, 8; Josefina Guevara de Castañeira, "Llevan a escena drama Salomé," *El Mundo*, April 30, 1948, 29, 32; Gaspar Gerena Brás, *Aljibe: Poemas* (San Juan: Editorial Club de la Prensa, 1959), 76–77.

121. Carmelo Ch.M., "Nota del club dramático," *El Despertar* 2, no. 2 (May 1950): 22.

122. "Big Show," *Realidad* 2, no. 1 (March-May 1957): 18.

123. Expediente del confinado Rufino Inglés Caraballo.

Chapter Six

1. Expediente del confinado Vicente Quiñones Ortiz, March-October 1954, Caja 460, SJLBP, FDJ, AGPR.

2. Expediente del confinado Vicente Quiñones Ortiz.

3. Expediente del confinado Vicente Quiñones Ortiz.

4. Peter M. Beattie, *Punishment in Paradise: Race, Slavery, Human Rights, and a Nineteenth-Century Brazilian Penal Colony* (Durham, NC: Duke University Press, 2015), 9.

5. María Elena Díaz, *The Virgin, the King, and the Royal Slaves of El Cobre: Negotiating Freedom in Colonial Cuba, 1670–1780* (Stanford, CA: Stanford University Press, 2000); Cynthia Milton, *The Many Meanings of Poverty: Colonialism, Social Compacts, and Assistance in Eighteenth-Century Ecuador* (Stanford, CA: Stanford University Press, 2007).

6. José Efraín Hernández Acevedo, "El poder exclusivo del indulto," *El Nuevo Día*, December 22, 2020, 29.

7. For example, see Expediente del confinado Benito Aponte, April 1929, Caja 180, SEC, FDJ, AGPR; Expediente del confinado Antolín Bones, April 1929, Caja 180, SEC, FDJ, AGPR; Expediente del confinado Juan Marrero, September 1932, Caja 223, SEC, FDJ, AGPR; Expediente del

confinado Pablo Muñiz Sepúlveda, December 1932, Caja 223, SEC, FDJ, AGPR; Expediente del confinado Emilio Torres Núñez, June 1942, Caja 227, SEC, FDJ, AGPR.

8. Carlos Rechaní Agrait, "Del Palacio al Capitolio," *El Universal*, December 29, 1947, 4.

9. "Editorial: La mente en acción de un confinado," *El Despertar* 1, no. 2 (June 1949): 1–3; Joaquín C.P., "Estadísticas," *El Despertar* 1, no. 2 (June 1949): 22; Florencio R.S., "¿Sabía ud. que?" *El Despertar* 1, no. 6 (October 1949): 21; "Editorial: Corazones Desiertos," *El Despertar* 1, no. 7 (November 1949): 1–4; Number of letters to and from prisoners, *El Despertar* 1, no. 10 (February 1950): inside front cover; Number of letters to and from prisoners, *El Despertar* 1, no. 11 (March 1950): inside front cover. Some letters offered inmates advice, encouraging them to make the most of their incarceration. "Buzón de El Despertar [carta de Arturo]," *El Despertar* 1, no. 11 (March 1950): 7–8. Marín Torres notes in *Eran ellos* that access to visits and letters was not automatic for incarcerated nationalists in the aftermath of the 1950 insurrection (42).

10. Expediente del confinado Roque González Cruz, October 1933, Caja 286, SEC, FDJ, AGPR.

11. Carta de R. Azpurún y otros del pueblo de Utuado al Hon. Gobernador de P.R., August 1931, Expediente del confinado Roque González Cruz, "Clemencia Ejecutiva," Caja 14, FOG, AGPR.

12. Carta de los escolares de Utuado al Hon. Teodoro Roosevelt, November 1931, Expediente del confinado Roque González Cruz, "Clemencia Ejecutiva," Caja 14, FOG, AGPR.

13. Carta del Comité Homenaje a la Vejez al Hon. Gobernador de P.R., April 1932; Carta de Luisa de Jesús al Honorable Gobernador de Puerto Rico, October 1932; Carta de Luisa de Jesús al Hon. Gobernador de Pto. Rico, November 1932; Carta de las damas de Utuado al Hon. Beverley, December 1932; Carta de la sociedad Utuadeña (caballeros), December 1932, Expediente del confinado Roque González Cruz, "Clemencia Ejecutiva," Caja 14, FOG, AGPR.

14. Carta de Luisa de Jesús al Honorable Gobernador de Puerto Rico, October 1932.

15. Carta de Luisa de Jesús al Hon. Gobernador de Pto. Rico, November 1932.

16. Carta de Luisa de Jesús al Hon. Gobernador de Pto. Rico, November 1932.

17. Carta de Luisa de Jesús al Hon. Gobernador de Pto. Rico, November 1932.

18. Asenjo, *Quién es quién en Puerto Rico*, 70–71.

19. Expediente del confinado José Sotero Ortiz Cruz.

20. Carta de José Sotero Ortiz al Hon. Blanton Winship, May 1934, Expediente del confinado José Sotero Ortiz Cruz, "Clemencia Ejecutiva," Caja 36, FOG, AGPR.

21. Carta del Dr. L. López de la Rosa al Sr. Sixto M. Saldaña, February 1934, Expediente del confinado José Sotero Ortiz Cruz, "Clemencia Ejecutiva," Caja 36, FOG, AGPR.

22. Carta de Benjamin J. Horton to the Hon., the Governor of Puerto Rico, August 1934, Expediente del confinado José Sotero Ortiz Cruz, "Clemencia Ejecutiva," Caja 36, FOG, AGPR.

23. Carta de José Sotero Ortiz al Hon. Blanton Winship, January 1935, Expediente del confinado José Sotero Ortiz Cruz, "Clemencia Ejecutiva," Caja 36, FOG, AGPR.

24. Carta de Beatriz Lassalle al Sr. Martín Ergui, May 9, 1935; Reporte de Isolina Peña Oms, May 8, 1935, Expediente del confinado José Sotero Ortiz Cruz, "Clemencia Ejecutiva," Caja 36, FOG, AGPR.

25. Carta de Jesús A. González to the Honorable, the Acting Governor of P.R., May 1935, Expediente del confinado José Sotero Ortiz Cruz, "Clemencia Ejecutiva," Caja 36, FOG, AGPR.

26. Carta de Beatriz Lassalle al Sr. Martín Ergui, May 27, 1935, Expediente del confinado José Sotero Ortiz Cruz, "Clemencia Ejecutiva," Caja 36, FOG, AGPR.

27. Winter, *Report of the Attorney General of Puerto Rico, 1933*, 14, 64; Expediente del confinado Santiago Aponte Vargas, November 1935, "Clemencia Ejecutiva," Caja 34, FOG, AGPR; Expediente del confinado Agustín Belmonte Benellán, August 1936, "Clemencia Ejecutiva," Caja

32, FOG, AGPR; Expediente del confinado Lino Rosario Báez, February 1939, "Clemencia Ejecutiva," Caja 64, FOG, AGPR; Expediente del confinado Francisco García Hornedo, June 1942, "Clemencia Ejecutiva," Caja 85, FOG, AGPR; Loveland, "Report on the Penal and Correctional Program of Puerto Rico," 2; Negrón Fernández, *Report of the Attorney General of Puerto Rico, 1947*, 40, 81; Gutiérrez Franqui, *Report of the Attorney General of Puerto Rico, 1951*, 71; Trías Monge, *Informe Anual del Secretario de Justicia, 1956*, 123–24.

28. Carta de empleados del Gobierno Insular en el Manicomio Insular al Hon. Rafael Menéndez Ramos, June 1937, Expediente del confinado Pablo Pacheco Cuevas, "Clemencia Ejecutiva," Caja 51, FOG, AGPR; Expediente del confinado Pablo Pacheco Cuevas, August 1937, Caja 328, SEC, FDJ, AGPR.

29. Carta de Laura Pacheco Mateu y Alberto Pacheco Mateu al Hon. Gobernador de Puerto Rico, June 1936; Carta de Providencia Trinidad y Virgilio Martínez (testigo) al Hon. Blanton Winship, June 1936, Expediente del confinado Pablo Pacheco Cuevas, "Clemencia Ejecutiva," Caja 51, FOG, AGPR.

30. Carta de empleados del Gobierno Insular en el Manicomio Insular al Hon. Rafael Menéndez Ramos, June 1937.

31. Picó refers to individual and community demands for the accountability of neighbors, peers, and others through the criminal-legal system in several of his works. See, for instance, Fernando Picó, *Santurce y las voces de su gente* (San Juan: Ediciones Huracán, 2014), ch. 5; Fernando Picó, *Realengos y residentes: Los menores en San Juan, 1918–1940* (San Juan: Centro de Investigaciones Históricas, 2019), chs. 5–6.

32. Expediente del confinado Graciano Arroyo Rivera, April 1945, Caja 416, SEC, FDJ, AGPR.

33. Carta de Graciano Arroyo Rivera al Hon. Blanton Winship, June 1938, Expediente del confinado Graciano Arroyo Rivera, "Clemencia Ejecutiva," Caja 55, FOG, AGPR.

34. Carta de Amelia Rivera de Arroyo al Hon. Gobernador de Puerto Rico, April 1940; Carta de Amelia Rivera de Arroyo al Hon. C. Gallardo, May 1940, Expediente del confinado Graciano Arroyo Rivera, "Clemencia Ejecutiva," Caja 55, FOG, AGPR.

35. Carta de José Culpeper al Hon. William D. Leahy, October 1940, Expediente del confinado Graciano Arroyo Rivera, "Clemencia Ejecutiva," Caja 55, FOG, AGPR.

36. Carta de Félix López Rodríguez al Hon. Rexford Guy Tugwell, October 1941, Expediente del confinado Graciano Arroyo Rivera, "Clemencia Ejecutiva," Caja 55, FOG, AGPR.

37. Carta de Dr. Carlos L. Massanet al Sr. Porfirio Díaz Santana, April 1942, Expediente del confinado Graciano Arroyo Rivera, "Clemencia Ejecutiva," Caja 55, FOG, AGPR.

38. Carta de vecinos de Río Piedras al Hon. Jesús T. Piñero, March 1947, Expediente del confinado Graciano Arroyo Rivera, "Clemencia Ejecutiva," Caja 55, FOG, AGPR.

39. Carta de Emilio Arroyo Rivera al Sr. Secretario Ejecutivo, July 1940, Expediente del confinado Emilio Arroyo Rivera, "Clemencia Ejecutiva," Caja 2, FOG, AGPR; Expediente del confinado Emilio Arroyo Rivera, March 1940, Caja 356, SEC, FDJ, AGPR.

40. Memorandum for Governor Winship, May 1937, Expediente del confinado Emilio Arroyo Rivera, "Clemencia Ejecutiva," Caja 2, FOG, AGPR.

41. Carta de Ramón Fontaine Morales al Hon. C. Gallardo, August 1940, Expediente del confinado Emilio Arroyo Rivera, "Clemencia Ejecutiva," Caja 2, FOG, AGPR.

42. Carta de Emilio Arroyo Rivera al Hon. Secretario Ejecutivo, December 1940, Expediente del confinado Emilio Arroyo Rivera, "Clemencia Ejecutiva," Caja 2, FOG, AGPR.

43. Benjamín Santana, "El pastor Crescencio Espinosa pasaría la vida en la prisión," *El Mundo*, March 21, 1950, 1.

44. Carta del Rdo. Carlos López Arellano al Honorable Don Luis Muñoz Marín, January 1951, Folder 646.1, "Petitions & Requests," Caja 119, FOG, AGPR.

45. Benjamín Santana, "Caso de Crescencio Espinosa fue referido a Junta Perdones," *El Mundo*, January 24, 1951, 7.

46. Benjamín Santana, "Gobernador no podría indultar a Pastor Espinosa," *El Mundo*, January 25, 1951, 7; "Piden Muñoz indulto para Pastor C. Espinosa," *El Mundo*, February 26, 1951, 7.

47. Benjamín Santana, "Preparan prueba recurso Coram Nobis en pro de Espinosa," *El Mundo*, March 28, 1951, 4; Benjamín Santana, "Recurso extraordinario," *El Mundo*, April 8, 1951, 6.

48. "Va al Supremo caso desacato de Espinosa," *El Mundo*, September 1, 1949, 1; Benjamín Santana, "Pastor Espinosa recurre ante la Suprema por cuarta vez," *El Mundo*, December 8, 1951, 3.

49. Benjamín Santana, "Juez se reserve fallo en el caso del Pastor Espinosa," *El Mundo*, July 31, 1951, 1.

50. "Excarcelan y en seguida encarcelan al Reverendo Espinosa en Humacao," *El Mundo*, August 9, 1951, 7.

51. "Pastor Espinosa fué vitoreado por fieles al salir de la cárcel," *El Mundo*, December 19, 1951, 22.

52. Benjamín Santana, "Pastor está en libertad tras decisión Supremo da fallo en caso Espinosa," *El Mundo*, January 18, 1954, 1.

53. See, e.g., Dr. José E. Igartua's medical certification, October 1933, Expediente del confinado Alberto Arce, "Clemencia Ejecutiva," Caja 34, FOG, AGPR; Dr. Martín O. de la Rosa's note of support, February 1934, Expediente del confinado Alberto Castro, "Clemencia Ejecutiva," Caja 34, FOG, AGPR; Rev. Aristides Villafañe's letter of support, June 1934, Expediente del confinado Joaquín Morales Orama, "Clemencia Ejecutiva," Caja 34, FOG, AGPR; Dr. Armando Antommattei's note of support, October 1940, Expediente del confinado José Santos Vélez, "Clemencia Ejecutiva," Caja 70, FOG, AGPR. Also see the letters of support submitted by technical unions and reconstruction administration officials in Expediente del confinado Rafael Márquez Maldonado, June 1939, "Clemencia Ejecutiva," Caja 64, FOG, AGPR; Expediente del confinado Fernando Leduc Ramos, July 1942–September 1942, "Clemencia Ejecutiva," Caja 78, FOG, AGPR; Expediente del confinado Salvador Morales Barrientos, June 1943, "Clemencia Ejecutiva," Caja 100, FOG, AGPR. Socialist and populist politicians such as José Berríos Berdecía and Jorge Gauthier, among others, wrote on behalf of incarcerated people. Expediente del confinado Juan Concepción Guerrido, March 1934, "Clemencia Ejecutiva," Caja 34, FOG, AGPR; Expediente del confinado Luis Millán Domey, January 1946, "Clemencia Ejecutiva," Caja 107, FOG, AGPR. It was not uncommon for social workers to be involved in clemency processes as well. Expediente del confinado Manuel Serrano Quiñones, February 1940, "Clemencia Ejecutiva," Caja 64, FOG, AGPR.

54. "Varios penados son indultados," *Listín Diario*, March 5, 1935, 2; "Con magnanimidad el Pdte. Trujillo indulta a varias personas," *Listín Diario*, August 16, 1935, 1, 5; "El Pdte. Trujillo Molina indulta a varios presos," *Listín Diario*, February 27, 1936, 1; "El Hon. Presidente de la República Dr. Trujillo Molina concede generosamente el indulto a diversos presos que sufrían condenas penales," *Listín Diario*, August 18, 1936, 1; "Magnánimo decreto del Hon. Pdte. Trujillo Molina concediendo el indulto a numerosos penados," *Listín Diario*, December 28, 1936, 1; "El Hon. Pdte. Trujillo concede el indulto a diversos presos," *Listín Diario*, February 26, 1938, 1; "El Hon. Pdte. de la República indulta a varios sentenciados," *Listín Diario*, February 27, 1939, 2; "Por medio de un decreto del Presidente de la República se indulta a varios presos," *Listín Diario*, August 16, 1940, 2; "Son indultados varios presos que cumplían condenas en la cárcel," *Listín Diario*, February 27, 1941, 2; "El poder ejecutivo concede el indulto a varios presos," *Listín Diario*,

December 24, 1941, 2; "Son indultados varios presos q. se hallaban cumpliendo condenas," *Listín Diario*, February 27, 1942, 2.

55. Garrido, *Memoria 1944*, 152–54.

56. Garrido, *Memoria 1945*, 86–87.

57. Mejías, *Memoria 1946*, 69–70; Mario Abreu Penzo, *Memoria 1947 Procuraduría General de la República* (Santiago, DR: Editorial El Diario, 1947), 65–66.

58. P. Santos, *La cárcel en República Dominicana* (Santiago, DR: Editora Teófilo, 2006); Yunior Andrés Castillo Silverio, *Origen, historia y formación del sistema penitenciario de la República Dominicana* (Santiago, DR: self-published, 2014), ch. 2.

59. "Una cárcel para menores," *Listín Diario*, June 17, 1937, 2; "Por disposición del Honorable Pte. Trujillo serán construidas varias cárceles modelo para mujeres," *Listín Diario*, July 30, 1937, 1; "El Reformatorio para menores se inaugura hoy en San Cristóbal" and J. Agustín Concepción, "El Reformatorio para menores," *Listín Diario*, February 26, 1938, 1, 6; "La cárcel provisional para mujeres se está construyendo en esta," *Listín Diario*, December 10, 1938, 3; "El Reformatorio para menores 'José Trujillo Valdez,'" *Listín Diario*, January 7, 1941, 2; "Inaugúrase hoy el Reformatorio 'José Trujillo Valdez,'" *Listín Diario*, April 9, 1941, 1, 4; "Por recomendación del Generalísimo Trujillo se aumenta notablemente la capacidad de nuestros Reformatorios," *Listín Diario*, April 22, 1941, 1; "Una nueva función de los reformatorios para menores," *Listín Diario*, April 24, 1941, 2; "El Reformatorio para niñas 'Julia Molina,'" *Listín Diario*, February 24, 1942, 2; "En un lucido acto fue inaugurado ayer tarde el Reformatorio para Niñas 'Julia Molina,' de Cambelén," *Listín Diario*, February 27, 1942, 2, 7.

60. Castillo Silverio, *Origen, historia y formación del sistema penitenciario de la República Dominicana*, ch. 5.

61. "Inauguran Penitenciaría Nacional en La Victoria," *El Caribe*, August 17, 1952, 16.

62. Ramón Alberto Ferreras, *Preso* (Santo Domingo: La Nación, 1962); José Antonio Tallaj, *Un médico en la 40: Recuerdos de una conspiración* (Santo Domingo: Editora Búho, 2006); Fredy Bonnelly Valverde, *Mi paso por la 40: Un testimonio* (Santo Domingo: Editora Mediabyte, 2009); Jimenes Grullón, *Una gestapo en América.*

63. Félix W. Bernardino, "Las cárceles de ayer y hoy," *Listín Diario*, May 31, 1937, 2.

64. "Cárceles para mujeres," *La Tribuna*, August 9, 1937, 2; Bernardino, "Las cárceles de ayer y hoy," 2.

65. Leoncio Ramos, *Yo pasé un día en Sing-Sing y otros escritos* (Santo Domingo: Pensamiento Criminológico Dominicano, 2001); Leoncio Ramos, *Trabajos penitenciarios: Reformas para el establecimiento de un nuevo sistema penitenciario dominicano* (Santo Domingo: Colección Pensamiento Criminológico, 2003).

66. Carta a Rafael Trujillo de Ramona Nolasco, December 1930, Caja 2037, IT: 2902037, SEJIP, PN, FP, AGN.

67. Carta al Secretario de Estado de la Presidencia, Solicitud de indulto elevada por el preso Luis F. Dorville Torres, August 1940, IT: 2902017, SEJIP, PN, FP, AGN.

68. Carta al Señor Secretario de Estado de la Presidencia, Solicitud de indulto a favor del preso Juan Humberto Tavarez, alias Juanito, April 1940, IT: 2902017, SEJIP, PN, FP, AGN.

69. Carta al Señor Secretario de E. de la Presidencia, Solicitud de indulto a favor del preso Luis A. Lockward (a) Danda, May 1940, IT: 2902017, SEJIP, PN, FP, AGN.

70. Solicitud de indulto a favor del preso Luis A. Lockward (a) Danda.

71. Carta al Generalísimo de Julio Pérez, November 1936, Caja 1039, no IT, Ref. Antigua 2728, SEJIP, PN, FP, AGN.

72. Carta al Generalísimo de Julio Pérez.

73. Carta al Señor Secretario de Estado de la Presidencia, Solicitud de indulto elevada en favor del preso Julio César Ricardo, en Pedernales, August 1940, IT: 2902017, SEJIP, PN, FP, AGN.

74. Carta al Señor Generalísimo de Julio César Ricardo, September 1940, IT: 2902017, SEJIP, PN, FP, AGN.

75. "Presenta el Honble. Pdte. Trujillo al Senado un Proyecto de Ley que clausura la Penitenciaría de Nigua: En tal sitio será instalado un Hospital," *Listín Diario*, April 27, 1938, 1; Virgilio Díaz Ordoñez, *Memoria de la Secretaría de Estado de Justicia, Educación Pública y Bellas Artes* (Ciudad Trujillo, DR: Editorial La Nación, 1939), 33; "Con un acto lleno de significación fue inaugurado el nuevo Manicomio 'Padre Billini' construido en Nigua," *Listín Diario*, March 10, 1940, 1, 5, 6; "La inauguración del nuevo 'Manicomio Padre Billini,'" *Listín Diario*, March 11, 1940, 2; Antonio Zaglul, *Mis 500 locos* (1966; Santo Domingo: Ediciones Taller, 1998), 18; Lino A. Romero, *Historia de la psiquiatría dominicana* (Santo Domingo: Editora Búho, 2005), 35, 41–47; Andrés Blanco Díaz, ed., *Obras selectas de Antonio Zaglul: Tomo I* (Santo Domingo: BanReservas, 2011), 33, 54, 84.

76. Carta al Generalísimo Dr. Rafael L. Trujillo M. de Víctor E. Puesan, February 1940, Caja 2016, IT: 2902016, SEJIP, PN, FP, AGN.

77. Carta al Señor Generalísimo Dr. Rafael L. Trujillo Molina de Leonte Martínez, November 1948, Caja 3709, no IT, Ref. Antigua 2660, SEJIP, PN, FP, AGN.

78. Carta al Honorable señor Presidente de la República de Felicita Recio, February 1940, Caja 2016, IT: 2902016, SEJIP, PN, FP, AGN.

79. Carta al Honorable señor Presidente de la República de Felicita Recio.

80. On the Dominican Republic's burgeoning biomedical health-care infrastructure during this period, see Alberto Ortiz Díaz, "Stepping through a Looking Glass: The Haitian Healer Mauricio Gastón on the Romana Sugar Mill in the Dominican Republic in 1938," in Armus and Gómez, *The Gray Zones of Medicine*, 166–67.

81. Carta al Generalísimo de Natividad Vázquez, February 1940, Caja 2016, IT: 2902016, SEJIP, PN, FP, AGN.

82. Carta al Generalísimo Dr. Don Rafael L. Trujillo M. de Juan Montalvo, sin fecha (likely November 1939 given placement in box), Caja 2016, IT: 2902016, SEJIP, PN, FP, AGN.

83. Carta al Señor Secretario de Estado de la Presidencia, Solicitud de indulto elevada por el preso Adón Mona, July 1940, IT: 2902017, SEJIP, PN, FP, AGN.

84. Carta a Rafael Trujillo de Eulalia Medina de Javier, September 1951, Caja 3711, IT: 2903711, SEJIP, PN, FP, AGN.

85. Carta a Rafael Trujillo de Lidia Adames, August 1951, Caja 3711, IT: 2903711, SEJIP, PN, FP, AGN.

86. Carta a Rafael Trujillo de Emilia Grullón Santana, August 1951, Caja 3711, IT: 2903711, SEJIP, PN, FP, AGN.

87. Carta al Señor Secretario de Estado de la Presidencia, Solicitud de indulto elevada en favor del preso Erasmo Rodríguez, August 1940, IT: 2902017, SEJIP, PN, FP, AGN.

88. Carta a Rafael Trujillo de Ramona Pontier, September 1951, Caja 3711, IT: 2903711, SEJIP, PN, FP, AGN.

89. Carta al Señor Secretario de Estado de la Presidencia, Solicitud de indulto [de Domingo González Gutiérrez], August 1940, IT: 2902017, SEJIP, PN, FP, AGN.

90. Carta al Señor Secretario de Estado de la Presidencia, Solicitud de indulto [de Domingo González Gutiérrez].

91. Carta al Generalísimo de Manuel Alberto Pérez a favor de Pedro Pablo Pérez, July 1934, Caja 1039, no IT, Ref. Antigua 2728, SEJIP, PN, FP, AGN; Carta al Generalísimo de los propietarios agricultores de la Piña, August 1934, Caja 1039, no IT, Ref. Antigua 2728, SEJIP, PN, FP, AGN; Carta al Sr. Generalísimo Rafael L. Trujillo M. del preso Ramón Polanco, August 1934, Caja 1039, no IT, Ref. Antigua 2728, SEJIP, PN, FP, AGN; Carta al Señor Secretario de Estado de la Presidencia, Solicitud de indulto [del Dr. Miguel A. Artiles L.], August 1940, IT: 2902017, SEJIP, PN, FP, AGN; Carta al Hon. Señor Presidente de la República de Adriana Filión de Rojas (Sociedad de Socorro Mutuo Santa Margarita), October 1948, Caja 3709, no IT, Ref. Antigua 2660, SEJIP, PN, FP, AGN; Carta al Generalísimo de la familia del preso Juan Francisco Reyes Volquez, December 1948, Caja 3709, no IT, Ref. Antigua 2660, SEJIP, PN, FP, AGN; Carta a Rafael Trujillo de Basilio Leonte Vásquez, September 1951, Caja 3711, IT: 2903711, SEJIP, PN, FP, AGN.

92. Paul Farmer, "On Suffering and Structural Violence: A View from Below," *Daedalus* 125, no. 1 (Winter 1996): 261–83.

Conclusion

1. Coll Cuchí, "Reforma penal," 57.

2. Edwards, *Carceral Ecology*; Edington, *Beyond the Asylum*.

3. "Campos del Toro se propone solicitar dos millones de dólares adicionales al actual presupuesto, para realizar reforma penal," *El Mundo*, December 11, 1945, 1, 20; "Escasa indumentaria dan a los reclusos en el Presidio Insular," *El Universal*, November 3, 1947, 22; "Escasez de agua afecta la higiene en el Presidio Insular," *El Universal*, November 3, 1947, 44; "Promulgan nuevas reglas para visitas a los presos," *El Universal*, December 26, 1947, 35; "Carta singular," *El Despertar* 1, no. 4 (August 1949): 10; Florencio R.S., "¿Sabía ud. que?," *El Despertar* (November 1949): 20; Frank M.Q., "Editorial," 3–4, 6; Joaquín B.V., Jr., "Problemas de actualidad," 17, 23.

4. Gil Ayala, *Del tratamiento jurídico de la locura*.

5. See, e.g., the twelve-part series published by Ramón M. Díaz in *El Imparcial* between February 14 and 25, 1955. Titled "The Truth about the Penitentiary," this fascinating series investigated whether Oso Blanco was a "paradise," a "hell," or a product of government negligence. The different articles cover Oso Blanco's extended lack of access to water; the institution's descent from order in the 1930s to rebellion by midcentury; the demoralizing security measures installed by Col. James M. Jones when he assumed the wardenship of the penitentiary in early 1951; the absence of transparent penal policy and the persistence of poor food quality and living conditions aggravated by overcrowding; the deleterious effects of a closed-door policy toward the press; improved conditions under expert creole leadership; the reversal of some of Jones's measures; a crackdown on the corruption of guards and cellblock bosses; an end to the privileges enjoyed by maximum-security prisoners at the expense of their minimum- and medium-security peers; the refinement of rehabilitative labor in penal encampments; and optimism for the future given government plans to make better use of penal encampments and the Parole Board.

6. Eugenio V.R., "Mas con la gracia de Dios," *Realidad* 2, no. 3 (September–November 1957): 16–17; Hilario R.A., "Sustituya el alcohol con la oración," *Realidad* 3, no. 1 (March–May 1958): 6–7.

7. Marcial, "Soy alcohólico," *Realidad* 1, no. 4 (December 1956–February 1957): 7–9; Juan P.R., "AA no solo es medicina para los alcóholicos, sino que puede aplicarse a otros males que aquejan a la humanidad," *Realidad* 4, no. 2 (May–August 1959): 13–14.

8. Nathan Leopold, "Características sicosociales de un grupo de miembros pertenecientes a la sociedad de Alcohólicos Anónimos en la Penitenciaría Estatal y su relación con las recaídas," *Revista de Servicio Social* 22, nos. 3–4 (July–October 1961): 35.

9. For example, consult Expediente del confinado Félix Valentín Cruz, October 1951, Caja 201, SJLBP, FDJ, AGPR; Expediente del confinado Cándido Cordero Ríos, March 1953, Caja 307, SJLBP, FDJ, AGPR; Rogelio M.C., "Impresiones de un recluso en libertad bajo palabra," *El Despertar* 2, nos. 3–4 (July-August 1950): 13–14.

10. Negrón Fernández, *Report of the Attorney General of Puerto Rico, 1948*, 38.

11. Expediente del confinado Luis Rodríguez Reyes, November 1953, Caja 395, SJLBP, FDJ, AGPR.

12. Pedro A. Vales, "El impacto de la libertad bajo palabra en la rehabilitación de confinados y las características sociales de los confinados, asociados con el éxito o fracaso en el disfrute de la misma," in Universidad de Puerto Rico, Centro de Investigaciones Sociales, *Primer ciclo de conferencias públicas sobre temas de investigación social* (Río Piedras, PR: Universidad de Puerto Rico, Centro de Investigaciones Sociales, 1969), 31, 40.

13. Teobaldo Casanova, *Estudios estadísticos del crimen: Con especial referencia a Puerto Rico* (San Juan: Casanova, 1967); Álvaro M. Rivera Ruiz, *Violencia política y subalternidad colonial: El caso de Filberto Ojeda y el MIRA, 1960–1972* (San Juan: Centro de Estudios Avanzados de Puerto Rico y el Caribe, 2020); Silvestrini, *Violencia y criminalidad en Puerto Rico*; LeBrón, *Policing Life and Death*, 6–8.

14. Picó, *El día menos pensado*, 73, 174.

15. LeBrón, *Policing Life and Death*, 8–9.

16. Josué Montijo, *Los Ñeta* (Río Piedras, PR: Centro de Investigaciones Históricas, Universidad de Puerto Rico–Río Piedras, 2011), 56–57.

17. Montijo, 7, 27–28.

18. Picó, *El día menos pensado*, 57.

19. Picó, 57.

20. Picó, 73.

21. Picó, 57; LeBrón, *Policing Life and Death*, 9–10.

22. Feliciano v. Barcelo, 497 F. Supp. 14 (DPR 1979).

23. Montijo, *Los Ñeta*, x, 23.

24. Picó, *El día menos pensado*, 73.

25. Montijo, *Los Ñeta*, 29–38.

26. Manuel Méndez Saavedra, *Mis experiencias en la Penitenciaría Insular*, 3rd ed. (Río Piedras, PR: Editorial Antillana, 1976); Luis Collazo, dir., *Casa sin ventanas* (San Juan: Zaga Films, 1988); Jorge L. Chaar Cacho, *Maldita sea la justicia* (Río Piedras, PR: Jay-Ce Printing, 1992); Miguel Serrano Arreche, *¡Convicto!* (Miami: Editorial Carisma, 1993); David Ortiz Rivera, *Entre el bien y el mal: Escrito en el complejo correccional de Río Piedras* (Hato Rey, PR: Publicaciones Puertorriqueñas, 1999); Elizam Escobar, *Cuadernos de cárcel* (San Juan: Instituto de Cultura Puertorriqueña, 2006); Ricardo Mercado, *Yo viví en el cementerio de los vivos* (Levittown, PR: Publicaciones Papyrus, 2007); Carmen Lydia Arcelay Santiago, *La dama del Oso Blanco* (San Juan: Publicaciones Puertorriqueñas, 2016).

27. Pablo Marcano García, *La criminalidad y la crisis de prisiones en Puerto Rico* (Chicago: Editorial El Coquí, 1985); Montijo, *Los Ñeta*, 36–38.

28. Montijo, *Los Ñeta*, 7, 62.

29. Martin Lamotte, "The Ñeta Law, the Ñeta World: Ethics and Imaginaries in Circulation between the South Bronx, Barcelona and Guayaquil," *Current Sociology* 65, no. 2 (March 2017): 302–14; Montijo, *Los Ñeta*, 62–128.

30. Christian Suau and Ramiro Millán, dirs., *Oso Blanco: Puerto Rico State Penitentiary* (Miami: Ondamax, Buena Americas, Tangram Films, 2008).

31. Noticel, "Muere histórico preso 'El Jíbaro,'" May 31, 2012, https://www.noticel.com/la-calle /20120531/muere-historico-preso-el-jibaro/; Gerardo Cordero, "Venganza y prisión de El Jíbaro," *Los secretos del Oso Blanco*, http://especiales.elnuevodia.com/osoblanco/nota1.html; Miranda Sánchez, *El Jíbaro.*

32. Alejandro J. García Padilla, "Deudas del pasado y deudas con el futuro," Mensaje del Gobernador del Estado Libre Asociado de Puerto Rico, April 29, 2014, 33, https://noticiasmicro juris.files.wordpress.com/2014/04/mensaje-estado-29-abril-20141.pdf.

Bibliography

Abreu Penzo, Mario. *Memoria 1947 Procuraduría General de la República.* Santiago, DR: Editorial El Diario, 1947.

Aguirre, Carlos. *The Criminals of Lima and Their Worlds: The Prison Experience, 1850–1935.* Durham, NC: Duke University Press, 2005.

Aguirre, Carlos, and Robert Buffington, eds. *Reconstructing Criminality in Latin America.* Wilmington, DE: Scholarly Resources Inc., 2000.

Aiken, Lewis R. *Tests psicológicos y evaluación.* 11th ed. Mexico City: Pearson, 2003.

Alexander, Franz, and William Healy. *Roots of Crime: Psychoanalytic Studies.* New York: Knopf, 1935.

Alexander, Michelle. *The New Jim Crow: Mass Incarceration in the Age of Colorblindness.* New York: New Press, 2010.

Allah, Wakeel. *In the Name of Allah.* Vol. 1, *A History of Clarence 13X and the Five Percenters.* Atlanta: A-Team Publishing, 2009.

Alonso, Francisco, ed. *Album 'X': Rari nantis in gurgite vasto.* N.p.: n.p., 1922–23.

Alper, Melvin G. "Three Pioneers in the Early History of Neuroradiology: The Snyder Lecture." *Documenta Ophthalmologica* 98, no. 1 (1999): 29–49.

Álvarez, Ana Isabel. "La enseñanza de la psicología en la Universidad de Puerto Rico, Recinto de Río Piedras: 1903–1950." *Revista Puertorriqueña de Psicología* 9, no. 1 (1993): 13–29.

Álvarez, Ernesto. *Manuel Zeno Gandía: Estética y sociedad.* San Juan: Editorial de la Universidad de Puerto Rico, 1987.

Amadeo y Antomarchi, Jesús María. *Una plaga social y la plegaria de una virgen.* San Juan: Tip. al vap. de "La Correspondencia," 1894.

Amador, Emma. *The Politics of Care: Puerto Ricans, Citizenship, and Migration after 1917.* Durham, NC: Duke University Press, forthcoming.

American Correctional Association. *State and National Correctional Institutions of the United States of America, Canada, England and Scotland.* New York: The Association, 1956.

American Prison Association. *Handbook on Classification in Correctional Institutions.* New York: American Prison Association, 1947.

American Psychological Association. *Directory.* Washington, DC: American Psychological Association, 1957.

Anderson, Clare, ed. *A Global History of Convicts and Penal Colonies*. London: Bloomsbury, 2018.

Anderson, Warwick. "Objectivity and Its Discontents." *Social Studies of Science* 43, no. 4 (August 2013): 557–76.

Aparicio Laurencio, Ángel. *La reforma penitenciaria en Cuba: Conferencia pronunciada en La Casa Cultural de Católicas, el día 5 de junio de 1956*. Havana: Ruiz-Castañeda, 1956.

Aponte Vázquez, Pedro I. *Locura por decreto*. San Juan: Publicaciones René, 1994.

Araujo, Lorenzo. *Muertos que viven: Cuentos con refranes, decires, creencias, y costumbres del alto sur de la República Dominicana*. Bloomington, IN: Palibrio, 2013.

Arcelay Santiago, Carmen Lydia. *La dama del Oso Blanco*. San Juan: Publicaciones Puertorriqueñas, 2016.

Arenal, Concepción. *La cárcel llamada Modelo*. Madrid: Imp. T. Fortanet, 1877.

———. *Cartas a los delincuentes*. La Coruña, Spain: Imp. del Hospicio, 1865.

———. *Estudios penitenciarios*. 2nd ed. Madrid: Impr. de T. Fortanet, 1877.

Armus, Diego, and Pablo Gómez, eds. *The Gray Zones of Medicine: Healers and History in Latin America*. Pittsburgh, PA: University of Pittsburgh Press, 2021.

Arnison, Nancy D. *Health Conditions in Haiti's Prisons*. Boston: Physicians for Human Rights, 1992.

Asenjo, Conrado, ed. *Quién es quién en Puerto Rico*. San Juan: Real Hermanos, 1933.

———. *Quién es quién en Puerto Rico*. 2nd ed. San Juan: Real Hermanos, 1936.

———. *Quién es quién en Puerto Rico*. 3rd ed. San Juan: Cantero Fernández and Co., 1942.

———. *Quién es quién en Puerto Rico*. 4th ed. San Juan: Imprenta Venezuela, 1947.

Ashford, Bailey K. *A Soldier in Science*. 1934; San Juan: Editorial de la Universidad de Puerto Rico, 1998.

Ashford, Bailey K., and Pedro Gutiérrez Igaravídez (Puerto Rico Anemia Commission). *Uncinariasis en Puerto Rico, un problema médico y económico*. San Juan: Bureau of Supplies, 1916.

Assmann, Jan. "Resurrection in Ancient Egypt." In *Resurrection: Theological and Scientific Assessments*, edited by Ted Peters, Robert John Russell, and Michael Welker, 124–35. Grand Rapids, MI: William B. Eerdmans Publishing, 2002.

Astol, Eugenio. "Men of the Past: Celio S. Rossy." In *El libro de Puerto Rico*, edited by Eugenio Fernández García, 1051. San Juan: El Libro Azul Publishing, 1923.

Auffant Vázquez, Vivian. *El concepto de crónicas en Crónicas de un Mundo Enfermo de Manuel Zeno Gandía*. San Juan: Publicaciones Puertorriqueñas, 1998.

Ayala, César J., and Rafael Bernabe. *Puerto Rico in the American Century: A History Since 1898*. Chapel Hill: University of North Carolina Press, 2007.

Babenco, Héctor, dir. *Carandiru*. Sony Pictures Classics/Globo Filmes, 2003.

"Back Matter." *Yearbook of the National Council on Measurements Used in Education*, no. 11 (1953–54): i–xviii.

Baerga Santini, María del Carmen. "History and the Contours of Meaning: The Abjection of Luisa Nevárez, First Woman Condemned to the Gallows in Puerto Rico, 1905." *Hispanic American Historical Review* 89, no. 4 (November 2009): 643–73.

Bascom Jones, Col. J. *Livre bleu d'Haïti*. New York: Klebold Press, 1919.

Bastian, Jeannette A., John A. Aarons, and Stanley H. Griffin. "Introduction: Decolonizing the Caribbean Record." In Jeannette A. Bastian, John A. Aarons, and Stanley H. Griffin, eds. *Decolonizing the Caribbean Record: An Archives Reader*. Sacramento, CA: Litwin Books, 2018. 1–7.

Bates, Victoria, Alan Bleakley, and Sam Goodman, eds. *Medicine, Health, and the Arts: Approaches to the Medical Humanities.* London: Routledge, 2015.

Beattie, Peter M. *Punishment in Paradise: Race, Slavery, Human Rights, and a Nineteenth-Century Brazilian Penal Colony.* Durham, NC: Duke University Press, 2015.

Beccaria, Cesare. *On Crimes and Punishments and Other Writings.* Edited by Jeremy Parzen and Aaron Thomas. Toronto: University of Toronto Press, 2006.

Becker, Peter, and Richard F. Wetzell, eds. *Criminals and Their Scientists: The History of Criminology in International Perspective.* New York: Cambridge University Press, 2006.

Belbenoît, René. *Dry Guillotine: Fifteen Years among the Living Dead.* New York: Blue Ribbon Books, 1938.

Benítez Laborde, Edna, ed. *Desde adentro: Entre la universidad y la cárcel.* 2nd ed. San Juan: Desde Adentro Editores, 2015.

Benson, S. G. (Trinidad and Tobago Prisons Department). *Administration Report of the Superintendent for the Year 1949.* Port of Spain: Government Printer, 1951.

———. *Administration Report of the Superintendent of Prisons for the Year 1950.* British West Indies: Government Printing Office, 1952.

Bentham, Jeremy. *Panopticon, or, The Inspection House.* 1791. Whithorn, UK: Anodos Books, 2017.

Berger, Dan, Mariame Kaba, and David Stein. "What Abolitionists Do." *Jacobin.* August 24, 2017. https://jacobinmag.com/2017/08/prison-abolition-reform-mass-incarceration.

Bernal, Guillermo. "La psicología clínica en Puerto Rico." *Revista Puertorriqueña de Psicología* 17, no. 1 (2006): 341–88.

———. "60 Years of Clinical Psychology in Puerto Rico." *Interamerican Journal of Psychology* 47, no. 2 (2013): 211–26.

Beverley, James R. *Report of the Attorney General of Porto Rico, 1928.* San Juan: Bureau of Supplies, Printing, and Transportation, 1929.

———. *Report of the Attorney General of Porto Rico, 1929.* San Juan: Bureau of Supplies, Printing, and Transportation, 1929–30.

———. *Report of the Attorney General of Porto Rico, 1931.* San Juan: Bureau of Supplies, Printing, and Transportation, 1931–32.

Bhattacharyya, Kalyan. "Walter Edward Dandy (1886–1946): The Epitome of Adroitness and Dexterity in Neurosurgery." *Neurology India* 66, no. 2 (March 1, 2018): 304–7.

Bingham, Walter V. "MacQuarrie Test for Mechanical Ability." *Occupations: The Vocational Guidance Journal* 14, no. 3 (December 1935): 202–5.

Birn, Anne-Emanuelle, and Raúl Necochea López, eds. *Peripheral Nerve: Health and Medicine in Cold War Latin America.* Durham, NC: Duke University Press, 2020.

Blackmon, Douglas A. *Slavery by Another Name: The Re-Enslavement of Black Americans from the Civil War to World War II.* New York: Random House, 2008.

Blanco Díaz, Andrés, ed. *Obras selectas de Antonio Zaglul.* Vol. 1. Santo Domingo: BanReservas, 2011.

"Blue Skies" (1929). *The Silent Film Still Archive.* https://www.silentfilmstillarchive.com/blue _skies.htm.

Boake, Corwin. "From the Binet-Simon to the Wechsler-Bellevue: Tracing the History of Intelligence Testing." *Journal of Clinical and Experimental Neuropsychology* 24, no. 3 (May 2002): 383–405.

Bonnelly Valverde, Fredy. *Mi paso por la 40: Un testimonio.* Santo Domingo: Editora Mediabyte, 2009.

Boulon-Díaz, Frances. "A Brief History of Psychological Testing in Puerto Rico: Highlights, Achievements, Challenges, and the Future." In *Psychological Testing of Hispanics: Clinical, Cultural, and Intellectual Issues*, 2nd ed., edited by Kurt F. Geisinger, 51–66. Washington, DC: American Psychological Association, 2015.

Boulon-Díaz, Frances, and Irma Roca de Torres. "School Psychology in Puerto Rico." In *The Handbook of International School Psychology*, edited by Shane R. Jimerson, Thomas Oakland, and Peter Thomas Farrell, 309–22. Thousand Oaks, CA: Sage, 2007.

Bradford Cannon, Walter. "Again the James-Lange and the Thalamic Theories of Emotion." *Psychological Review* 38, no. 4 (1931): 281–95.

Brau, Salvador. *Ensayos: Disquisiciones sociológicas*. Río Piedras, PR: Editorial Edil, 1972.

Briggs, Laura. *Reproducing Empire: Race, Sex, Science, and US Imperialism in Puerto Rico*. Berkeley: University of California Press, 2003.

Bronfman, Alejandra M. *Measures of Equality: Social Science, Citizenship, and Race in Cuba, 1902–1940*. Chapel Hill: University of North Carolina Press, 2004.

Brown, Vincent. *The Reaper's Garden: Death and Power in the World of Atlantic Slavery*. Cambridge, MA: Harvard University Press, 2010.

Buffington, Robert. *Criminal and Citizen in Modern Mexico*. Lincoln: University of Nebraska Press, 2000.

Bulhan, Hussein Abdilahi. *Frantz Fanon and the Psychology of Oppression*. New York: Plenum, 1985.

Burgos Ortiz, Nilsa M. *Pioneras de la profesión de trabajo social en Puerto Rico*. San Juan: Publicaciones Puertorriqueñas, 2013.

Burns, Kathryn. *Into the Archive: Writing and Power in Colonial Peru*. Durham, NC: Duke University Press, 2010.

Burrows, Geoff G. "The New Deal in Puerto Rico: Public Works, Public Health, and the Puerto Rico Reconstruction Administration, 1935–1955." PhD diss., Graduate Center, City University of New York, 2014.

Butte, George C. *Report of the Attorney General of Porto Rico, 1927*. San Juan: Bureau of Supplies, Printing, and Transportation, 1927.

Cabán, Pedro A. *Constructing a Colonial People: Puerto Rico and the United States, 1898–1932*. Boulder, CO: Westview Press, 1999.

Caimari, Lila M. *Apenas un delincuente: Crimen, castigo y cultura en la Argentina, 1880–1955*. Buenos Aires: Siglo Veintiuno Editores, 2004.

———. "The Archive's Moment." *Histories* 1 (July 2021): 100–107.

———. "Psychiatrists, Criminals, and Bureaucrats: The Production of Scientific Biographies in the Argentine Penitentiary System." In *Argentina on the Couch: Psychiatry, State, and Society, 1880 to the Present*, edited by Mariano Plotkin, 113–38. Albuquerque: University of New Mexico Press, 2003.

———. "Remembering Freedom: Life as Seen from the Prison Cell (Buenos Aires Province, 1930–1950)." In *Crime and Punishment in Latin America: Law and Society Since Late Colonial Times*, edited by Ricardo D. Salvatore, Carlos Aguirre, and Gilbert M. Joseph, 391–414. Durham, NC: Duke University Press, 2001.

———. "Whose Criminals Are These? Church, State, and Patronatos and the Rehabilitation of Female Convicts (Buenos Aires, 1890–1940)." *The Americas* 54, no. 2 (October 1997): 185–208.

Campos del Toro, Enrique. *Report of the Attorney General of Puerto Rico, 1945*. San Juan: Service Office of the Government of Puerto Rico, Printing Division, 1946.

———. *Report of the Attorney General of Puerto Rico, 1946*. San Juan: Administración General de Suministros, Oficina de Servicios, División de Imprenta, 1947.

Camuñas, Manuel. "Executive Departments of the Government of Porto Rico and Functions of Same." In *El libro de Puerto Rico*, edited by Eugenio Fernández García, 163–77. San Juan: El Libro Azul Publishing, 1923.

Cancelli, Elizabeth. *Carandiru: A prisão, o psiquiatria e o preso*. Brasília: Ed. UnB, 2005.

Cancio, Hiram R. *Informe Anual del Secretario de Justicia al Gobernador del Estado Libre Asociado de Puerto Rico, 1963–64*. San Juan: Departamento de Hacienda, Servicio de Compra y Suministro, División de Imprenta, 1966.

Candelario, Ginetta E. B., Elizabeth S. Manley, and April J. Mayes, eds. *Cien años de feminismos dominicanos*. Vol. 2. Santo Domingo: Archivo General de la Nación, 2016.

Carlo Altieri, Gerardo A. *Justicia y gobierno: La Audiencia de Puerto Rico, 1831–1861*. Seville: Consejo Superior de Investigaciones Científicas, Academia Puertorriqueña de la Historia, 2007.

———. *El sistema legal y los litigios de esclavos en Indias: Puerto Rico, siglo XIX*. Sevilla: Consejo Superior de Investigaciones Científicas, 2010.

Carrafiello, Susan B. *"The Tombs of the Living": Prisons and Prison Reform in Liberal Italy*. New York: Peter Lang Publishing, 1998.

Carreras, Gerónimo. "Board of Medical Examiners." In *El libro de Puerto Rico*, edited by Eugenio Fernández García, 259–60. San Juan: El Libro Azul Publishing, 1923.

Carson, John. "Mental Testing in the Early Twentieth Century: Internationalizing the Mental Testing Story." *History of Psychology* 17, no. 3 (August 2014): 249–55.

Casanova, Teobaldo. *Estudios estadísticos del crimen: Con especial referencia a Puerto Rico*. San Juan: Casanova, 1967.

Castillo Silverio, Yunior Andrés. *Origen, historia y formación del sistema penitenciario de la República Dominicana*. Santiago, DR: Self-published, 2014. https://www.monografias.com/trabajos 102/origen-historia-y-formacion-del-sistema-penitenciario-republica-dominicana/origen -historia-y-formacion-del-sistema-penitenciario-republica-dominicana.shtml.

Castro Arroyo, María de los Ángeles. *Arquitectura en San Juan de Puerto Rico, siglo XIX*. San Juan: Editorial de la Universidad de Puerto Rico, 1980.

Celeste Marín, Rosa, Awilda Paláu de López, and Gloria P. Barbosa de Chardón. *La efectividad de la rehabilitación en los delincuentes de Puerto Rico*. San Juan: Universidad de Puerto Rico, 1959.

Chaar Cacho, Jorge L. *Maldita sea la justicia*. Río Piedras, PR: Jay-Ce Printing, 1992.

Chakravorty Spivak, Gayatri. "Can the Subaltern Speak?" In *Marxism and the Interpretation of Culture*, edited by Cary Nelson and Lawrence Grossberg, 271–313. Urbana: University of Illinois Press, 1988.

Charleroy, Margaret Lynn. "Penitentiary Practice: Healthcare and Medicine in Minnesota State Prison, 1855–1930." PhD diss., University of Minnesota, 2013.

Chase, Robert T. *We Are Not Slaves: State Violence, Coerced Labor, and Prisoners' Rights in Postwar America*. Chapel Hill: University of North Carolina Press, 2020.

Chazkel, Amy. "Social Life and Civic Education in the Rio de Janeiro City Jail." *Journal of Social History* 42, no. 3 (Spring 2009): 697–731.

Chelala, José. *Reacciones mentales, psíquicas y sexuales en nuestras prisiones*. Havana: Editorial "La República," 1941.

Chenault, Price, and George Jennings. *Institutional and Parole Problems of Inmates*. New York: State Department of Corrections, Sing Sing School of Printing, 1945.

Childs, Dennis. *Slaves of the State: Black Incarceration from the Chain Gang to the Penitentiary.* Minneapolis: University of Minnesota Press, 2015.

Chitwood, Ken. "Los Musulmanes Boricuas: Puerto Rican Muslims and the Idea of Cosmopolitanism." PhD diss., University of Florida, 2019.

Coats, Herbert P. *Report of the Attorney General of Porto Rico, 1923.* Washington, DC: Government Printing Office, 1925.

Cole, Thomas, Nathan Carlin, and Ronald Carson. *Medical Humanities: An Introduction.* New York: Cambridge University Press, 2015.

Collazo, Luis, dir. *Casa sin ventanas.* San Juan: Zaga Films, 1988.

Colombán Rosario, José. *Problema de la criminalidad en Puerto Rico.* Río Piedras, PR: Universidad de Puerto Rico, Colegio de Pedagogía, 1952.

Congreso Médico Dominicano. *Memoria del Congreso Médico Dominicano del Centenario.* Vol. 3. Santiago, DR: Editorial El Diario, 1945.

Connerton, Winifred C. "Working towards Health, Christianity and Democracy: American Colonial and Missionary Nurses in Puerto Rico, 1900–30." In *Colonial Caring: A History of Colonial and Post-Colonial Nursing,* edited by Helen Sweet and Sue Hawkins, 126–44. Manchester, UK: Manchester University Press, 2015.

Connolly, Margaret. *The Life Story of Orison Swett Marden: A Man Who Benefitted Men.* New York: Thomas Crowell Co., 1925.

Cope, R. Douglas. *The Limits of Racial Domination: Plebeian Society in Colonial Mexico City, 1660–1720.* Madison: University of Wisconsin Press, 1994.

Cordero, Gerardo. "Venganza y prisión de El Jíbaro." *Los secretos del Oso Blanco.* http://especiales.elnuevodia.com/osoblanco/nota1.html.

Cordero Gómez, José Ignacio. "La obra literaria de Eduardo Zamacois." PhD diss., Universidad Complutense de Madrid, 2007.

Córdoba Chirino, Jacobo. *Los que murieron en la horca: Historia del crimen, juicio y ajusticiamento de los que en Puerto Rico murieron en la horca desde las Partidas Sediciosas a Pascual Ramos.* 1954. San Juan: Editorial Cordillera, 2007.

Costa Mandry, Oscar. *Apuntes para la historia de la medicina en Puerto Rico: Reseña histórica de las ciencias de la salud.* San Juan: Departamento de Salud, 1971.

Cruz, Mara Daisy, ed. *Cicatrices de mi encierro: Antología de cuentos y otros escritos desde las prisiones.* San Juan: Editorial Otros, Instituto de Formación Literaria, 2018.

———. *De adentro hacia afuera: Antología de cuentos y cartas desde las prisiones.* San Juan: Divinas Letras, Instituto de Formación Literaria, 2015.

Cunha Miranda, Carlos Alberto. "A fatalidade biológica: A medição dos corpos, de Lombroso aos biotipologistas." In *História das prisões no Brasil,* edited by Clarissa Nunes Maia, Flávio de Sá Neto, Marcos Costa, and Marcos Luiz Bretas, 2:277–317. Rio de Janeiro: Editora Rocco, 2009.

Dahm, Clair. "Community Corrections: The Rise and Fall of the Rehabilitative Ideal in Postwar St. Louis." PhD diss., Brandeis University, 2017.

Dalgleish, Tim. "The emotional brain." *Nature Reviews Neuroscience* 5, no. 7 (July 2004): 582–89.

Da Mota Gomes, Marleide. "From the Wax Cast of Brain Ventricles (1508–9) by Leonardo da Vinci to Air Cast Ventriculography (1918) by Walter E. Dandy." *Neurologique* 176, no. 5 (May 2020): 393–96.

Danziger, Kurt. *Constructing the Subject: Historical Origins of Psychological Research.* New York: Cambridge University Press, 1994.

Datta, Amaresh. *The Encyclopedia of Indian Literature, Volume Two: Devraj to Jyoti*. 1988. New Delhi: Sahitya Akademi, 1996.

Davis, Angela Y. *Are Prisons Obsolete?* New York: Seven Stories Press, 2003.

De la Torriente Brau, Pablo. *Presidio Modelo*. Havana: Instituto del Libro, Editorial de Ciencias Sociales, 1969.

Delano, Jack. *Puerto Rico mío: Cuatro décadas de cambio*. Washington, DC: Smithsonian Institution Press, 1990.

Del Carmen Baerga, María. "Routes to Whiteness, or How to Scrub Out the Stain: Hegemonic Masculinity and Racialization in Nineteenth-Century Puerto Rico." *Translating the Americas* 3 (2015): 109–47.

Del Moral, Solsiree. "Street Children, Crime, and Punishment in Puerto Rico, 1940–1965." Unpublished manuscript.

Del Valle Atiles, Francisco. *El campesino puertorriqueño: Sus condiciones físicas, intelectuales y morales, causas que las determinan y medios para mejorarlas*. San Juan: Tip. de José González Font, 1887.

Díaz, María Elena. *The Virgin, the King, and the Royal Slaves of El Cobre: Negotiating Freedom in Colonial Cuba, 1670–1780*. Stanford, CA: Stanford University Press, 2000.

Díaz Ordóñez, Virgilio. *Memoria de la Secretaría de Estado de Justicia, Educación Pública y Bellas Artes*. Ciudad Trujillo, DR: Editorial La Nación, 1939.

Dietz, James L. *Economic History of Puerto Rico: Institutional Change and Capitalist Development*. Princeton, NJ: Princeton University Press, 1986.

Dikötter, Frank. *Crime, Punishment, and the Prison in Modern China*. New York: Columbia University Press, 2002.

Domínguez Navarro, Ofelia. *De 6 a 6: La vida en las prisiones cubanas*. Mexico City: n.p., 1937.

Dostoyevsky, Fyodor. *The House of the Dead*. Translated by Constance Garnett. Mineola, NY: Dover, 2004.

Douglas, Andy. *Redemption Songs: A Year in the Life of a Community Prison Choir*. San Germán, PR: Innerworld Publications, 2019.

Dow Burkhead, Michael. *The Treatment of Criminal Offenders: A History*. Jefferson, NC: McFarland, 2007.

Drescher, Seymour, and Stanley L. Engerman, eds. *A Historical Guide to World Slavery*. New York: Oxford University Press, 1998.

Drucker, Ernest. *A Plague of Prisons: The Epidemiology of Mass Incarceration in America*. New York: New Press, 2014.

Duffy Burnett, Christina, and Burke Marshall, eds. *Foreign in a Domestic Sense: Puerto Rico, American Expansion, and the Constitution*. Durham, NC: Duke University Press, 2001.

Edington, Claire E. *Beyond the Asylum: Mental Illness in French Colonial Vietnam*. Ithaca, NY: Cornell University Press, 2019.

Edwards, Ryan C. *A Carceral Ecology: Ushuaia and the History of Landscape and Punishment in Argentina*. Oakland: University of California Press, 2021.

Eghigian, Greg. *The Corrigible and the Incorrigible: Science, Medicine, and the Convict in Twentieth-Century Germany*. Ann Arbor: University of Michigan Press, 2015.

Ellenbogen, Josh. *Reasoned and Unreasoned Images: The Photography of Bertillon, Galton, and Marey*. University Park, PA: Pennsylvania State University Press, 2012.

Embade Neyra, José E. *El gran suicida (apuntes de una época revolucionaria): Obra escrita en el Presidio Modelo.* Havana: Imp. y Lib. "La Propagandista," 1934.

Emre, Merve. *The Personality Brokers: The Strange History of Myers-Briggs and the Birth of Personality Testing.* New York: Doubleday, 2018.

Enscore, Susan I., Suzanne P. Johnson, Julie L. Webster, and Gordon L. Cohen. *Guarding the Gates: The Story of Fort Clayton.* Champaign, IL: US Army Corp of Engineers, 2000.

Equipo T[elemundo]. "Yo era Alex Trujillo." *Telemundo Puerto Rico.* April 5, 2021. https://www.telemundopr.com/noticias/puerto-rico/equipo-t-yo-era-alex-trujillo-2/2198786/.

Ergui, Martín. "Penal Institutions and Reform School." In *El libro de Puerto Rico,* edited by Eugenio Fernández García, 278–82. San Juan: El Libro Azul Publishing, 1923.

Erman, Sam. *Almost Citizens: Puerto Rico, the US Constitution, and Empire.* New York: Cambridge University Press, 2019.

Escobar, Elizam. *Cuadernos de cárcel.* San Juan: Instituto de Cultura Puertorriqueña, 2006.

Espaillat de la Mota, R. *Memoria 1950 Secretaría de Estado de Sanidad y Asistencia Pública.* Ciudad Trujillo, DR: Editora del Caribe, 1957.

Espinosa, Mariola. *Epidemic Invasions: Yellow Fever and the Limits of Cuban Independence, 1878–1930.* Chicago: University of Chicago Press, 2009.

Essex Wynter, W. "Four Cases of Tubercular Meningitis in which Paracentesis of the Theca Vertebralis Was Performed for the Relief of Fluid Pressure." *Lancet* 137, no. 3531 (May 2, 1891): 981–82.

Etain, Bruno, and Laurence Roubaud. "Jean Delay, M.D., 1907–1987." *American Journal of Psychiatry* 159, no. 9 (September 2002): 1489.

Experiencias cortas escogidas del ministerio de Sally Olsen: "El ángel de los prisioneros." San Juan: Rose of Sharon Foundation, 1976.

Farmer, Paul. "On Suffering and Structural Violence: A View from Below." *Daedalus* 125, no. 1 (Winter 1996): 261–83.

Farquhar Fulton, John. *Frontal Lobotomy and Affective Behavior: A Neurophysiological Analysis.* New York: W. W. Norton & Co., 1951.

Fenton, Norman. *Manual sobre el uso de la consejería en grupos en las instituciones correccionales.* Translated by Porfirio Díaz Santana. Río Piedras, PR: Centro de Investigaciones Sociales, Facultad de Ciencias Sociales, Universidad de Puerto Rico, 1967; Sacramento, CA: Instituto para el Estudio del Crimen y la Delincuencia, 1967.

Fernández Badillo, Juan B. *Informe Anual del Secretario de Justicia para el año que terminó el 30 de junio de 1957.* San Juan: Departamento de Hacienda, Servicio de Compra y Suministro, División de Imprenta, 1959.

———. *Informe Anual del Secretario de Justicia para el año económico 1957–58.* San Juan: Departamento de Hacienda, Servicio de Compra y Suministro, División de Imprenta, 1964.

Fernández García, Benigno. *Report of the Attorney General of Puerto Rico, 1936.* San Juan: Bureau of Supplies, Printing, and Transportation, 1936.

———. *Report of the Attorney General of Puerto Rico, 1937.* San Juan: Justice Department, 1937–38.

———. *Report of the Attorney General of Puerto Rico, 1938.* San Juan: Justice Department, 1938–39.

———. *Report of the Attorney General of Puerto Rico, 1939.* San Juan: Justice Department, 1939–40.

Fernández García, Eugenio, ed. *El libro de Puerto Rico*. San Juan: El Libro Azul Publishing, 1923.

Fernández Olmos, Margarite, and Lizabeth Paravisini, eds. *Healing Cultures: Art and Religion as Curative Practices in the Caribbean and its Diaspora*. New York: Palgrave, 2001.

Fernós Isern, Antonio. *Report of the Commissioner of Health of Puerto Rico, 1942–43*. San Juan: Insular Procurement Office, Printing Division, 1944.

Ferracuti, Franco, and G. B. Rizzo. "Signos sobresalientes de la homosexualidad en una población penitenciaria femenina, obtenidos mediante la aplicación de técnicas de proyección." *Revista de Ciencias Sociales* 2, no. 4 (December 1958): 469–79.

Ferracuti Franco, and Maria Christina Giannini. *L'incesto padre-figlia: Studio clinico-criminológico*. Río Piedras, PR: University of Puerto Rico, 1968.

Ferreras, Ramón Alberto. *Preso*. Santo Domingo: La Nación, 1962.

Fessler, Daniel. "El delito con rostro: Los comienzos de la identificación de delincuentes en Uruguay." *Passagens: Revista Internacional de História Política e Cultura Jurídica* 7, no. 1 (January-April 2015): 15–39.

Fielding Reid, Harry, and Stephen Taber. *The Porto Rico Earthquake of 1918: Report of the Earthquake Investigation Commission*. Washington, DC: Government Printing Office, 1919.

Findlay, Eileen J. *Imposing Decency: The Politics of Sexuality and Race in Puerto Rico, 1870–1920*. Durham, NC: Duke University Press, 2000.

First Annual Report of Charles H. Allen, Governor of Porto Rico. Washington, DC: Government Printing Office, 1901.

Flores, Juan. *From Bomba to Hip-Hop: Puerto Rican Culture and Latino Identity*. New York: Columbia University Press, 2000.

Forrai, Judit. "History of Different Therapeutics of Venereal Disease before the Discovery of Penicillin." In *Syphilis: Recognition, Description, and Diagnosis*, edited by Neuza Satomi Sato, 37–58. Rijeka, Croatia: InTech, 2011.

Foucault, Michel. *The Birth of the Clinic: An Archeology of Medical Perception*. 1973. Translated by A. M. Sheridan Smith. New York: Vintage, 1994.

———. *Discipline and Punish: The Birth of the Prison*. 1975. Translated by Alan Sheridan. New York: Vintage, 1995.

———. *Madness and Civilization: A History of Insanity in the Age of Reason*. 1965. Translated by Richard Howard. New York: Vintage, 1988.

———. "Panopticism" from *Discipline and Punish: The Birth of the Prison*. *Race/Ethnicity: Multidisciplinary Global Contexts* 2, no. 1 (Autumn 2008): 1–12.

Friedman, Bruce H. "Feelings and the Body: The Jamesian Perspective on Autonomic Specificity of Emotion." *Biological Psychology* 84, no. 3 (July 2010): 383–93.

Frith, John. "Syphilis—Its Early History and Treatment Until Penicillin, and the Debate on Its Origins." *Journal of Military and Veterans' Health* 20, no. 4 (November 2012): 49–56.

Fuentes, Marisa J. *Dispossessed Lives: Enslaved Women, Violence, and the Archive*. Philadelphia: University of Pennsylvania Press, 2016.

Galindo, Naomi. "Decolonización de los espacios de reclusión." December 13, 2016. http://umbral.uprrp.edu/archivo-de-la-palabra/conferencia/jornada/segunda-jornada-de-refle xion-sobre-educacion-universitaria-en-la-carcel/de-colonizacion-de-los-espacios-de -reclusion/.

Galindo-Malavé, Nahomi. "Cuerpos truculentos y 'desviados': Las confinadas de la Escuela Industrial para Mujeres de Vega Alta." *Identidades* 8 (November 2010): 11–34.

García González, Armando, and Consuelo Naranjo Orovio. "Antropología, 'raza' y población en Cuba en el último cuarto del siglo XIX." *Anuario de Estudios Americanos* 55, no. 1 (1998): 267–89.

García Leduc, José Manuel. *Intolerancia y heterodoxias en Puerto Rico (siglo XIX): Protestantes, masones y espiritistas-kardecianos reclaman su espacio social, c. 1869–1898*. San Juan: Isla Negra Editores, 2009.

García Padilla, Alejandro J. "Deudas del pasado y deudas con el futuro." Mensaje del Gobernador del Estado Libre Asociado de Puerto Rico. April 29, 2014. 1–34. https://noticiasmicro juris.files.wordpress.com/2014/04/mensaje-estado-29-abril-20141.pdf.

García Rodríguez, Francisco J. "Conformación y evolución de los sistemas administrativos de la cárcel de San Juan en la transición del régimen español al régimen estadounidense en Puerto Rico (1888 a 1910)." PhD diss., Centro de Estudios Avanzados de Puerto Rico y el Caribe, 2012.

Gard, Raymond L. *Rehabilitation and Probation in England and Wales, 1876–1962*. London: Bloomsbury, 2016.

Garland, David. *Punishment and Modern Society: A Study in Social Theory*. Chicago: University of Chicago Press, 1990.

———. *Punishment and Welfare: A History of Penal Strategies*. Aldershot, England: Gower, 1985.

Garrido, Víctor. *Memoria 1944 Procuraduría General de la República*. Santiago, DR: Editorial El Diario, 1944.

———. *Memoria 1945 Procuraduría General de la República*. Santiago, DR: Editorial El Diario, 1945.

Garton, Stephen. "Crime, Prisons, and Psychiatry: Reconsidering Problem Populations in Australia, 1890–1930." In *Criminals and Their Scientists: The History of Criminology in International Perspective*, edited by Peter Becker and Richard F. Wetzell, 231–51. New York: Cambridge University Press, 2006.

Gerena Brás, Gaspar. *Aljibe: Poemas*. San Juan: Editorial Club de la Prensa, 1959.

Gibby, Robert E., and Michael E. Zickar. "A History of the Early Days of Personality Testing in American Industry: An Obsession with Adjustment." *History of Psychology* 11, no. 3 (September 2008): 164–84.

Gibson, Mary. "Global Perspectives on the Birth of the Prison." *American Historical Review* 116, no. 4 (October 2011): 1040–63.

———. *Italian Prisons in the Age of Positivism, 1861–1914*. London: Bloomsbury, 2019.

Gil Ayala, Carlos C. *Del tratamiento jurídico de la locura: Proyecto psiquiátrico y gobernabilidad en Puerto Rico*. San Juan: Editorial Posdata, 2009.

Gilbert, Jane. *Living Death in Medieval French and English Literature*. New York: Cambridge University Press, 2014.

Ginzburg, Carlo. *The Cheese and the Worms: The Cosmos of a Sixteenth-Century Miller*. Baltimore: Johns Hopkins University Press, 1980.

Goffman, Erving. "On the Characteristics of Total Institutions." In *Asylums: Essays on the Social Situation of Mental Patients and Other Inmates*. New York: Anchor, 1961.

Goldstein, Jan E. "Toward an Empirical History of Moral Thinking: The Case of Racial Theory in Mid-Nineteenth-Century France." *American Historical Review* 120, no. 1 (February 2015): 1–27.

Gómez, Pablo. *The Experiential Caribbean: Creating Knowledge and Healing in the Early Modern Atlantic*. Chapel Hill: University of North Carolina Press, 2017.

González, José Luis. *Puerto Rico: The Four-Storeyed Country and Other Essays*. Translated by Gerald Guinness. Princeton, NJ: Markus Wiener Publishers, 1993.

González Ascencio, Gerardo. *Los orígenes de la criminología en México: La recepción del positivismo y los gabinetes antropométricos en las cárceles de la Ciudad de México, 1867–1910*. Saarbrücken, Germany: Editorial Académica Española, 2012.

González García, María D. *El negro y la negra libres, Puerto Rico: 1800–1873, su presencia y contribución a la identidad puertorriqueña*. San Juan: MGG Editorial, 2014.

Geary, Patrick J. *Living with the Dead in the Middle Ages*. Ithaca, NY: Cornell University Press, 1994.

Green, Cecilia A. "Local Geographies of Crime and Punishment in a Plantation Colony: Gender and Incarceration in Barbados, 1878–1928." *New West Indian Guide* 86, nos. 3–4 (2012): 263–90.

Grupo Espírita Apoyo Fraterno Sin Fronteras. "Personalidades relevantes a través de la história espírita en Cuba." *La Siembra: Revista Espírita* (June 2010): 9–10.

Guenther, Lisa. *Solitary Confinement: Social Death and its Afterlives*. Minneapolis: University of Minnesota Press, 2013.

Guerra, Lillian. *Popular Expression and National Identity in Puerto Rico: The Struggle for Self, Community, and Nation*. Gainesville: University Press of Florida, 1998.

Gutiérrez Franqui, Víctor. *Report of the Attorney General of Puerto Rico, 1951*. San Juan: Justice Department, 1951–52.

Hall, Clarence Jefferson, Jr. *A Prison in the Woods: Environment and Incarceration in New York's North Country*. Amherst: University of Massachusetts Press, 2020.

Hall, Douglas. "A population of free persons." In *General History of the Caribbean*, vol. 4, *The Long Nineteenth-Century: Nineteenth-Century Transformations*, edited by K. O. Laurence and Jorge Ibarra Cuesta, 35–61. London: Macmillan; Paris: UNESCO, 2011.

Hallowell, A. Irving. "The Rorschach Technique in the Study of Personality and Culture." *American Anthropologist* 47, no. 2 (1945): 195–210.

Hammett, A. B. J. *Miracle within the Walls: The Texas Prison Story*. Corpus Christi, TX: South Texas Pub. Co., 1963.

Harrington, Nicola. *Living with the Dead: Ancestor Worship and Mortuary Ritual in Ancient Egypt*. Oakville, CT: Oxbow Books, 2013.

Harris, Dawn P. *Punishing the Black Body: Marking Social and Racial Structures in Barbados and Jamaica*. Athens, GA: University of Georgia Press, 2017.

Harrison, Patti L., and Alan S. Kaufman. "History of Intelligence Testing." In *Encyclopedia of Special Education*, 3rd ed., edited by Cecil R. Reynolds and Elaine Fletcher-Janzen, 1127–30. New York: John Wiley & Sons, 2007.

Healy, David. *The Creation of Psychopharmacology*. Cambridge, MA: Harvard University Press, 2002.

Hemarajata, Peera. "Revisiting the Great Imitator: The Origin and History of Syphilis." American Society for Microbiology. June 17, 2019. https://asm.org/Articles/2019/June/Revisiting-the-Great-Imitator,-Part-I-The-Origin-a.

Herman, Ellen. *The Romance of American Psychology: Political Culture in the Age of Experts*. Berkeley: University of California Press, 1995.

Hernández, Francisco. "The Insular Biological Laboratory." In *El libro de Puerto Rico*, edited by Eugenio Fernandez García, 347–52. San Juan: El Libro Azul Publishing, 1923.

Hindus, Michael S. *Prison and Plantation: Crime, Justice, and Authority in Massachusetts and South Carolina, 1767–1878*. Chapel Hill: University of North Carolina Press, 1980.

Hornblum, Allen M. *Acres of Skin: Human Experiments at Holmesburg Prison*. New York: Routledge, 1998.

Horton, Benjamin J. *Report of the Attorney General of Puerto Rico, 1934*. San Juan: Negociado de Materiales, Imprenta y Transporte, 1934.

———. *Report of the Attorney General of Puerto Rico, 1935*. San Juan: Bureau of Supplies, Printing, and Transportation, 1935.

Huertas, Luz E., Bonnie Lucero, and Gregory J. Swedburg, eds. *Voices of Crime: Constructing and Contesting Social Control in Modern Latin America*. Tucson: University of Arizona Press, 2016.

Imada, Adria L. *An Archive of Skin, An Archive of Kin: Disability and Life-Making during Medical Incarceration*. Oakland: University of California Press, 2022.

Jacó-Vilela, Ana María. "Psychological Measurement in Brazil in the 1920s and 1930s." *History of Psychology* 17, no. 3 (August 2014): 237–48.

Janssen, Volker. "Convict Labor, Civic Welfare: Rehabilitation in California's Prisons, 1941–1971." PhD diss., University of California–San Diego, 2005.

Jimenes Grullón, Juan Isidro. *Una gestapo en América: Vida, tortura, agonía y muerte de presos políticos bajo la tiranía de Trujillo*. 1948; Santo Domingo: Editora Montalvo, 1962.

Johnson, Suzanne P. *An American Legacy in Panama*. Washington, DC: Department of Defense, 1995.

Kaba, Mariame. *We Do This 'Til We Free Us: Abolitionist Organizing and Transforming Justice*. Chicago: Haymarket, 2021.

Kandel, Eric R. *In Search of Memory: The Emergence of a New Science of Mind*. New York: W. W. Norton and Co., 2007.

Keller, Richard C. *Colonial Madness: Psychiatry in French North Africa*. Chicago: University of Chicago Press, 2007.

Kerley, Kent R., ed. *Finding Freedom in Confinement: The Role of Religion in Prison Life*. Santa Barbara, CA: Praeger, 2018.

Kern, Howard L. *Report of the Attorney General of Porto Rico, 1919*. Washington, DC: Government Printing Office, 1919.

Kim, Sonja M. *Imperatives of Care: Women and Medicine in Colonial Korea*. Honolulu: University of Hawai'i Press, 2019.

Kinsbruner, Jay. *Not of Pure Blood: The Free People of Color and Racial Prejudice in Nineteenth-Century Puerto Rico*. Durham, NC: Duke University Press, 1996.

Koenig, Harold G., Dana E. King, and Verna Benner Carson, eds. *Handbook of Religion and Health*. Second edition. New York: Oxford University Press, 2012.

Koss, Joan D. "Religion and Science Divinely Related: A Case History of Spiritism in Puerto Rico." *Caribbean Studies* 16, no. 1 (April 1976): 22–43.

Koss-Chioino, Joan. *Women as Healers, Women as Patients: Mental Health Care and Traditional Healing in Puerto Rico*. Boulder, CO: Westview Press, 1992.

Laboy Pérez, Suset L. "Minor Problems: Juvenile Delinquents and the Construction of a Puerto Rican Subject, 1880–1938." PhD diss., University of Pittsburgh, 2014.

Lagrange, Francis. *Flag on Devil's Island: The Autobiography of One of the Great Counterfeiters and Art Forgers of Modern Times*. Garden City, NY: Doubleday, 1961.

Lalo, Eduardo. *El deseo del lápiz: Castigo, urbanismo, escritura*. San Juan: Editorial Tal Cual, 2010.

Lambe, Jennifer L. *Madhouse: Psychiatry and Politics in Cuban History*. Chapel Hill: University of North Carolina Press, 2017.

Lambelet, Kyle B. T. *¡Presente! Nonviolent Politics and the Resurrection of the Dead*. Washington, DC: Georgetown University Press, 2019.

Lamotte, Martin. "The Ñeta Law, the Ñeta World: Ethics and Imaginaries in Circulation between the South Bronx, Barcelona and Guayaquil." *Current Sociology* 65, no. 2 (March 2017): 302–14.

Lanauze Rolón, José A. *Por los caminos de la violencia: La idea comunista*. Ponce: Casa Editorial América, 1932.

Lapp, Michael. "The Rise and Fall of Puerto Rico as a Social Laboratory, 1945–1965." *Social Science History* 19, no. 2 (Summer 1995): 169–99.

Lauro, Sarah Juliet. *The Transatlantic Zombie: Slavery, Rebellion, and Living Death*. New Brunswick, NJ: Rutgers University Press, 2015.

Law, Victoria. *"Prisons Make Us Safer": And 20 Other Myths about Mass Incarceration*. Boston: Beacon, 2021.

Leake, Chauncey D. "Eloge: John Farquhar Fulton, 1899–1960." *Isis* 51, no. 4 (December 1960): 486, 560–62.

LeBrón, Marisol. *Policing Life and Death: Race, Violence, and Resistance in Puerto Rico*. Oakland: University of California Press, 2019.

———. "Puerto Rico, Colonialism, and the US Carceral State." *Modern American History* 2, no. 2 (July 2019): 169–73.

Lecouteux, Claude. *The Return of the Dead: Ghosts, Ancestors, and the Transparent Veil of the Pagan Mind*. Rochester, VT: Inner Traditions, 2009.

Lederer, Susan E. *Subjected to Science: Human Experimentation in America Before the Second World War*. Baltimore: Johns Hopkins University Press, 1997.

Lee Borges, José. *Los chinos en Puerto Rico*. San Juan: Ediciones Callejón, 2015.

LeFlouria, Talitha. *Chained in Silence: Black Women and Convict Labor in the New South*. Chapel Hill: University of North Carolina Press, 2015.

Leys Stepan, Nancy. *"The Hour of Eugenics": Race, Gender, and Nation in Latin America*. Ithaca, NY: Cornell University Press, 1996.

Lichtenstein, Alex. *Twice the Work of Free Labor: The Political Economy of Convict Labor in the New South*. New York: Verso, 1996.

Lira, Natalie. *Laboratory of Deficiency: Sterilization and Confinement in California, 1900–1950s*. Oakland: University of California Press, 2021.

Litsios, Socrates. "John Black Grant: A 20th-Century Public Health Giant." *Perspectives in Biology and Medicine* 54, no. 4 (Autumn 2011): 532–49.

Lockward, Yoryi. *Acúcheme uté: Cuentos típicos dominicanos*. Puerto Plata, DR: Imp. El Porvenir, A. Rodríguez D., 1941.

Lombroso, Cesare. *Criminal Man*. Edited by Mary Gibson and Nicole Hahn Rafter. Durham, NC: Duke University Press, 2006.

Loveman, Mara, and Jeronimo O. Muniz. "How Puerto Rico Became White: Boundary Dynamics and Intercensus Racial Reclassification." *American Sociological Review* 72, no. 6 (December 2007): 915–39.

Lucas, Ashley E. *Prison Theatre and the Global Crisis of Incarceration*. London: Bloomsbury, 2020.

Lytle Hernández, Kelly. *City of Inmates: Conquest, Rebellion, and the Rise of Human Caging in Los Angeles, 1771–1965*. Chapel Hill: University of North Carolina Press, 2017.

Malaret, Márel, dir. *Todos íbamos a ser reyes*. San Juan: Producciones Damiana, 2020.

Malavet Vega, Pedro. *El sistema de justicia criminal en Puerto Rico*. Ponce: Ediciones Lorena, 2005.

Malcolm, George A. *Report of the Attorney General of Puerto Rico, 1940*. San Juan: Bureau of Supplies, Printing, and Transportation, 1940.

———. *Report of the Attorney General of Puerto Rico, 1941*. San Juan: Justice Department, 1941–42.

———. *Report of the Attorney General of Puerto Rico, 1942*. San Juan: Bureau of Supplies, Printing, and Transportation, 1942.

Maldonado, Alex W. *Teodoro Moscoso and Puerto Rico's Operation Bootstrap*. Gainesville: University Press of Florida, 1997.

Marcano García, Pablo. *La criminalidad y la crisis de prisiones en Puerto Rico*. Chicago: Editorial El Coquí, 1985.

Marín Torres, Heriberto. *Coabey: El valle heróico*. San Juan: Editorial Patria, 2019.

———. *Eran ellos*. San Juan: Editorial Patria, 2018.

Martin, William G., and Joshua M. Price, eds. *After Prisons? Freedom, Decarceration, and Justice Disinvestment*. Lanham, MD: Lexington Books, 2016.

Marturano, Jorge. *Narrativas de encierro en la República cubana*. Madrid: Editorial Verbum, 2017.

Mathews, Thomas. *Puerto Rican Politics and the New Deal*. Gainesville: University of Florida Press, 1960.

Mayo Santana, Raúl, Annette B. Ramírez de Arellano, and José G. Rigau-Pérez, eds. *A Sojourn in Tropical Medicine: Francis W. O'Connor's Diary of a Puerto Rican Trip, 1927*. San Juan: Editorial de la Universidad de Puerto Rico, 2008.

Mayo Santana, Raúl, Silvia E. Rabionet, and Ángel A. Román Franco. *Historia de la medicina tropical en Puerto Rico en el siglo XX*. San Juan: Ediciones Laberinto, 2022.

Mbembe, Joseph-Achille. *Necropolitics*. Durham, NC: Duke University Press, 2019.

McCoy, Alfred W. *Policing America's Empire: The United States, the Philippines, and the Rise of the Surveillance State*. Madison: University of Wisconsin Press, 2009.

Mejías, Félix. *De la crisis económica del 86 al año terrible del 87*. Río Piedras, PR: Ediciones Puerto, 1972.

Mejías, J. Tomás. *Memoria 1946 Procuraduría General de la República*. Santiago, DR: Editorial El Diario, 1946.

Meléndez, Edwin, and Jennifer Hinojosa. *Estimates of Post–Hurricane Maria Exodus from Puerto Rico: Research Brief*. New York: Centro de Estudios Puertorriqueños, 2017.

Meléndez Badillo, Jorell A. *The Lettered Barriada: Workers, Archival Power, and the Politics of Knowledge in Puerto Rico*. Durham, NC: Duke University Press, 2021.

Melossi, Dario, and Massimo Pavarini. *The Prison and the Factory: Origins of the Penitentiary System*. Basingstoke, UK: Palgrave Macmillan, 2018.

Memorias de la cuarta convención de trabajo social de Puerto Rico, marzo 1947. Santurce: Imprenta Soltero, 1949.

Méndez, José Luis. *Las ciencias sociales y el proceso político puertorriqueño*. San Juan: Ediciones Puerto, 2005.

Méndez Saavedra, Manuel. *Mis experiencias en la Penitenciaría Insular*. 3rd ed. Río Piedras, PR: Editorial Antillana, 1976.

Mercado, Ricardo. *Yo viví en el cementerio de los vivos*. Levittown, PR: Publicaciones Papyrus, 2007.

Mestre, Salvador. *Report of the Attorney General of Porto Rico, 1921*. Washington, DC: Government Printing Office, 1923.

Milton, Cynthia. *The Many Meanings of Poverty: Colonialism, Social Compacts, and Assistance in Eighteenth-Century Ecuador*. Stanford, CA: Stanford University Press, 2007.

Mintz, Sidney. "Slave Life on Caribbean Sugar Plantations: Some Unanswered Questions." In *Slave Cultures and the Cultures of Slavery*, edited by Stephan Palmié, 12–22. Knoxville: University of Tennessee Press, 1995.

Miranda Sánchez, Nelson. *El Jíbaro: Víctima o culpable del sistema correccional*. Naguabo, PR: Extreme Graphics, 2008.

Monnais, Laurence. "From Colonial Medicines to Global Pharmaceuticals? The Introduction of Sulfa Drugs in French Vietnam." *East Asian Science, Technology, and Society: An International Journal* 3, nos. 2–3 (2009): 257–85.

Montijo, Josué. *Los Ñeta*. Río Piedras, PR: Centro de Investigaciones Históricas, Universidad de Puerto Rico–Río Piedras, 2011.

Morales, Luis M. *Psiquiatría, neurología e higiene mental*. San Juan: Secretaría de Instrucción Pública del Estado Libre Asociado de Puerto Rico, 1953.

Moreno Vega, Marta. "Kongo Presence in the Espiritismo of Puerto Rico." In *Actualidad de las tradiciones espirituales y culturas africanas en el Caribe y Latinoamérica*, edited by María Elba Torres Muñoz, Mónica Cortés, and Marta Moreno Vega, 169–87. San Juan: Centro de Estudios Avanzados de Puerto Rico y el Caribe, 2010.

Mörner, Magnus. *Race Mixture in the History of Latin America*. Boston: Little, Brown, 1967.

"Muere histórico preso 'El Jíbaro.'" *Noticel*. May 31, 2012. https://www.noticel.com/la-calle/2012 0531/muere-historico-preso-el-jibaro/.

Negrón Fernández, Luis. *Report of the Attorney General of Puerto Rico, 1947*. San Juan: Real Hermanos, 1950.

———. *Report of the Attorney General of Puerto Rico, 1948*. San Juan: Real Hermanos, 1950.

Niles, Blair. *Condemned to Devil's Island: The Biography of an Unknown Convict*. New York: Harcourt, Brace, and Co., 1928.

Nistal Moret, Benjamín. *Esclavos, prófugos y cimarrones: Puerto Rico, 1770–1870*. 1984. San Juan: Editorial de la Universidad de Puerto Rico, 2004.

Noll, Steven. *Feeble-Minded in Our Midst: Institutions for the Mentally Retarded in the South, 1900–1940*. Chapel Hill: University of North Carolina Press, 1994.

Nunes Maia, Clarissa, Flávio de Sá Neto, Marcos Costa, and Marcos Luiz Bretas, eds. *História das prisões no Brasil*. 2 vols. Rio de Janeiro: Editora Rocco, 2009.

Núñez Molina, Mario A. "Toward an Experiential Approach for Researching Religious Experiences." *Revista Puertorriqueña de Psicología* 10, no. 1 (1995): 247–65.

Olguín, Ben V. *Violentologies: Violence, Identity, and Ideology in Latina/o Literature*. New York: Oxford University Press, 2021.

Ordoñez y Fernández, Fernando. *Influencia del instinto sexual sobre las facultades psíquicas, ensayo*. N.p.: n.p., 1936.

Ortiz, Armando. "Colonia psiquiátrica." In *Memoria del Congreso Médico Dominicano del Centenario*, by Congreso Médico Dominicano, 3:216–17. Santiago, DR: Editorial El Diario, 1945.

Ortiz, Fernando. *Hampa afro-cubana: Los negros brujos, apuntes para un estudio de etnología criminal*. 1906. Miami: Ediciones Universal, 1973.

Ortiz Díaz, Alberto. "Pathologizing the *Jíbaro*: Mental and Social Health in Puerto Rico's *Oso Blanco* (1930s to 1950s)." *The Americas* 77, no. 3 (July 2020): 409–41.

———. "Redeeming Bodies and Souls: Penitentiary Science and Spirituality in Twentieth-Century Puerto Rico and the Dominican Republic." PhD diss., University of Wisconsin–Madison, 2017.

———. "Stepping through a Looking Glass: The Haitian Healer Mauricio Gastón on the Romana Sugar Mill in the Dominican Republic in 1938." In *The Gray Zones of Medicine: Healers and History in Latin America*, edited by Diego Armus and Pablo Gómez, 155–69. Pittsburgh, PA: University of Pittsburgh Press, 2021.

Ortiz-Minaya, Reynaldo. "From Plantation to Prison: Visual Economies of Slave Resistance, Criminal Justice, and Penal Exile in the Spanish Caribbean (1820–1886)." PhD diss., State University of New York–Binghamton, 2014.

Ortiz Rivera, David. *Entre el bien y el mal: Escrito en el complejo correccional de Río Piedras*. Hato Rey, PR: Publicaciones Puertorriqueñas, 1999.

Osborn, Tommy Lee. *Personal Diary Notes: The Ponce, Puerto Rico Crusade and Its Significance*. Tulsa, OK: Osborn Publishers, 2007.

———. *Puerto Rico: Revival Harvest, With Miracles of Healing*. Tulsa, OK: Voice of Faith Ministries, 1951.

O'Shea, J. G. "'Two Minutes with Venus, Two Years with Mercury'—Mercury as an Antisyphilitic Chemotherapeutic Agent." *Journal of the Royal Society of Medicine* 83, no. 6 (June 1990): 392–95.

Oshinsky, David M. *"Worse Than Slavery": Parchman Farm and the Ordeal of Jim Crow Justice*. New York: Free Press, 1997.

Palau de López, Awilda, and Ernesto Ruiz Ortiz. *En la calle estabas: La vida en una institución de menores*. Río Piedras, PR: Editorial Universitaria, Universidad de Puerto Rico, 1976.

Pantojas-García, Emilio. "Puerto Rican Populism Revisited: The PPD during the 1940s." *Journal of Latin American Studies* 21, no. 3 (October 1989): 521–57.

Paralitici, Ché. *Sentencia impuesta: 100 años de encarcelamientos por la independencia de Puerto Rico*. San Juan: Ediciones Puerto, 2004.

Parascandola, John. *Sex, Sin, and Science: A History of Syphilis in America*. Westport, CT: Praeger, 2008.

Parker, James D. A. "From the Intellectual to the Non-Intellectual Traits: A Historical Framework for the Development of American Personality Research." MA thesis, York University, Toronto, 1986.

Paton, Diana. *No Bond but the Law: Punishment, Race, and Gender in Jamaican State Formation, 1780–1870*. Durham, NC: Duke University Press, 2004.

Patterson, Orlando. *Slavery and Social Death: A Comparative Study*. Cambridge, MA: Harvard University Press, 1982.

Paulino Ramos, Alejandro. "Los centros de torturas de la dictadura de Trujillo: La cárcel de Nigua." *Acento*. January 20, 2018. https://acento.com.do/politica/los-centros-torturas-la-dictadura -trujillo-la-carcel-nigua-2-8528544.html.

Peña Beltrán, Lydia. *30 años en las cárceles de Puerto Rico*. Río Piedras, PR: Boriкén, 1995.

Pérez, Gina M. *The Near Northwest Side Story: Migration, Displacement, and Puerto Rican Families*. Berkeley: University of California Press, 2004.

Pérez, José G. *Puerto Rico: US Colony in the Caribbean*. New York: Pathfinder Press, 1976.

Pérez-Pérez, Roberto. "A Survey of the Insular Industrial School for Boys at Mayagüez, Puerto Rico." MA thesis, Ohio State University, 1951.

Peters, Edward M. "Prison before the Prison: The Ancient and Medieval Worlds." In *The Oxford History of the Prison: The Practice of Punishment in Western Society*, edited by Norval Morris and David J. Rothman, 3–43. New York: Oxford University Press, 1995.

Picart, Juan B. "Validation of the WBIS for a Disabled Puerto Rican Veteran College Population." *Vocational Rehabilitation and Education Quarterly Information Bulletin* (January 1960): 14–15.

Piccato, Pablo. *City of Suspects: Crime in Mexico City, 1900–1931*. Durham, NC: Duke University Press 2001.

Picó, Fernando. "La caducidad de la cárcel." *Revista del Colegio de Abogados de Puerto Rico* 60, no. 2 (April–June 1999): 6–15.

———. *El día menos pensado: Historia de los presidiarios en Puerto Rico, 1793–1993*. Río Piedras, PR: Ediciones Huracán, 1994.

———. "Esclavos y convictos: Esclavos de Cuba y Puerto Rico en el presidio de Puerto Rico en el siglo XIX." In *Al filo del poder: Subalternos y dominantes en Puerto Rico, 1739–1910*, 115–32. San Juan: Editorial de la Universidad de Puerto Rico, 1996.

———. *Al filo del poder: Subalternos y dominantes en Puerto Rico, 1739–1910*. San Juan: Editorial de la Universidad de Puerto Rico, 1996.

———. *Los gallos peleados*. 1983. Río Piedras, PR: Ediciones Huracán, 2003.

———. *Libertad y servidumbre en el Puerto Rico del siglo XIX: Los jornaleros utuadeños en vísperas del auge del café*. Río Piedras, PR: Ediciones Huracán, 1983.

———. "Por una historia en que la gente encuentre sus apellidos." In *Una historia de servicio*, by Universidad Interamericana de Puerto Rico, 55–64. San Juan: Universidad Interamericana, 1979.

———. *Realengos y residentes: Los menores en San Juan, 1918–1940*. San Juan: Centro de Investigaciones Históricas, 2019.

———. *Santurce y las voces de su gente*. San Juan: Ediciones Huracán, 2014.

Piñero, Jesús T. *Forty-Seventh Annual Report of the Governor of Puerto Rico for the Fiscal Year 1946–1947*. San Juan: Service Office of the Government of Puerto Rico, Printing Division, 1948.

Pisciotta, Alexander W. *Benevolent Repression: Social Control and the American Reformatory-Prison Movement*. New York: New York University Press, 1994.

Pons, Juan A. *Annual Report of the Commissioner of Health for the Fiscal Year 1948–1949*. San Juan: Health Department, 1949.

Portocarrero, Jesús A. *Proyecciones de la ciencia penitenciaria en Cuba*. Havana: Editorial Lex, 1945.

Proceedings of the Seventy-Sixth Annual Congress of the American Prison Association, Detroit, Michigan. New York: The Association, 1946.

Promey, Sally, ed. *Sensational Religion: Sensory Cultures in Material Practice*. New Haven, CT: Yale University Press, 2017.

Puerto Rico Health Department. *Annual Report*. San Juan: Health Department, 1959.

Puerto Rico Justice Department (Charles E. Winter). *Reglamento para el régimen y gobierno de la Penitenciaría de Puerto Rico en Río Piedras*. San Juan: Negociado de Materiales, Imprenta y Transporte, 1933.

Puerto Rico Justice Department (Office of the Attorney General). *Special Report of the Attorney General of Porto Rico to the Governor of Porto Rico Concerning the Suppression of Vice and Prostitution in Connection with the Mobilization of the National Army at Camp Las Casas, February 1, 1919*. San Juan: Bureau of Supplies, Printing and Transportation, 1919.

Purnell, Derecka. *Becoming Abolitionists: Police, Protests, and the Pursuit of Freedom*. New York: Astra House, Penguin Random House, 2021.

Quétel, Claude. *History of Syphilis*. Cambridge: Polity, 1990.

Quiles Rodríguez, Edwin R. *San Juan tras la fachada: Una mirada desde sus espacios ocultos, 1508–1900*. San Juan: Instituto de Cultura Puertorriqueña, 2003.

Quincke, Heinrich. *Die Technik der Lumbalpunction*. Berlin: Urban & Schwarzenberg, 1902.

Quintero Rivera, Ángel. "La ideología populista y la institucionalización universitaria de las ciencias sociales." In *Del nacionalismo al populismo: Cultura y política en Puerto Rico*, edited by Silvia Álvarez Curbelo and María Elena Rodríguez Castro, 122–45. Río Piedras, PR: Ediciones Huracán, 1993.

Rama, Ángel. *The Lettered City*. Translated by John Charles Chasteen. Durham, NC: Duke University Press, 1996.

Ramos, Leoncio. *Trabajos penitenciarios: Reformas para el establecimiento de un nuevo sistema penitenciario dominicano*. Santo Domingo: Colección Pensamiento Criminológico, 2003.

———. *Yo pasé un día en Sing-Sing y otros escritos*. Santo Domingo: Pensamiento Criminológico Dominicano, 2001.

Rappaport, Joanne. *The Disappearing Mestizo: Configuring Difference in the Colonial New Kingdom of Granada*. Durham, NC: Duke University Press, 2014.

R. de Goenaga, Francisco. *Antropología médica y jurídica*. San Juan: Imprenta Venezuela, 1934.

———. *Desarrollo histórico del Asilo de beneficencia y manicomio de Puerto Rico desde su creación hasta julio 31, 1929, y circulares relativas a hospitales*. San Juan: Cantero, Fernández & Co., 1929.

Restall, Matthew. *The Black Middle: Africans, Mayas, and Spaniards in Colonial Yucatan*. Stanford, CA: Stanford University Press, 2009.

Rieber, Robert W., ed. *Encyclopedia of Psychological Theories*. New York: Springer, 2012.

Rivera Ruiz, Álvaro M. *Violencia política y subalternidad colonial: El caso de Filberto Ojeda y el MIRA, 1960–1972*. San Juan: Centro de Estudios Avanzados de Puerto Rico y el Caribe, 2020.

Roberts, Peter A. *The Roots of Caribbean Identity: Language, Race and Ecology*. New York: Cambridge University Press, 2008.

Robiou, Manuel A. *Memoria 1949 Secretaría de Estado de Sanidad y Asistencia Pública*. Ciudad Trujillo, DR: Editora del Caribe, 1956.

Roca de León, Pablo. *Escala de inteligencia Stanford-Binet para niños*. San Juan: Departamento de Instrucción Pública, 1953.

———. *Manual escala de inteligencia Wechsler para niños*. San Juan: Departamento de Instrucción Pública, 1951.

Roca de Torres, Irma. "Algunos precursores/as de la psicología en Puerto Rico: Reseñas biográficas." *Revista Puertorriqueña de Psicología* 17, no. 1 (2006): 63–88.

———. "Perspectiva histórica sobre la medición psicológica en Puerto Rico." *Revista Puertorriqueña de Psicología* 19, no. 1 (2008): 11–48.

Rocklin, Alexander. *The Regulation of Religion and the Making of Hinduism in Colonial Trinidad*. Chapel Hill: University of North Carolina Press, 2019.

Rodríguez, Julia. *Civilizing Argentina: Science, Medicine, and the Modern State*. Chapel Hill: University of North Carolina Press, 2006.

Rodríguez, Manuel. *A New Deal for the Tropics: Puerto Rico during the Depression Era*. Princeton, NJ: Markus Wiener, 2010.

Rodríguez Bou, Ismael. *El analfabetismo en Puerto Rico*. San Juan: Universidad de Puerto Rico, Consejo Superior de Enseñanza, 1945.

Rodríguez Castro, José. *La embriaguez y la locura, o, Consecuencias del alcoholismo.* San Juan: Imp. del Boletín Mercantil, 1889.

Rodríguez Juliá, Edgardo. *Una noche con Iris Chacón.* Carolina, PR: Editorial Antillana, 1986.

Rodríguez Ramos, Manuel. *Report of the Attorney General of Puerto Rico, 1943.* San Juan: Insular Procurement Office, Printing Division, 1943.

Rodríguez Silva, Ileana. *Silencing Blackness: Disentangling Race, Colonial Regimes, and National Struggles in Post-Emancipation Puerto Rico, 1850–1920.* New York: Palgrave, 2012.

Rogers, H. E. *Yearbook of the Seventh-Day Adventist Denomination.* Washington, DC: Review and Herald Publishing, 1933.

Román, Reinaldo L. *Governing Spirits: Religion, Miracles, and Spectacles in Cuba and Puerto Rico, 1898–1956.* Chapel Hill: University of North Carolina Press, 2009.

Romero, Lino A. *Historia de la psiquiatría dominicana.* Santo Domingo: Editora Búho, 2005.

Ross, J. E., and M. Tomkins. "The British reception of salvarsan." *Journal of the History of Medicine and Allied Sciences* 52, no. 4 (October 1997): 398–423.

Rosselló, Juan A. *Historia de la psiquiatría en Puerto Rico, 1898–1988.* San Juan: Instituto de Relaciones Humanas, 1988.

Ruiz Rivera, Eloy A. "La 'gran agenda del porvenir': Ruta de la reforma educativa, 1949–1960." *Revista Magisterio* 5, no. 1 (December 2015): 13–39.

Sáez, Florencio. *Río Piedras: Estampas de mi pueblo, 1898–1945.* 1988. San Juan: Editorial Palma Real, 1996.

Sáez, José Luis, ed. *La sumisión bien pagada: La iglesia dominicana bajo la era de Trujillo, 1930–1961.* Vol. 1. Santo Domingo: Archivo General de la Nación, 2008.

Salcedo Chirinos, César Augusto. *Las negociaciones del arte de curar: Los orígenes de la regulación de las prácticas sanitarias en Puerto Rico, 1816–1846.* Lajas, PR: Editorial Akelarre, 2016.

Salla, Fernando. *As prisões de São Paulo, 1822–1940.* São Paulo: Annablume, 1999.

Salvatore, Ricardo D., and Carlos Aguirre, eds. *The Birth of the Penitentiary in Latin America: Essays on Criminology, Prison Reform, and Social Control, 1830–1940.* Austin: University of Texas Press, 1996.

———. "The Birth of the Penitentiary in Latin America: Toward an Interpretive Social History of Prisons." In *The Birth of the Penitentiary in Latin America: Essays on Criminology, Prison Reform, and Social Control, 1830–1940,* edited by Ricardo D. Salvatore and Carlos Aguirre, 1–43. Austin: University of Texas Press, 1996.

Salvatore, Ricardo D., Carlos Aguirre, and Gilbert M. Joseph, eds. *Crime and Punishment in Latin America: Law and Society Since Late Colonial Times.* Durham, NC: Duke University Press, 2001.

San Miguel, Pedro L. "Economic activities other than sugar: Part One The Agrarian Economies." In *General History of the Caribbean,* vol. 4, *The Long Nineteenth-Century: Nineteenth-Century Transformations,* edited by K. O. Laurence and Jorge Ibarra Cuesta, 104–34. London: Macmillan; Paris: UNESCO, 2011.

Santiago-Valles, Kelvin. "American Penal Forms and Colonial Spanish Custodial-Regulatory Practices in Fin de Siècle Puerto Rico." In *Colonial Crucible: Empire and the Making of the Modern American State,* edited by Alfred W. McCoy and Francisco A. Scarano, 87–94. Madison: University of Wisconsin Press, 2009.

———. "'Bloody Legislations,' 'Entombment,' and Race Making in the Spanish Atlantic: Differentiated Spaces of General(ized) Confinement in Spain and Puerto Rico, 1750–1840." *Radical History Review* 96 (Fall 2006): 33–57.

———. "'Forcing Them to Work and Punishing Whoever Resisted': Servile Labor and Penal Servitude under Colonialism in Nineteenth-Century Puerto Rico." In *The Birth of the Penitentiary in Latin America: Essays on Criminology, Prison Reform, and Social Control, 1830–1940*, edited by Ricardo D. Salvatore and Carlos Aguirre, 123–59. Austin: University of Texas Press, 1996.

———. *"Subject People" and Colonial Discourses: Economic Transformation and Social Disorder in Puerto Rico, 1898–1947.* Albany: State University of New York Press, 1994.

Santos, P. *La cárcel en República Dominicana.* Santiago: Editora Teófilo, 2006.

Saumell, Rafael. *La cárcel letrada.* Madrid: Editorial Betania, 2012.

Scarano, Francisco A. "In a Sea of Colonial Cane: Caribbean History as Autobiography." Unpublished paper delivered at "Caribbean Pasts, Presents, and Futures: An Interdisciplinary Conference in Honor of Francisco Scarano." University of Wisconsin–Madison, April 13, 2019.

———. "The *Jíbaro* Masquerade and the Subaltern Politics of Creole Identity Formation in Puerto Rico, 1745–1823." *American Historical Review* 101, no. 5 (December 1996): 1398–1431.

———. *Puerto Rico: Cinco siglos de historia.* Cuarta edición. San Juan: McGraw-Hill, 2015.

———. *Sugar and Slavery in Puerto Rico: The Plantation Economy of Ponce, 1800–1850.* Madison: University of Wisconsin Press, 1984.

Scheper-Hughes, Nancy. *Death without Weeping: The Violence of Everyday Life in Brazil.* Berkeley: University of California Press, 1993.

Schilling, Rebecca, and Stephen T. Casper. "Of Psychometric Means: Starke R. Hathaway and the Popularization of the Minnesota Multiphasic Personality Inventory." *Science in Context* 28, no. 1 (March 2015): 77–98.

Scott, Linda H. "Measuring Intelligence with the Goodenough-Harris Drawing Test." *Psychological Bulletin* 89, no. 3 (May 1981): 483–505.

Scott, Rebecca J. *Slave Emancipation in Cuba: The Transition to Free Labor, 1860–1899.* Pittsburgh, PA: University of Pittsburgh Press, 2000.

Searls, Damion. *The Inkblots: Hermann Rorschach, His Iconic Test, and the Power of Seeing.* New York: Crown, 2017.

Second Annual Report of the Governor of Porto Rico. Washington, DC: Government Printing Office, 1902.

Serrano Arreche, Miguel. *¡Convicto!* Miami: Editorial Carisma, 1993.

Sheller, Mimi. *Consuming the Caribbean: From Arawaks to Zombies.* London: Routledge, 2003.

Sheppard, Cassandra. "The Neuroscience of Singing." *Uplift: Science.* December 11, 2016. https://upliftconnect.com/neuroscience-of-singing/.

Siegel, Eleanor. "Arthur Sinton Otis and the American Mental Testing Movement." PhD diss., University of Miami, 1992.

Silva Gotay, Samuel. *Protestantismo y política en Puerto Rico, 1898–1930: Hacia una historia del protestantismo evangélico en Puerto Rico.* San Juan: Editorial de la Universidad de Puerto Rico, 1997.

Silvestrini, Blanca G. *Violencia y criminalidad en Puerto Rico, 1898–1973: Apuntes para un estudio de historia social.* Río Piedras, PR: Editorial Universitaria, Universidad de Puerto Rico, 1980.

Simey, T. S. *Principles of Prison Reform: Development and Welfare in the West Indies, Bulletin No. 10.* Bridgetown, Barbados: n.p., 1944.

Sinclair, Gordon. *Loose among Devils: A Voyage from Devil's Island to Those Jungles of West Africa Labelled "the White Man's Grave."* Toronto: Doubleday, Doran & Gundy, 1935.

Smith, Caleb. *The Prison and the American Imagination.* New Haven, CT: Yale University Press, 2009.

Smith, Philip. *Punishment and Culture*. Chicago: University of Chicago Press, 2008.

Smith, Roger. *The Fontana History of the Human Sciences*. London: Fontana Press, 1997.

Snodgrass, Jon. "William Healy (1869–1963): Pioneer Child Psychiatrist and Criminologist." *Journal of the History of the Behavioral Sciences* 20, no. 4 (October 1984): 332–39.

Speckman Guerra, Elisa. "La identificación de criminales y los sistemas ideados por Alphonse Bertillon: Discursos y prácticas (Ciudad de México 1895–1913)." *Historia y grafía* 17 (2001): 99–129.

Spieler, Miranda F. *Empire and Underworld: Captivity in French Guiana*. Cambridge, MA: Harvard University Press, 2012.

Stern, Alexandra M. *Eugenic Nation: Faults and Frontiers of Better Breeding in Modern America*. Chapel Hill: University of North Carolina Press, 2005.

Stoddard, Brad. *Spiritual Entrepreneurs: Florida's Faith-Based Prisons and the American Carceral State*. Chapel Hill: University of North Carolina Press, 2021.

Stoler, Ann Laura. *Along the Archival Grain: Epistemic Anxieties and Colonial Common Sense*. 2008; Princeton, NJ: Princeton University Press, 2010.

———. *Carnal Knowledge and Imperial Power: Race and the Intimate in Colonial Rule*. Berkeley: University of California Press, 2010.

Suárez Findlay, Eileen J. *We Are Left without a Father Here: Masculinity, Domesticity, and Migration in Postwar Puerto Rico*. Durham, NC: Duke University Press, 2014.

Suau, Christian, and Ramiro Millán, directors. *Oso Blanco: Puerto Rico State Penitentiary*. Miami: Ondamax, Buena Americas, Tangram Films, 2008.

Sub-Committee of the Howard League of Jamaica. *The After-Care of Discharged Prisoners in Jamaica*. Kingston: Farquharson Institute of Public Affairs, 1968.

Sued Badillo, Jalil, and Ángel López Cantos. *Puerto Rico negro*. 1986; San Juan: Editorial Cultural, 2007.

Sweeney, Megan. *Reading Is My Window: Books and the Art of Reading in Women's Prisons*. Chapel Hill: University of North Carolina Press, 2010.

Sweet, James. *Domingos Álvares, African Healing, and the Intellectual History of the Atlantic World*. Chapel Hill: University of North Carolina Press, 2011.

Tallaj, José Antonio. *Un médico en la 40: Recuerdos de una conspiración*. Santo Domingo: Editora Búho, 2006.

Tampa, Mircea, I. Sarbu, C. Matei, V. Benea, and S. R. Georgescu. "Brief History of Syphilis." *Journal of Medicine and Life* 7, no. 1 (March 15, 2014): 4–10.

Tauch, Kunlyna. "Life Inside: I Am Not Your 'Other.'" Marshall Project. July 9, 2020. https://www.themarshallproject.org/2020/07/09/i-am-not-your-other.

Tejada Vega, Josefina V. *Vagos, desertores y presos políticos en el Presidio Provincial de Puerto Rico, siglo XIX*. Las Vegas, NV: Ediciones Nóema, 2021.

Thomas, Deborah A. "Caribbean Studies, Archive Building, and the Problem of Violence." *Small Axe* 17, no. 2 (July 2013): 27–42.

Thomen, Luis F. *Memoria 1944 Secretaría de Estado de Sanidad y Asistencia Pública*. Santiago, DR: Editorial El Diario, 1944.

———. *Memoria 1945 Secretaría de Estado de Sanidad y Asistencia Pública*. Vol. 2. Ciudad Trujillo, DR: Impresora Dominicana, 1947.

———. *Memoria 1946 Secretaría de Estado de Sanidad y Asistencia Pública*. Tomo I. Ciudad Trujillo, DR: Editorial Arte y Cine, 1947.

Thurston, Herbert. *The Stations of the Cross: An Account of Their History and Devotional Purpose*. Charleston, SC: Nabu Press, 2010.

Tiadmin. "The Salvarsan Wars." *Proto Magazine* (Massachusetts General Hospital). May 3, 2010. https://protomag.com/infectious-disease/paul-ehrlich-and-the-salvarsan-wars/.

Tinajero, Araceli. *El Lector: A History of the Cigar Factory Reader.* Translated by Judith E. Grasberg. Austin: University of Texas Press, 2010.

Toro Calder, Jaime. "Personal Crime in Puerto Rico: A Study of the Cultural Elements in Personal Crime." MA thesis, University of Wisconsin–Madison, 1950.

Torregrosa, Ángel M. *Luis Muñoz Marín: Su vida y su patriótica obra.* San Juan: Editorial Esther, 1944.

Torregrosa, José Luis. *Historia de la radio en Puerto Rico.* San Juan: Publicaciones Gaviota, 1991.

Towner, Horace M. *Twenty-Fifth Annual Report of the Governor of Porto Rico, for the Fiscal Year Ended June 30, 1925.* Washington, DC: Government Printing Office, 1926.

Trautmann Banks, Joanne. *Healing Arts in Dialogue: Medicine and Literature.* Carbondale, IL: Southern Illinois University Press, 1981.

Travisono, Anthony P. *Arts in Corrections.* Washington, DC: American Correctional Association, 1978.

Trent, James W. *Inventing the Feeble Mind: A History of Mental Retardation in the United States.* Berkeley: University of California Press, 1995.

Trías Monge, José. *El sistema judicial de Puerto Rico.* San Juan: Editorial de la Universidad de Puerto Rico, 1988.

———. *Informe Anual del Secretario de Justicia para el año que terminó el 30 de junio de 1956.* San Juan: Departamento de Hacienda, Servicio de Compra y Suministro, División de Imprenta, 1961.

———. *Report of the Attorney General of Puerto Rico, 1954.* San Juan: Department of the Treasury, Purchase and Supply Service, Printing Division, 1958.

Trouillot, Michel-Rolph. *Silencing the Past: Power and the Production of History.* Boston: Beacon, 1995.

Trujillo-Pagán, Nicole. *Modern Colonization by Medical Intervention: US Medicine in Puerto Rico.* Chicago: Haymarket, 2014.

Tuck, Eve, and K. Wayne Yang. "R-Words: Refusing Research." In *Humanizing Research: Decolonizing Qualitative Inquiry with Youth and Communities,* edited by Django Paris and Maisha T. Winn, 223–47. Thousand Oaks, CA: Sage Publications, 2014.

Tugwell, Rexford G. *Puerto Rican Public Papers.* San Juan: Service Office of the Government of Puerto Rico, Printing Division, 1945.

Twitchell, James B. *The Living Dead: A Study of the Vampire in Romantic Literature.* 1981. Durham, NC: Duke University Press, 1997.

US Children's Bureau. *Directory of Public Training Schools Serving Delinquent Children.* Washington, DC: US Department of Health, Education, and Welfare Administration, 1958.

———. *Public Training Schools for Delinquent Children: Directory.* Washington, DC: Government Printing Office, 1955.

US Department of Health, Education, and Welfare. *Bulletin No. 12: Research Relating to Children.* Washington, DC: Government Printing Office, February 1960–July 1960.

Vales, Pedro A. "El impacto de la libertad bajo palabra en la rehabilitación de confinados y las características sociales de los confinados, asociados con el éxito o fracaso en el disfrute de la misma." In *Primer ciclo de conferencias públicas sobre temas de investigación social,* 29–44. Río Piedras, PR: Universidad de Puerto Rico, Centro de Investigaciones Sociales, 1969.

Vega, Bernardo. "Juan Bosch narra sobre su experiencia en una prisión en 1934." *Hoy.* July 16, 2007. https://hoy.com.do/juan-bosch-narra-sobre-su-experiencia-en-una-prision-en-1934/.

Vélez, Carlos, Raquel Colón, and Hiram Arroyo. *Desde uncinariasis hasta estilos de vida: Crónicas de la educación para la salud en Puerto Rico.* San Juan: Delta, 1994.

Vemer Andrzejewski, Anna. *Building Power: Architecture and Surveillance in Victorian America.* Knoxville: University of Tennessee Press, 2008.

Vergetti de Menezes, Mozart. "A Escola Correcional do Recife (1909–1929)." In *História das prisões no Brasil,* edited Clarissa Nunes Maia, Flávio de Sá Neto, Marcos Costa, and Marcos Luiz Bretas, 2:249–76. Rio de Janeiro: Editora Rocco, 2009.

Vetö, Silvana. "Child Delinquency and Intelligence Testing at Santiago's Juvenile Court, Chile, 1929–1942." *History of Psychology* 22, no. 3 (August 2019): 244–65.

Viera Lozada, David Joel. "Deusdedid Marrero: La criminalización del ideario comunista en Puerto Rico, 1947–1957." MA thesis, Centro de Estudios Avanzados de Puerto Rico y el Caribe, 2018.

Virgili López, Goretti. *Guía medicinal y espiritual de plantas tropicales.* Barcelona, Spain: Angels Fortune Editions, 2017.

Wall, E. D. (Trinidad and Tobago Prisons Department). *Administration Report of the Superintendent of Prisons for the Year 1951.* Trinidad, British West Indies: Government Printing Office, 1953.

———. *Administration Report of the Superintendent of Prisons for the Year 1952.* Trinidad, British West Indies: Government Printing Office, 1953.

Walsh, Ellen. "'Advancing the Kingdom': Missionaries and Americanization in Puerto Rico, 1898–1930s." PhD diss., University of Pittsburgh, 2008.

Weber, Benjamin David. "America's Carceral Empire: Confinement, Punishment, and Work at Home and Abroad, 1865–1946." PhD diss., Harvard University, 2017.

Weegels, Julienne. "Beyond the Cemetery of the Living: An Exploration of Disposal and the Politics of Visibility in the Nicaraguan Prison System." In *Carceral Communities in Latin America: Troubling Prison Worlds in the 21st Century,* edited by Sacha Darke, Chris Garces, Luis Duno-Gottberg, and Andrés Antillano, 295–320. Cham, Switzerland: Palgrave Macmillan, 2021.

Welch, Michael. *Escape to Prison: Penal Tourism and the Pull of Punishment.* Oakland: University of California Press, 2015.

Weld, Kirsten. *Paper Cadavers: The Archives of Dictatorship in Guatemala.* Durham, NC: Duke University Press, 2014.

Whalen, Carmen Teresa, and Víctor Vázquez Hernández, eds. *The Puerto Rican Diaspora: Historical Perspectives.* Philadelphia: Temple University Press, 2005.

Williams, K. J. "The Introduction of 'Chemotherapy' Using Arsphenamine—The First Magic Bullet." *Journal of the Royal Society of Medicine* 102, no. 8 (August 2009): 343–48.

Williford, Miriam. *Jeremy Bentham on Spanish America: An Account of His Letters and Proposals to the New World.* Baton Rouge: Louisiana State University Press, 1980.

Wilson Gilmore, Ruth. *Abolition Geography: Essays Towards Liberation.* Brooklyn, NY: Verso, 2022.

———. *Golden Gulag: Prisons, Surplus, Crisis, and Opposition in Globalizing California.* Berkeley: University of California Press, 2007.

Winship, Blanton. *Thirty-Sixth Annual Report of the Governor of Puerto Rico.* San Juan: Bureau of Supplies, Printing, and Transportation, 1936.

Winter, Charles E. *Report of the Attorney General of Puerto Rico, 1932.* San Juan: Bureau of Supplies, Printing, and Transportation, 1932–33.

————. *Report of the Attorney General of Puerto Rico, 1933.* San Juan: Negociado de Materiales, Imprenta, y Transporte, 1934.

Zaffiri, Lorenzo, Jared Gardner, and Luis H. Toledo-Pereyra. "History of Antibiotics: From Salvarsan to Cephalosporins." *Journal of Investigative Surgery* 25, no. 2 (April 2012): 67–77.

Zaglul, Antonio. *Mis 500 locos.* 1966; Santo Domingo: Ediciones Taller, 1998.

Zamacois, Eduardo. *Los vivos muertos.* Madrid: Compañía Ibero-Americana de Publicaciones, 1929.

Zayas Bazán, Rogerio. *El Presidio Modelo.* La Habana: publisher not identified, 1928.

Zayas León, Else. "La presencia de pardos en Toa Alta." In *Thoa Arriba, Toa Alta: Una Historia,* edited by Gloria Tapia Ríos, 79–85. Toa Alta, PR: Ediciones Magna Cultura, 2021.

Zemon Davis, Natalie. *Fiction in the Archives: Pardon Tales and Their Tellers in Sixteenth-Century France.* Stanford, CA: Stanford University Press, 1987.

Zenderland, Leila. *Measuring Minds: Henry Goddard and the Intelligence Testing Movement.* New York: Cambridge University Press, 1998.

Zeno Gandía, Manuel. *La charca: Crónicas de un mundo enfermo.* Ponce, PR: Est. Tip. de M. López, 1894.

Index

Page numbers in italics refer to figures.